T0205670

ADOLESCENT MENTAL HEALTH

CONNECTIONS TO THE COMMUNITY

ADOLESCENT
MENTAL HEALTH
CONNECTIONS TO THE COMMUNITY

Edited by
Areej Hassan, MD

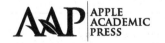

Apple Academic Press Inc. | Apple Academic Press Inc.
3333 Mistwell Crescent | 9 Spinnaker Way
Oakville, ON L6L 0A2 | Waretown, NJ 08758
Canada | USA

© 2015 by Apple Academic Press, Inc.

First issued in paperback 2021

Exclusive worldwide distribution by CRC Press, a member of Taylor & Francis Group

No claim to original U.S. Government works

ISBN 13: 978-1-77463-377-9 (pbk)
ISBN 13: 978-1-77188-103-6 (hbk)

Library of Congress Control Number: 2014952126

Library and Archives Canada Cataloguing in Publication

Adolescent mental health: connections to the community/edited by Areej Hassan, MD.

Includes bibliographical references and index.
ISBN 978-1-77188-103-6 (bound)
1. Social psychiatry. 2. Adolescent psychopathology. 3. Community mental health services. I. Hassan, Areej, editor

RC455.A36 2015   362.20835   C2014-906652-X

Apple Academic Press also publishes its books in a variety of electronic formats. Some content that appears in print may not be available in electronic format. For information about Apple Academic Press products, visit our website at **www.appleacademicpress.com** and the CRC Press website at **www.crcpress.com**

ABOUT THE EDITOR

AREEJ HASSAN, MD

Areej Hassan MD, MPH, is an attending physician at Boston Children's Hospital. She completed her pediatric residency at Hasbro Children's Hospital prior to training in adolescent medicine at Boston Children's. In addition to primary care, her clinical interests include reproductive endocrinology and international health. She also maintains an active role in medical education and has particular interest in building and developing innovative teaching tools through open educational resources. She currently teaches, consults, and is involved in pediatric and adolescent curricula development at multiple sites abroad in Central America and Southeast Asia.

CONTENTS

ACKNOWLEDGMENT AND HOW TO CITE

The editor and publisher thank each of the authors who contributed to this book, whether by granting their permission individually or by releasing their research as open source articles or under a license that permits free use, provided that attribution is made. The chapters in this book were previously published in various places in various formats. To cite the work contained in this book and to view the individual permissions, please refer to the citation at the beginning of each chapter. Each chapter was read individually and carefully selected by the editor; the result is a book that provides a nuanced study of adolescent mental health. The chapters included examine the following topics:

- The novel study in Chapter 1 lays a foundation for connecting adolescent mental health with communities and neighborhoods.
- Low socioeconomic status, lack of adequate housing, food security, domestic violence, and other social issues all play a role in mental health. In adults, this can then lead to increased morbidity and mortality, while adolescents and children are more likely to experience ongoing, long-term psychological issue. Chapter 2 provides a well-written review that encompasses these factors by looking at multiple social determinants, including poverty, child care, access to education, and availability of medical resources.
- Chapter 3 is a simple and easy-to-follow study. Although it relies only on cross-sectional data, meaning that causal relationships are hard to determine, nevertheless, the author finds significant associations. These are valuable as a way to encourage school systems and educational personnel to be more sensitive to signs of depression and suicidal ideation among female-dominated classes and in vocational programs.
- Chapter 4 studies a unique question with well-validated data-collection instruments, while nicely controlling for other variables that can impact mental health functioning.
- Clinicians and educators have long known that mental health problems impact educational attainment—but in order to change policy, we have needed concrete data to prove it. The amazingly well-designed study in Chapter 5, with great longitudinal data, speaks to how critical it is to address mental health early on. It is truly a landmark paper that should be brought to the attention of policymakers.

- When mental health services are available in a school setting, it is easier for students to get care during the school year, which increases compliance with visits. The large US sample used by the authors of Chapter 6 makes this case convincingly.
- All of us—the media, educators, clinicians, and parents—pay a lot of attention lately to bullying, while we overlook the affect that being socially isolated can have on adolescents. Chapter 7 indicates that in fact, loneliness has the most powerful effect on school well being.
- So much in the media looks at bullying from an anecdotal viewpoint. Chapter 8 is a key paper that connects both traditional and cyber bullying with concrete mental health outcomes such as suicidal ideation.
- Chapter 9 is a well done study that indicates that the relationship between parents and adolescents is especially significant in the context of negative life events, while not as significant for those adolescents who have no negative life events.
- Chapter 10 offers a strong conclusion to this section, controlling for substance use while looking at the connections between family relationship and depression
- One of the authors of Chapter 11, Vikram Patel, is the most prominent expert in this area of study. He and his co-authors offer convincing research that training community members to give mental health interventions will not only empower ordinary people to care for others but will also have more powerful and widespread effect than any other form of intervention.
- As with the previous TRAILS paper included in chapter 5, Chapter 12 is a very well-designed paper. The results were disturbing but offer a great starting point for new research and discussion.
- Chapter 13 is an excellent study that focuses not only on efficacy of the intervention but also its feasibility. A detailed intervention that is impossible to implement has little practical use.
- Chapter 14 provides a strong conclusion to this compendium, with qualitative data from the people taking part in the particular interventions.

LIST OF CONTRIBUTORS

Olayinka Atilola
Department of Behavioural Medicine, Lagos State University College of Medicine, Ikeja, Lagos 10001, Nigeria

Rienke Bannink
Department of Public Health, Erasmus University Medical Center Rotterdam, Rotterdam, the Netherlands

Margaret M. Barry
WHO Collaborating Centre for Health Promotion Research, National University of Ireland Galway, University Road, Galway, Ireland

Angelo Belardi
Department of Psychology, Division of Clinical Psychology and Psychiatry, University of Basel, Basel, Switzerland

Melanie D. Bertino
Centre for Mental Health and Wellbeing Research, School of Psychology, Faculty of Health, Deakin University, Melbourne, VIC 3125, Australia

Suzanne Broeren
Department of Public Health, Erasmus University Medical Center Rotterdam, Rotterdam, the Netherlands

Ute Bültmann
University Medical Center Groningen, University of Groningen, Department of Health Sciences, Community & Occupational Medicine, Groningen, The Netherlands

Aleisha M. Clarke
WHO Collaborating Centre for Health Promotion Research, National University of Ireland Galway, University Road, Galway, Ireland

David Cohen
Department of Child and Adolescent Psychiatry, GH Pitié-Salpêtrière, APHP, Paris, F-75013, France and CNRS UMR 7222, Institut des Systèmes Intelligents et Robotiques, University Pierre et Marie Curie, Paris, France

Angèle Consoli
Department of Child and Adolescent Psychiatry, GH Pitié-Salpêtrière, APHP, Paris, F-75013, France, INSERM U-669, PSIGIAM, Paris, F-75679, France, and Univ. Paris-Sud, Univ. Paris-Descartes, Paris, F-75005, France

Joakim D. Dalen
NTNU Social Research, Trondheim, Norway, and Department of Sociology and Political science, Norwegian University of Science and Technology, Trondheim, Norway

Frouwkje G. de Waart
Municipal Public Health Service Rotterdam area, Rotterdam, the Netherlands

Suzanne Dziurawiec
School of Psychology and Exercise Science, Murdoch University, Murdoch, WA 6150, Australia

Bruno Falissard
Département de Santé Publique, Hôpital Paul Brousse, APHP, Villejuif, F-94804, France, INSERM U-669, PSIGIAM, Paris, F-75679, France, and Univ. Paris-Sud, Univ. Paris-Descartes, Paris, F-75005, France

Marita Falkmer
School of Occupational Therapy and Social Work, Curtin Health Innovation Research Institute, Curtin University, Perth, Western Australia, Australia and School of Education and Communication, CHILD programme, Institution of Disability Research Jönköping University, Jönköping, Sweden

Torbjörn Falkmer
School of Occupational Therapy and Social Work, Curtin Health Innovation Research Institute, Curtin University, Perth, Western Australia, Australia, School of Occupational Therapy, La Trobe University, Melbourne, Victoria, Australia, and Rehabilitation Medicine, Department of Medicine and Health Sciences (IMH), Faculty of Health Sciences, Linköping University & Pain and Rehabilitation Centre, UHL, County Council, Linköping, Sweden

J. Dennis Fortenberry
Department of Pediatrics, Indiana University School of Medicine, Indianapolis, Indiana, United States of America

Keren Geddes
Rockingham Kwinana Child and Adolescent Mental Health Service, P.O. Box 288, Rockingham, WA 6968, Australia

Christine Hassler
INSERM U-669, PSIGIAM, Paris, F-75679, France and Univ. Paris-Sud, Univ. Paris-Descartes, Paris, F-75005, France

Odin Hjemdal
Department of Psychology, Norwegian University of Science and Technology, Trondheim, Norway

Daniëlle E. M. C. Jansen
Department of Health Sciences, University Medical Centre Groningen, University of Groningen, Groningen, The Netherlands

Rachel Jenkins
WHO Collaborating Centre for Research and Training for Mental Health, Institute of Psychiatry, King's College London, 16 De Crespigny Park, London SE5 8AF, UK

Frederike Jörg
Interdisciplinary Centre Psychopathology and Emotion regulation, University Medical Centre Groningen, University of Groningen, Groningen, The Netherlands

Tess Knight
Centre for Mental Health and Wellbeing Research, School of Psychology, Faculty of Health, Deakin University, Melbourne, VIC 3125, Australia

Marianne N. Kvande
Research Centre for Health Promotion and Resources, Trondheim, Norway and Department of Social Work and Health Sciences, Norwegian University of Science and Technology, Trondheim, Norway

Mei-Po Kwan
Department of Geography and Geographic Information Science, University of Illinois, Urbana-Champaign, Illinois, United States of America

Christopher William Lee
School of Psychology and Exercise Science, Murdoch University, Murdoch, WA 6150, Australia

Andrew J. Lewis
Centre for Mental Health and Wellbeing Research, School of Psychology, Faculty of Health, Deakin University, Melbourne, VIC 3125, Australia

Monica Lillefjell
Research Centre for Health Promotion and Resources, Trondheim, Norway, Department of Social Work and Health Sciences, Norwegian University of Science and Technology, Trondheim, Norway, and Department of Occupational Therapy, Sør-Trøndelag University College, Trondheim, Norway

Audhild Løhre
Research Centre for Health Promotion and Resources, Trondheim, Norway and Department of Social Work and Health Sciences, Norwegian University of Science and Technology, Trondheim, Norway

Gunther Meinlschmidt
Department of Psychology, Division of Clinical Psychology and Epidemiology, University of Basel, Basel, Switzerland and Faculty of Medicine, Ruhr-University Bochum, Bochum, Germany

Marie-Rose Moro
Maison de Solenn, Hôpital Cochin, APHP, Paris, F-75014, France, INSERM U-669, PSIGIAM, Paris, F-75679, France, and, Univ. Paris-Sud, Univ. Paris-Descartes, Paris, F-75005, France

Albertine J. Oldehinkel
Interdisciplinary Centre Psychopathology and Emotion regulation, University Medical Centre Groningen, University of Groningen, Groningen, The Netherlands

Johan Ormel
University Medical Center Groningen, University of Groningen, Interdisciplinary Center for Psychopathology and Emotion Regulation, Groningen, The Netherlands

Richard Parsons
School of Pharmacy, Curtin Health Innovation Research Institute, Curtin University, Perth, Western Australia, Australia and School of Occupational Therapy and Social Work, Curtin Health Innovation Research Institute, Curtin University, Perth, Western Australia, Australia

Anne Elizabeth Passmore
School of Occupational Therapy and Social Work, Curtin Health Innovation Research Institute, Curtin University, Perth, Western Australia, Australia

Vikram Patel
Centre for Global Mental Health, London School of Hygiene & Tropical Medicine, Keppel Street, London WC1E 7HT, UK and Sangath, Goa, India

Hugo Peyre
Department of Child and Adolescent Psychiatry, GH Pitié-Salpêtrière, APHP, Paris, F-75013, France, INSERM U-669, PSIGIAM, Paris, F-75679, France, and Univ. Paris-Sud, Univ. Paris-Descartes, Paris, F-75005, France

Hein Raat
Department of Public Health, Erasmus University Medical Center Rotterdam, Rotterdam, the Netherlands

Sijmen A. Reijneveld
University Medical Center Groningen, University of Groningen, Department of Health Sciences, Community & Occupational Medicine, Groningen, The Netherlands

Anne Révah-Lévy
Centre de Soins Psychothérapeutiques de Transition pour Adolescents, Hôpital d'Argenteuil, Argenteuil, Argenteuil, France, INSERM U-669, PSIGIAM, Paris, F-75679, France, and Univ. Paris-Sud, Univ. Paris-Descartes, Paris, F-75005, France

Narelle Robertson
Centre for Mental Health and Wellbeing Research, School of Psychology, Faculty of Health, Deakin University, Melbourne, VIC 3125, Australia

Mario Speranza
Department of Child and Adolescent Psychiatry, Centre Hospitalier de Versailles, Le Chesnay, France, INSERM U-669, PSIGIAM, Paris, F-75679, France, and Univ. Paris-Sud, Univ. Paris-Descartes, Paris, F-75005, France

Esther Stalujanis
Department of Psychology, Division of Clinical Psychology and Psychiatry, University of Basel, Basel, Switzerland

Roy E. Stewart
University Medical Center Groningen, University of Groningen, Department of Health Sciences, Community & Occupational Medicine, Groningen, The Netherlands

Marion Tegethoff
Department of Psychology, Division of Clinical Psychology and Psychiatry, University of Basel, Basel, Switzerland

Evelyne Touchette
Research Unit on Children's Psychosocial Maladjustment, University of Montreal, Montreal, Canada

John W. Toumbourou
Centre for Mental Health and Wellbeing Research, School of Psychology, Faculty of Health, Deakin University, Melbourne, VIC 3125, Australia

Petra M. van de Looij-Jansen
Municipal Public Health Service Rotterdam area, Rotterdam, the Netherlands

Sharmila Vaz
School of Occupational Therapy and Social Work, Centre for Research into Disability and Society, Curtin Health Innovation Research Institute, Curtin University, Perth, Western Australia, Australia

Karin Veldman
University Medical Center Groningen, University of Groningen, Department of Health Sciences, Community & Occupational Medicine, Groningen, The Netherlands

Frank C. Verhulst
Erasmus Medical Center, Department of Child and Adolescent Psychiatry, Rotterdam, The Netherlands

Sarah E. Wiehe
Department of Pediatrics, Indiana University School of Medicine, Indianapolis, Indiana, United States of America

Jeff Wilson
Department of Geography, School of Liberal Arts, Indiana University-Purdue University Indianapolis, Indianapolis, Indiana, United States of America

INTRODUCTION

Mental health illness often emerges during childhood and adolescence, and it accounts for a large portion of the global burden of disease among youth. These illnesses are often rooted in the community, making them a social worker's challenge, even while they are more commonly expected to be treated by the medical and counseling communities. In addition, mental health disorders interface with numerous other social and health problems; youth with mental illness are more likely to drop out of school, engage in high-risk behaviors, and sustain injuries from accidents.

Despite the high prevalence, there are many barriers for treatment, including lack of government policy, inadequate funding for services, and lack of trained clinicians. Protective factors have been well studied and include positive family attachment, educational attainment, positive role models, positive cultural experiences, and connectedness to the community.

This collection of scholarly articles gives the reader insight into the interface between mental health disease in adolescents with 1) their community, 2) their school, 3) their peers and families; it ends with a series of successful community interventions, with applications for the social worker, as well as educators, counselors, and medical clinicians. It is our sincere hope that the protective factors, risk factors, and interventions described here can also lead to policy development focused on prevention and early treatment.

Areej Hassan

Various forms of community disorder are associated with health outcomes but little is known about how dynamic context where an adolescent spends time relates to her health-related behaviors. The goal of Chapter 1, by Wiehe and colleagues, was to assess whether exposure to contexts associated with crime (as a marker of community disorder) correlates with self-reported health-related behaviors among adolescent girls. Girls (N = 52), aged 14–17, were recruited from a single geographic urban area and monitored for 1 week using a GPS-enabled cell phone. Adolescents completed an audio computer-assisted self-administered interview survey on substance use (cigarette, alcohol, or marijuana use) and sexual intercourse in the last 30 days. In addition to recorded home and school address, phones transmitted location data every 5 minutes (path points). Using ArcGIS, we defined community disorder as aggregated point-level Unified Crime Report data within a 200-meter Euclidian buffer from home, school and each path point. Using Stata, the authors analyzed how exposures to areas of higher crime prevalence differed among girls who reported each behavior or not. Participants lived and spent time in areas with variable crime prevalence within 200 meters of their home, school and path points. Significant differences in exposure occurred based on home location among girls who reported any substance use or not (p 0.04) and sexual intercourse or not (p 0.01). Differences in exposure by school and path points were only significant among girls reporting any substance use or not (p 0.03 and 0.02, respectively). Exposure also varied by school/non-school day as well as time of day. Adolescent travel patterns are not random. Furthermore, the crime context where an adolescent spends time relates to her health-related behavior. These data may guide policy relating to crime control and inform time- and space-specific interventions to improve adolescent health.

Efforts at improving child-health and development initiatives in sub-Saharan Africa had focused on the physical health of children due to the neglect of child and adolescent mental health (CAMH) policy initiatives. A thorough and broad-based understanding of the prevalent child mental-health risk and vulnerability factors is needed to successfully articulate CAMH policies. In Chapter 2, Atilola presents a narrative on the child mental-health risk and vulnerability factors in sub-Saharan Africa. Through an ecological point of view, the author identified widespread family poverty, poor availability and uptake of childcare resources, inadequate community and institutional childcare systems, and inadequate framework for social protection for vulnerable children as among the risk and vulnerability factors for CAMH in the region. Others are poor workplace policy/practice that does not support work-family life balance, poor legislative framework for child protection, and some harmful traditional practices. The article concludes that an ecological approach shows that child mental-health risks are diverse and cut across different layers of the care environment. The approach also provides a broad and holistic template from which appropriate CAMH policy direction in sub-Saharan Africa can be understood.

Few studies have explored the association between social context and suicidal ideation using multilevel models. Chapter 3, by Dalen, examines how suicidal ideation in adolescence is related to school class composition. Data were obtained from the Young-HUNT 3 study (2006–2008), a population study of adolescents attending secondary school in the Norwegian county of Nord-Trøndelag. The final sample included 2923 adolescents distributed among 379 school classes in 13 schools. Multilevel logistic regression was used to estimate the contribution of various factors at the individual and school class levels. The results indicate that 5.3 percent of the variation in suicidal ideation can be attributed to differences between school classes. However, a substantial part of this variation can be explained by an unequal distribution of students at risk as a result of individual factors. After controlling for individual-level variables, the results show a higher probability of suicidal ideation in school classes having higher proportions of girls as well as in those following a vocational education programme. Targeting classes that either follow a vocational education programme or have a high proportion of girls can be an effective approach to intervention because such classes may include a greater number of students at risk for having suicidal thoughts compared to classes with a high proportion of boys or classes following a general education programme.

Students negotiate the transition to secondary school in different ways. While some thrive on the opportunity, others are challenged. In Chapter 4, Vaz and colleagues used a prospective longitudinal design to determine the contribution of personal background and school contextual factors on academic competence (AC) and mental health functioning (MHF) of 266 students, 6-months before and after the transition to secondary school. Data from 197 typically developing students and 69 students with a disability were analysed using hierarchical linear regression modelling. Both in primary and secondary school, students with a disability and from socially disadvantaged backgrounds gained poorer scores for AC and MHF than their typically developing and more affluent counterparts. Students who attended independent and mid-range sized primary schools had the highest concurrent AC. Those from independent primary schools had the lowest MHF. The primary school organisational model significantly influenced post-transition AC scores; with students from Kindergarten - Year 7 schools reporting the lowest scores, while those from the Kindergarten - Year 12 structure without middle school having the highest scores. Attending a school which used the Kindergarten - Year 12 with middle school structure was associated with a reduction in AC scores across the transition. Personal background factors accounted for the majority of the variability in post-transition AC and MHF. The contribution of school contextual factors was relatively minor. There is a potential opportunity for schools to provide support to disadvantaged students before the transition to secondary school, as they continue to be at a disadvantage after the transition.

Chapter 5, by Veldman and colleagues, examines if mental health problems at age 11 and changes in mental health problems between age 11 and 16 predict educational attainment of adolescents at age 19, overall and stratified by gender. Data from 1711 adolescents (76.8% from initial cohort) of the Tracking Adolescents' Individual Lives Survey (TRAILS), a Dutch prospective cohort study with 9year follow-up, were used. Mental health problems (externalizing, internalizing and attention problems) were measured by the Youth Self Report and the Child Behavior Checklist at ages 11 and 16. Difference scores for mental health problems between age 11 and 16 were calculated. Educational attainment was assessed at age 19. Externalizing, internalizing and attention problems at age 11 were significantly associated with low educational attainment at age 19 (crude model). When adjusted for demographic variables and the other mental health problems, only the association for attention problems remained significant (odds ratio (OR), 95% confidence interval: 3.19, 2.11–4.83). Increasing externalizing problems between age 11 and 16 also predicted low educational attainment at age 19 (OR 3.12, 1.83–5.32). Among girls, increasing internalizing problems between age 11 and 16 predicted low educational attainment (OR 2.21, 1.25–3.94). For boys, no significant association was found for increasing internalizing problems and low educational attainment. For increasing attention problems between age 11 and

16 no significant association with low educational attainment was found. Externalizing, internalizing and attention problems at age 11 and an increase of these problems during adolescence predicted low educational attainment at age 19. Early treatment of these mental health problems may improve educational attainment, and reduce socioeconomic health differences in adulthood.

School mental health services are important contact points for children and adolescents with mental disorders, but their ability to provide comprehensive treatment is limited. The main objective in Chapter 6, by Tegethoff and colleagues, was to estimate in mentally disordered adolescents of a nationally representative United States cohort the role of school mental health services as guide to mental health care in different out-of-school service sectors. Analyses are based on weighted data (N = 6483) from the United States National Comorbidity Survey Replication Adolescent Supplement (participants' age: 13–18 years). Lifetime DSM-IV mental disorders were assessed using the fully structured WHO CIDI interview, complemented by parent report. Adolescents and parents provided information on mental health service use across multiple sectors, based on the Service Assessment for Children and Adolescents. School mental health service use predicted subsequent out-of-school service utilization for mental disorders i) in the medical specialty sector, in adolescents with affective (hazard ratio (HR) = 3.01, confidence interval (CI) = 1.77–5.12), anxiety (HR = 3.87, CI = 1.97–7.64), behavior (HR = 2.49, CI = 1.62–3.82), substance use (HR = 4.12, CI = 1.87–9.04), and eating (HR = 10.72, CI = 2.31–49.70) disorders, and any mental disorder (HR = 2.97, CI = 1.94–4.54), and ii) in other service sectors, in adolescents with anxiety (HR = 3.15, CI = 2.17–4.56), behavior (HR = 1.99, CI = 1.29–3.06), and substance use (HR = 2.48, CI = 1.57–3.94) disorders, and any mental disorder (HR = 2.33, CI = 1.54–3.53), but iii) not in the mental health specialty sector. The findings indicate that in the United States, school mental health services may serve as guide to out-of-school service utilization for mental disorders especially in the medical specialty sector across various mental disorders, thereby highlighting the relevance of school mental health services in the trajectory of mental care. In light of the missing link between school mental health services and mental health specialty services, the promotion of a stronger collaboration between these sectors should be considered regarding the potential to improve and guarantee adequate mental care at early life stages.

Loneliness is negatively related to good health and wellbeing, especially among girls. There is little research, however, on factors that may ease the burdens of loneliness in the school setting. Thus, in Chapter 7, Løhre and colleagues explored the relationship between girls' loneliness and later school wellbeing adjusted for other adversities. Furthermore, the authors assessed the significance of having someone whom the girl trusted by investigating possible modifying influences on the addressed association. Altogether, 119 girls in grades 1–8 provided baseline data and answered the same set of questions two years later. Logistic regression models including perceived academic problems, victimisation by bullying, loneliness and trusted others were tested with bad versus good school wellbeing two years later as outcome using SPSS. In the multivariable analysis of loneliness, academic problems, and victimisation, loneliness was the only variable showing a strong and negative contribution to later school wellbeing. Next, demonstrated in separate models; the inclusion of having a trusted class advisor fully attenuated the association of loneliness with later school wellbeing. In contrast, other trusted teachers, trusted parents, or trusted students did not affect the association. Loneliness in girls strongly predicted school wellbeing two years later. However, having a class advisor whom the girl trusted to contact in hurtful situations clearly reduced the burden of loneliness. This finding highlights the clinical importance of stability, long-lasting relations, and trust that main teachers may represent for lonely girls.

The goal in Chapter 8, by Bannink and colleagues, was to examine whether traditional and cyber bullying victimization were associated with adolescent's mental health problems and suicidal ideation at two-year follow-up. Gender differences were explored to determine whether bullying affects boys and girls differently. A two-year longitudinal study was conducted among first-year secondary school students (N = 3181). Traditional and cyber bullying victimization were assessed at baseline, whereas mental health status and suicidal ideation were assessed at baseline and follow-up by means of self-report questionnaires. Logistic regression analyses were conducted to assess associations between these variables while controlling for baseline problems. Additionally, the authors tested whether gender differences in mental health and suicidal ideation were present for the two types of bullying. There was a significant interaction between gender and traditional bullying victimization and between gender and cyber bullying victimization on mental health problems. Among boys, traditional and cyber bullying victimization were not related to mental health problems after controlling for baseline mental health. Among girls, both traditional and cyber bullying victimization were associated with mental health problems after controlling for baseline mental health. No significant interaction between gender and traditional or cyber bullying victimization on suicidal ideation was found. Traditional bullying victimization was associated with suicidal ideation, whereas cyber bullying victimization was not associated with suicidal ideation after controlling for baseline suicidal ideation. Traditional bullying victimization is associated with an increased risk of suicidal ideation, whereas traditional, as well as cyber bullying victimization is associated with an increased risk of mental health problems among girls. These findings stress the importance of programs aimed at reducing bullying behavior, especially because early-onset mental health problems may pose a risk for the development of psychiatric disorders in adulthood.

The aim of Chapter 9, by Bannink and colleagues, was to examine the association of negative life events and parent-adolescent attachment relationship quality with mental health problems and to explore an interaction between the parent-adolescent attachment relationship and one or multiple negative life events on the mental health of adolescents. A two-year longitudinal study was conducted among first-year secondary school students (N = 3181). The occurrence of life events and the quality of parent-adolescent attachment were assessed at baseline and mental health status at two-year follow-up by means of self-report questionnaires. Binary logistic regression analyses were conducted to assess associations between life events, parent-adolescent attachment and mental health problems. Relative Excess Risk due to Interaction techniques were used to determine the interaction effects on the additive scale. Life events were related to mental health status, as was parent-adolescent attachment. The combined effect of an unfavourable parent-adolescent attachment with life events on mental health was larger than the sum of the two individual effects. Among adolescents with one life event or multiple life events, an unfavourable parent-adolescent attachment increased the risk of mental health problems at follow-up compared to the group without life events. Results supported an interaction effect between parent-adolescent attachment and negative life events on mental health. Especially adolescents with one or multiple life events and an unfavourable parent-adolescent attachment seems to be a vulnerable group for mental health problems. Implications for further research are discussed.

Suicide is the second leading cause of death in adolescents and young adults in Europe. Reducing suicides is therefore a key public health target. Previous studies have shown associations between suicidal behaviors, depression and family factors. In Chapter 10, Consoli and colleagues aimed to assess the role of family factors in depression and suicidality in a large community-based sample of adolescents and to explore specific contributions (e.g. mother vs. father; conflict vs. no conflict; separation vs. no separation) taking into account other risk factors. A cross-sectional sample of adolescents aged 17 years was recruited in 2008. 36,757 French adolescents (18,593 girls and 18,164 boys) completed a questionnaire including socio-demographic characteristics, drug use, family variables, suicidal ideations and attempts. Current depression was assessed with the Adolescent Depression Rating Scale (ADRS). Adolescents were divided into 4 groups according to suicide risk severity (grade 1=depressed without suicidal ideation and without suicide attempts, grade 2=depressed with suicidal ideations and grade 3=depressed with suicide attempts; grade 0=control group). Multivariate regressions were applied to assess the Odds Ratio of potential risk factors comparing grade 1, 2 or 3 risk with grade 0. 7.5% of adolescents (10.4% among girls vs. 4.5% among boys) had ADRS scores compatible with depression; 16.2% reported suicidal ideations in the past 12 months and 8.2% reported lifetime suicide attempts. Repeating a year in school was significantly associated to severity grade of suicide risk (1 and 3), as well as all substance use, tobacco use (severity grades 2 and 3) and marijuana use (severity grade 3), for girls and boys. After adjustment, negative relationships with either or both parents, and parents living together but with a negative relationship were significantly associated with suicide risk and/or depression in both genders (all risk grades), and Odds Ratios increased according to risk severity grade. Family discord and negative relationship with parents were associated with an increased suicide risk in depressed adolescents. So it appears essential to take intrafamilial relationships into account in depressed adolescents to prevent suicidal behaviours.

In Chapter 11, Barry and colleagues provide a systematic review that gives a narrative synthesis of the evidence on the effectiveness of mental health promotion interventions for young people in low and middle-income countries (LMICs). Commissioned by the WHO, a review of the evidence for mental health promotion interventions across the lifespan from early years to adulthood was conducted. This paper reports on the findings for interventions promoting the positive mental health of young people (aged 6–18 years) in school and community-based settings. Searching a range of electronic databases, 22 studies employing RCTs (N = 11) and quasi-experimental designs conducted in LMICs since 2000 were identified. Fourteen studies of school-based interventions implemented in eight LMICs were reviewed; seven of which included interventions for children living in areas of armed conflict and six interventions of multicomponent lifeskills and resilience training. Eight studies evaluating out-of-school community interventions for adolescents were identified in five countries. Using the Effective Public Health Practice Project (EPHPP) criteria, two reviewers independently assessed the quality of the evidence. The findings from the majority of the school-based interventions are strong. Structured universal interventions for children living in conflict areas indicate generally significant positive effects on students' emotional and behavioural wellbeing, including improved self-esteem and coping skills. However, mixed results were also reported, including differential effects for gender and age groups, and two studies reported nonsignficant findings. The majority of the school-based lifeskills and resilience programmes received a moderate quality rating, with findings indicating positive effects on students' self-esteem, motivation and self-efficacy. The quality of evidence from the community-based interventions for adolescents was moderate to strong with promising findings concerning the potential of multicomponent interventions to impact on youth mental health and social wellbeing. The review findings indicate that interventions promoting the mental health of young people can be implemented effectively in LMIC school and community settings with moderate to strong evidence of their impact on both positive and negative mental health outcomes. There is a paucity of evidence relating to interventions for younger children in LMIC primary schools. Evidence for the scaling up and sustainability of mental health promotion interventions in LMICs needs to be strengthened.

The increased use and costs of specialist child and adolescent mental health services (MHS) urge us to assess the effectiveness of these services. The aim of Jörg and colleagues in Chapter 12 is to compare the course of emotional and behavioural problems in adolescents with and without MHS use in a naturalistic setting. Participants are 2230 (pre)adolescents that enrolled in a prospective cohort study, the TRacking Adolescents' Individual Lives Survey (TRAILS). Response rate was 76%, mean age at baseline 11.09 (SD 0.56), 50.8% girls. We used data from the first three assessment waves, covering a six year period. Multiple linear regression analysis, propensity score matching, and data validation were used to compare the course of emotional and behavioural problems of adolescents with and without MHS use. The association between MHS and follow-up problem score (β 0.20, SE 0.03, p-value<0.001) was not confounded by baseline severity, markers of adolescent vulnerability or resilience nor stressful life events. The propensity score matching strategy revealed that follow-up problem scores of non-MHS-users decreased while the problem scores of MHS users remained high. When taking into account future MHS (non)use, it appeared that problem scores decreased with limited MHS use, albeit not as much as without any MHS use, and that problem scores with continuous MHS use remained high. Data validation showed that using a different outcome measure, multiple assessment waves and multiple imputation of missing values did not alter the results. A limitation of the study is that, although we know what type of MHS participants used, and during which period, we lack information on the duration of the treatment. The benefits of MHS are questionable. Replication studies should reveal whether a critical examination of everyday care is necessary or an artefact is responsible for these results.

The literature suggests a link between childhood trauma and maladaptive emotion regulation strategies, including nonsuicidal self-injury (NSSI) and suicidality. In Chapter 13, Geddes and colleagues assessed the impact of a pilot dialectical behaviour therapy (DBT) programme on reducing trauma-related symptoms and improving emotional regulation, suicidality, and NSSI in adolescents. Six adolescents attending a community mental health service received 26 weeks of DBT, together with a parent. Independent assessors collected measures on each participant at baseline, posttreatment, and three-month followup. The authors implemented further improvements over past research with the use of adolescent-specific outcome measures as well as independent assessment of treatment integrity, noted as problematic in previous studies, using videotapes. Results. Firstly, adolescents reported a decrease in trauma-based symptoms, suicidality, and NSSI following participation in the DBT programme that was maintained at the three-month followup. Secondly, adolescents also reported improved emotion regulation immediately following treatment, and this was maintained, albeit more moderately, three months later. Given the burgeoning demand on mental health services, it is notable that five of the six adolescents were discharged from the service following the DBT intervention. The results of this pilot programme suggest that DBT has the potential to improve the symptoms of this at-risk population.

Chapter 14, by Lewis and colleagues, presents findings derived from consumer feedback, following a multicentre randomised controlled trial for adolescent mental health problems and substance misuse. The paper focuses on the implementation of a family-based intervention, including fidelity of delivery, family members' experiences, and their suggestions for program improvements. Methods. Qualitative and quantitative data (n = 21) were drawn from the Deakin Family Options trial consumer focus groups, which occurred six months after the completion of the trial. Consumer focus groups were held in both metropolitan and regional locations in Victoria, Australia. Findings. Overall reductions in parental isolation, increases in parental self-care, and increased separation/individuation were the key therapeutic features of the intervention. Sharing family experiences with other parents was a key supportive factor, which improved parenting confidence and efficacy and potentially reduced family conflict. Consumer feedback also led to further development of the intervention, with a greater focus on aiding parents to engage adolescents in services and addressing family factors related to adolescent's mood and anxiety symptoms. Conclusions. Participant feedback provides valuable qualitative data, to monitor the fidelity of treatment implementation within a trial, to confirm predictions about the effective mechanisms of an intervention, and to inform the development of new interventions.

PART I

THE INTERACTION OF ADOLESCENT MENTAL HEALTH WITH THE CULTURAL AND SOCIOECONOMIC COMMUNITY

PART 2

CHAPTER 1

ADOLESCENT HEALTH-RISK BEHAVIOR AND COMMUNITY DISORDER

SARAH E. WIEHE, MEI-PO KWAN, JEFF WILSON, AND J. DENNIS FORTENBERRY

1.1 INTRODUCTION

Though the physical and emotional resources within homes clearly influence adolescent health and well-being, the surrounding physical area and its social milieu, loosely understood as the residential neighborhood, also plays a role. In fact, poor health outcomes cluster at various levels of area aggregation from country to census block group [1], [2]. Characteristics of these contextual areas (such as collective efficacy and poverty rates) based on or derived with various schemes of area aggregation are often observed to spatially correlate with health outcomes [3], [4]. Although past research tends to identify a general correlation between the qualities

Adolescent Health-Risk Behavior and Community Disorder. © Wiehe SE, Kwan M-P, Wilson J, and Fortenberry JD. PLoS ONE, 8,11 (2013). doi:10.1371/journal.pone.0077667. Licensed under Creative Commons Attribution 3.0 Unported License, http://creativecommons.org/licenses/by/3.0/.

of neighborhoods where adolescents live and their health, how specific sociogeographic contexts outside their homes influence this relationship remains unclear [5].

This limited understanding of how adolescents interact with the physical and social spaces of their neighborhoods is an important barrier to the success of health promotion and disease prevention efforts. Previous studies of context primarily use arbitrary administrative areas (e.g., census tracts or block groups) or buffers surrounding participants' residential addresses to assess neighborhood contextual exposure. However, these areal units often do not fully or accurately characterize where adolescents spend time and interact with others at the micro-geographic level (e.g., spending time on the front stoop, street corners, vacant lots, or other places without adult supervision). They also cannot differentiate contextual influences that adolescents experienced at various distances from home (e.g., area immediately surrounding the home versus areas farther away from home but that are normally considered part of their residential neighborhood). As contextual influences on adolescents' health behaviors (e.g., community disorder) may vary at the micro-geographic level even within their residential neighborhoods, using arbitrary buffers or administrative units to assess their exposure seriously constrains our understanding of how specific contexts affect health outcomes [4], [6], [7]. A few studies include path data (data that capture the locations and routes taken over time) [8]–[12], but most do not examine how health behaviors vary by micro sociogeographic context within a neighborhood or by where an individual spends time.

Path data are particularly important in mobile populations where the exposure of interest occurs outside the home. Adolescence is developmentally characterized by increasing autonomy and mobility, and adolescents have a great deal of latitude to choose and use the environments where they spend time. Since adolescents spend only about half their time at home [13], environments outside the home may exert substantial influence on adolescents' health-related behaviors. In particular, behaviors such as cigarette smoking, alcohol and other drug use, and partnered sexual activity are associated with substantial morbidity in adolescence and have been linked to neighborhood and community influences, independent of those found in the home and family [14]–[17].

In order to better understand potential mechanisms by which neighborhood contexts outside but near the home might influence adolescent health-related behaviors, we asked if time spent in areas with higher prevalence of reported crimes (as an indicator of community disorder) was correlated with self-reported health-related behaviors among adolescent girls living in one area of Indianapolis, Indiana. This relatively homogenous neighborhood was chosen to specifically evaluate health-related behaviors associated with adolescent path exposures, in addition to those directly associated with areas immediately surrounding the home.

1.2 MATERIALS AND METHODS

1.2.1 ETHICS STATEMENT

This research was reviewed and approved by the Indiana University Institutional Review Board. We obtained written consent from each participant and her parent/guardian.

1.2.2 STUDY DESIGN AND POPULATION

The Pearl Grlz study is a prospective study of adolescent girls (N = 52), aged 14–17 years, living in one area of Indianapolis, Indiana. Girls were recruited from this area by approaching potential participants in clinic settings and in neighborhood venues as well as through flyers and announcements in the target community and a website/Facebook site. The racial-ethnic composition of our cohort reflected the larger community, with 63% self-identified Black, 31% White, and 6% Latina participants. Inclusion criteria in addition to age, gender and residence was the ability to speak and understand English.

Each participant was monitored for 4 one-week periods over the course of a year using a GPS-enabled cell phone during the study period of 2008–2011. Participants took a baseline audio computer-assisted self-administered interview (ACASI) survey indicating demographic characteristics as well as self-reported health-related behaviors. The first of the 4 one-week periods for all participants were used for this analysis.

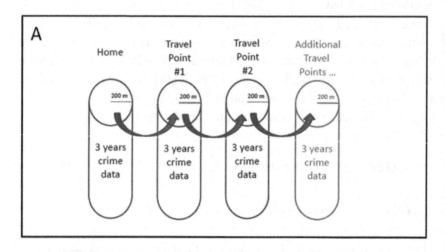

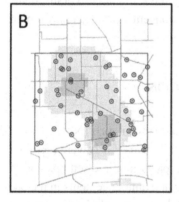

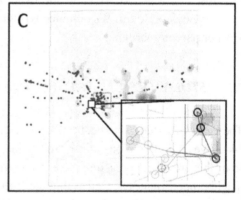

FIGURE 1: Methodology and measurement of areas of crime prevalence. (A) Conceptual depiction of path pattern exposure data to areas of crime prevalence. Each 5 minute path point includes the 3-year crime data within a 200-meter (~1 block) buffer of this point. (B) Location of participant homes and 200-meter buffers (black) within the study recruitment area with background levels of crime 'hot-spots' (grey shading) and Census block groups (grey lines). (C) Path points of 1 participant within and outside of the study area with the inset indicating a zoomed area of path with points linked using color coding (red in the morning to blue in the evening), 200-meter buffers (black) and crime hot-spots (grey shading) and Census block groups (grey lines).

1.2.3 QUANTITATIVE DATA ON CONTEXT

Path data were collected using a global positioning system (GPS)-enabled cell phone which each participant carried during monitoring periods. The cell phone used assisted GPS signaling to determine longitude and latitude using both cell tower and satellite triangulation (accuracy: 20 feet horizontally, 36 feet vertically). The phones transmitted a device ID, time-stamp, and GPS coordinates every 5 minutes to a secure server. Location was not assessed when the phone was off. In some cases, a location was identified only using cell tower triangulation when GPS satellites were not accessible by the phone. We assessed the data quality of locations identified only from cell towers by comparing the distance between cell tower locations and prior/following satellite locations. We determined that cell tower data were not reliable. Several points identified by cell tower data indicated implausible travel speeds to another location and were not always consistent with more accurate satellite locations. As a result, we interpolated data using only satellite-derived locations. For points with missing data (due to phone being off or no satellite data available, 15% of path points), location data were interpolated using the most recent satellite location under several stringent assumptions. The closest satellite location was used if the missing data period was less than 8 hours and data points before and after the missing period were at the same location (<30 meters apart). Straight-line imputation was used if missing data comprised less than a one hour period and data points before and after the missing period were not at the same location (>30 meters apart). Remaining missing data were excluded from analyses (<7% of path points). Sensitivity analyses were performed using less stringent criteria (100 and 200 m distances reducing missing data to 6% and 5%, respectively) with no differences in reported outcomes.

We used crime as an indicator of neighborhood disorder because it has been correlated with adverse health outcomes [18] and point-level crime data were readily available for our study area. In this study, crime was measured using geocoded locations of Unified Crime Reports (UCR) Part 1 Offenses filed in the study area. UCR Part 1 Offenses, as classified by the Federal Bureau of Investigation, include violent crime (i.e., criminal homicide, aggravated assault, robbery, forcible rape) and property crime (i.e., burglary, larceny-theft, motor vehicle theft, arson). Point-level crime data for a 3-year period (2007–2009) were aggregated in a 200-meter radius around each GPS path point (Figure 1). A 3-year period was used to provide a more stable indicator of prevalence of crime in an area. A 200-meter (approximately 1 city-block) radius was selected because we hypothesized that mobile adolescents could visually and aurally perceive the social context within this area. We used crime counts within buffers rather than crimes per capita as a proxy for social disorder based on recommendations from the criminology and crime mapping literature that caution against bias caused by the use of population-based crime rates for small areas [19]. In addition, we specifically do not state "crime" as the exposure in this paper as the 3-year crime count was intended solely as an indicator of the type of area the girls were spending time in. Thus, we refer to this measure more generally as "community disorder."

Geocoded crime report location data were available for Marion County, which encompasses the city of Indianapolis, Indiana (USA). Point-level crime data were not available for neighboring counties. For 200-meter buffers around girl's path points which had at least 50% of the area falling within Marion County, the total crime count within the buffer was estimated based on the available data and an assumption of uniformity. Specifically, the total number of crimes within buffers with <100% but ≥50% of their area in Marion County was estimated as: (observed crime count in known data area/area of buffer in Marion County) * total buffer area. Less than 0.01% of the total path points had buffers that overlapped the border of Marion County by <50%. Buffers around girls' path point that had >50% of their area outside of Marion County were excluded from analyses (3% of path points).

1.2.4 OUTCOME MEASURES

Participants completed an ACASI capturing demographic characteristics and self-reported health behaviors that correlate closely with primary causes of adult morbidity and mortality [20]. Substance use (including cigarette, alcohol and marijuana use) and sexual intercourse within the last 30 days were coded as binary variables. Questions were drawn from the CDC Youth

Risk Behavior Survey which has shown good reliability for substance use questions [21]. A comparable recall period was used for sexual behavior. Questions on sensitive behaviors such as sexual activity, using ACASI and a short recall period, has been shown to have reliable recall [22]–[24].

1.2.5 ANALYSIS

We described the number and percent of participants with various demographic and behavior characteristics overall and by reported health-related behavior. We assessed the time spent at home as well as various distances from home by health-related behavior. We presented mean crime exposures within 200-meters by reported health-related behavior, using home and path data and during school and non-school days. We compared mean crime exposures between each risk group (any substance use and any sexual intercourse) and a referent group reporting neither behavior using t tests.

Contextual exposure to prevalence of crime was compared among participants reporting engaging or not engaging in each of the health-related behaviors of interest. Using Stata/MP, we created average crime counts within 200-meters of each participant's path points based on time of day and day of week (school and non-school days). Exposure by time of day is displayed in 100 increments, each increment representing 14.4 minutes of the day (e.g., 12:00–12:14am). These path points can be considered as a representative sample of all the locations a participant visited or passed through during the monitoring periods. We took the mean crime count surrounding each GPS point for participants reporting each health-related behavior: substance use or no substance use, sexual intercourse or no sexual intercourse.

1.3 RESULTS

Twelve percent of participants reported cigarette use, 8% alcohol use and 10% marijuana use in the last 30 days (Table 1). Seventeen percent reported sexual intercourse in the last 30 days. Demographic characteristics varied among adolescents reporting no substance use or sex, substance use but no sex, sex but no substance use, and both behaviors.

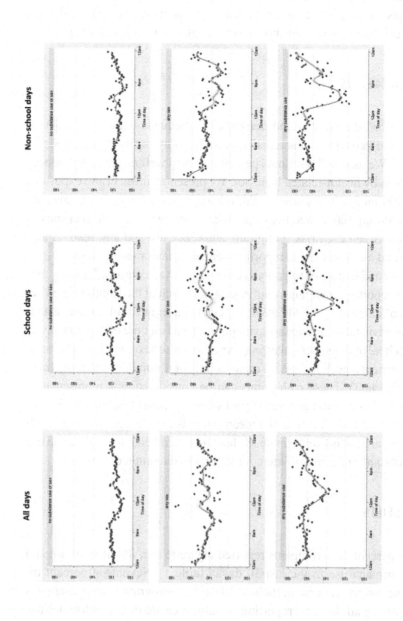

FIGURE 2: Average 200/day of week and self-reported health-related behavior in the last 30 days.

TABLE 1: Cohort characteristics.

	Total	Behaviors, last 30 days			
		no substance use	substance use	no substance use	substance use
		no sex	no sex	sex	sex
N	52	36	7	5	4
Race/ethnicity					
black	63%	64%	71%	100%	0%
white	31%	28%	29%	0%	100%
Latina	6%	8%	0%	0%	0%
Grade in school					
7	6%	6%	0%	20%	0%
8	21%	19%	14%	0%	75%
9	31%	33%	43%	20%	0%
10	21%	19%	29%	20%	25%
11	21%	22%	14%	40%	0%
Behavior in last 30 days					
cigarettes	12%		43%	0%	75%
alcohol	8%		43%	0%	25%
marijuana	10%		57%	0%	25%
sex	17%		0%	100%	100%
Percent of time spent					
home	54%	57%	59%	34%	42%
within 200 m, not at home	13%	12%	25%	16%	2%
between 200 m–1 km	8%	7%	2%	7%	25%
between 1 km–5 km	12%	11%	9%	17%	17%
more than 5 km away	14%	14%	5%	27%	14%

Participants spent about half their time at home during the monitoring period, and the majority of time in areas surrounding their home when not at home (Table 1). Participants who reported sexual intercourse in the last month spent less time at home; at least a quarter of their points occurred 5 kilometers or more away from home.

Prevalence of crime within 200 meters (one block) of a participant's home varied by her reported health behaviors (Table 2). Participants reporting substance use lived in areas of higher crime prevalence, compared to those reporting neither sexual intercourse nor substance use (p = 0.02). Similarly, participants who reported engaging in any sexual intercourse had greater prevalence of crime around their homes, compared to those reporting neither sexual intercourse nor substance use (p<0.001). When analyzing path locations, exposure to areas with greater prevalence of crime was significantly higher among girls reporting substance use, compared to those reporting neither behavior (p = 0.04). Though exposures were also higher among girls reporting sexual intercourse (compared to those reporting neither behavior), these differences were not statistically significant (p = 0.17).

TABLE 2: Mean and standard deviation (sd) exposure to areas of crime prevalence (3 year aggregate) by reported behavior among all participants for exposure only based on home or using all path data*.

	home			path		
	mean	sd	p	mean	sd	p
no sexual intercourse, no substance use	122.9	57.0	ref	119.0	50.8	ref
any substance use	174.5	61.6	0.02	154.6	43.8	0.04
any sexual intercourse	193.7	61.3	0.00	144.7	44.2	0.17

P values compare participants reporting either any substance use or any sexual intercourse to participants reporting no sexual intercourse or substance use. Home represents 200 meters surrounding the residential parcel.

Patterns of exposure to crime prevalence varied by time of day and day of week between participants reporting no substance use or sex compared to participants reporting each of these behaviors (Figure 2). As reflected in the mean and standard deviation of exposures (Table 2), participants reporting neither substance use nor sexual intercourse had lower overall exposure to crime prevalence and this varied less by time of day and day of week than girls reporting substance use or sexual intercourse. Participants reporting substance use had the most dramatic difference by time of day, reflecting higher exposures in the evening and early morning which did not vary substantially by school and non-school days.

1.4 DISCUSSION

These data demonstrate clear differences in terms of within-neighborhood variability of adolescent women's health behaviors relating to differing exposure to the area's crime (as a marker for community disorder). Participants spent only approximately half their time at home, and substance use and sexual behaviors were significantly associated with crime characteristics of the area surrounding the home. Our adolescent participants, however, spent substantial time outside of the home, and the crime prevalence within one block of where they spent time when not at home was independently associated with their behavior. In short, participants reporting either substance use or sexual intercourse live and spend time in areas of higher crime prevalence.

Multiple studies of adolescent health behaviors consider the role of contextual influence [25]–[36]. The vast majority of studies measure contextual exposure based on a larger area and often using arbitrary administrative boundaries. A census tract, block group, or other arbitrary geographic area surrounding a residential address does not fully characterize where adolescents spend time and interact with others [37]. It is difficult to accurately assess contextual influences on individuals through using different aggregations of census tracts or other arbitrary areal units—what contextual area best represents a neighborhood, community, or significant space may influence the health outcome of interest [6], [7]. In this study, we hypothesized that a relatively small area of contextual exposure would be relevant—within a 1-block radius—and that crime as a proxy for community disorder might be a relevant contextual measure. Given adolescent girls reporting substance use lived and spent time in areas of highest crime prevalence, perhaps this represents increased access to illicit substances or increased exposure to social norms accepting substance use among minors. The relationship was weaker among girls reporting sex in the last 30 days and might indicate that crime as an indicator of community disorder is not the most salient measure of contextual influence on adolescents' sexual behavior. A different measure relating to sexual risk such as teen pregnancy prevalence may be more relevant. Adolescents reporting risk behaviors spent time in areas with lower crime prevalence when not at home which may highlight the lack of specificity or relevance of this measure or the fact that these adolescents are in fact at less risk than those who are not able to leave home. In a larger sample, it would be interesting to make this direct comparison. Regardless, this is one of the first studies to assess within-neighborhood contextual exposure and indicate relative differences in reported health-risk behaviors.

There is little understanding of the mechanisms by which neighborhoods affect health. In an article entitled "Putting People into Place," [4] Barbara Entwisle outlines criticisms of the conceptualization and measurement of neighborhoods and their health effects. These include: (1) theories that "neighborhoods are exogenous and predetermined, and individuals are passive recipients of their effects," (2) narrow characterization of neighborhoods with two thirds of studies focusing on measures of poverty and the remaining generally incorporating only one or two characteristics, and (3) reliance on cross sectional analyses with little attention to change within neighborhoods over time or lagged effects. Using methods and analyses similar to those in this study could start to address some of the concerns raised in her first point. Future studies incorporating a longitudinal design and multiple measures may help to further identify mechanisms and perhaps uncover causal associations between context and health.

Many studies do not report smaller area variability due to the large area of contextual measure aggregation. For many contextual measures, only aggregated data are available due to confidentiality risk, sampling methodology, or other reasons. Even when point-level data are available, they are often aggregated to census block group or tract for unclear reasons. In this study, we purposefully recruited from the same geographic area to assess within-neighborhood variability in both residential and path-related exposures. Given the significance of our findings with even a small sample, additional studies should consider smaller areas of exposure in the future.

Evidence suggests that a narrower view of context may increase our understanding of its relationship with health. In the Moving to Opportunity (MTO) program in which families in public housing were randomized to either stay in public housing, move to another location of their choice, or a low-poverty neighborhood, 5-year outcomes were mixed with respect to adolescent health behaviors [38]. One interesting finding was that girls were less likely to smoke in the intervention groups than girls in the control group, whereas boys in the intervention groups were more likely to smoke than their control counterparts. In a follow-up qualitative study in 1 of the 5 sites, researchers found that the gender differences were not due to variability in general where girls and boys generally spent time but rather where girls and boys specifically spent time [39]. Girls in intervention groups were more likely to spend time closer to home, on the front stoop, for example. Boys were more likely to congregate on street corners, parks, vacant lots, and other places without adult supervision. This suggests that within neighborhoods, and perhaps even between neighborhoods, specific areas where (and specific times when) individuals experienced contextual influences are volitionally chosen or somehow determined in a non-random way. Reasons for these choices, however, are not well understood.

This study has several limitations. First, this is a small sample of a single area of Indianapolis. We purposefully sampled in one area due to our interest in within-neighborhood variation but further study is needed to assess whether similar associations are present in other areas. Second, our analysis was limited by the availability of point-level crime report data, which was only available within Marion County. However, we employed a straightforward, conservative method to estimate crime counts in buffers with <100% but ≥50% of their area within the study area and excluded observations exceeding this threshold. Overall, this affected a very small proportion of the total path points and we have no reason to believe that there is significant difference in crime patterns across county boundaries that would be manifested within the relatively small buffer size we used. Third, this is a cross-sectional analysis in which we did not control for potentially confounding variables. These variables might include individual (such as school failure, self-esteem), family (such as family conflict, parent connectedness) and neighborhood characteristics (such as alcohol or drug availability, poverty, neighborhood norms) known to be associated with substance use and sex [36], [40]–[42]. Likewise, this study cannot differentiate whether these contexts contribute to girls' behavior choices or whether girls engaging in particular behaviors seek different environments. Given our interests, however, in primarily identifying associations for the purposes of future interventions, this study shows promise that similar analyses may identify adolescent girls at times and places where these behaviors are more likely to occur. Again, further longitudinal study is needed to assess causal relationships and, specifically, if these behaviors of interest are in fact occurring when they are in areas of high crime.

In sum, this analysis of space-time patterns for adolescent health behaviors is particularly important given the strong and consistent association between social context and health outcomes. The micro-sociogeographic context where adolescents spend time while away from home influence their health-related behaviors. Moreover, there is variability within neighborhoods in terms of exposure to community disorder and reported behaviors. Thus, more specific measurements of contextual exposures and individual-level analyses are warranted. In addition, there may be differences in the relationship between community disorder with either substance use or sex, indicating the complexity of the person-environment interaction with respect to each behavior. Our hope is that this within-neighborhood and path-specific contextual data collection and analysis may better inform future crime-control policy and time- and space-specific interventions to improve adolescent health. For instance, we may be able to use GPS technology to identify times and places where various health-risk behaviors are likely to occur (based on their association with more micro-measures of context such as community disorder) in order to better target health messages or other health-promoting interventions. Adolescents may be more receptive and responsive to these space- and time-specific interventions, though this assertion merits further study.

REFERENCES

1.   Cohen DA, Mason K, Bedimo A, Scribner R, Basolo V, et al. (2003) Neighborhood physical conditions and health. Am J Public Health 93: 467–471. doi: 10.2105/ajph.93.3.467

2.   Diez Roux AV, Merkin SS, Arnett D, Chambless L, Massing M, et al. (2001) Neighborhood of residence and incidence of coronary heart disease. N Engl J Med 345: 99–106. doi: 10.1056/nejm200107123450205

3.   Sampson RJ (2003) The neighborhood context of well-being. Perspect Biol Med 46: S53–64. doi: 10.1353/pbm.2003.0059

4.   Entwisle B (2007) Putting people into place. Demography 44: 687–703. doi: 10.1353/dem.2007.0045

5.   Leventhal T, Brooks-Gunn J (2003) Children and youth in neighborhood contexts. Current Directions in Psychological Science 12: 27–31. doi: 10.1111/1467-8721.01216

6. Kwan MP (2009) From place-based to people-based exposure measures. Soc Sci Med 69: 1311–1313. doi: 10.1016/j.socscimed.2009.07.013

7. Kwan MP (2012) The Uncertain Geographic Context Problem. Annals of the Association of American Geographers 102: 958–968. doi: 10.1080/00045608.2012.687349

8. Elgethun K, Fenske RA, Yost MG, Palcisko GJ (2003) Time-location analysis for exposure assessment studies of children using a novel global positioning system instrument. Environ Health Perspect 111: 115–122. doi: 10.1289/ehp.5350

9. Troped PJ, Wilson JS, Matthews CE, Cromley EK, Melly SJ (2010) The built environment and location-based physical activity. Am J Prev Med 38: 429–438. doi: 10.1016/j.amepre.2009.12.032

10. Maddison R, Jiang Y, Vander Hoorn S, Exeter D, Mhurchu CN, et al. (2010) Describing patterns of physical activity in adolescents using global positioning systems and accelerometry. Pediatr Exerc Sci 22: 392–407.

11. Basta LA, Richmond TS, Wiebe DJ (2010) Neighborhoods, daily activities, and measuring health risks experienced in urban environments. Soc Sci Med 71: 1943–1950. doi: 10.1016/j.socscimed.2010.09.008

12. Wiehe SE, Carroll AE, Liu GC, Haberkorn KL, Hoch SC, et al. (2008) Using GPS-enabled cell phones to track the travel patterns of adolescents. Int J Health Geogr 7: 22. doi: 10.1186/1476-072x-7-22

13. Larson RW, Richards MH, Sims B, Dworkin J (2001) How urban African American young adolescents spend their time: time budgets for locations, activities, and companionship. Am J Community Psychol 29: 565–597.

14. Chassin L, Presson CC, Pitts SC, Sherman SJ (2000) The natural history of cigarette smoking from adolescence to adulthood in a midwestern community sample: multiple trajectories and their psychosocial correlates. Health Psychol 19: 223–231. doi: 10.1037//0278-6133.19.3.223

15. Hawkins JD, Catalano RF, Kosterman R, Abbott R, Hill KG (1999) Preventing adolescent health-risk behaviors by strengthening protection during childhood. Arch Pediatr Adolesc Med 153: 226–234. doi: 10.1001/archpedi.153.3.226

16. Zapert K, Snow DL, Tebes JK (2002) Patterns of substance use in early through late adolescence. Am J Community Psychol 30: 835–852. doi: 10.1023/a:1020257103376

17. Cavazos-Rehg PA, Krauss MJ, Spitznagel EL, Schootman M, Bucholz KK, et al. (2009) Age of sexual debut among US adolescents. Contraception 80: 158–162. doi: 10.1016/j.contraception.2009.02.014

18. Lorenc T, Clayton S, Neary D, Whitehead M, Petticrew M, et al. (2012) Crime, fear of crime, environment, and mental health and wellbeing: mapping review of theories and causal pathways. Health Place 18: 757–765. doi: 10.1016/j.healthplace.2012.04.001

19. Zhang H, Peterson M (2007) A spatial analysis of neighbourhood crime in Omaha, Nebraska using alternative measures of crime rates. Internet Journal of Criminology

20. Mokdad AH, Marks JS, Stroup DF, Gerberding JL (2004) Actual causes of death in the United States, 2000. JAMA 291: 1238–1245. doi: 10.1001/jama.291.10.1238

21. Centers for Disease C, Prevention (2013) Brener ND, Kann L, Shanklin S, et al. (2013) Methodology of the Youth Risk Behavior Surveillance System–2013. MMWR Recomm Rep 62: 1–20.

22. Brener ND, Billy JO, Grady WR (2003) Assessment of factors affecting the validity of self-reported health-risk behavior among adolescents: evidence from the scientific literature. J Adolesc Health 33: 436–457. doi: 10.1016/s1054-139x(03)00052-1

23. Fenton KA, Johnson AM, McManus S, Erens B (2001) Measuring sexual behaviour: methodological challenges in survey research. Sex Transm Infect 77: 84–92. doi: 10.1136/sti.77.2.84

24. Turner CF, Ku L, Rogers SM, Lindberg LD, Pleck JH, et al. (1998) Adolescent sexual behavior, drug use, and violence: increased reporting with computer survey technology. Science 280: 867–873. doi: 10.1126/science.280.5365.867

25. Averett SL, Rees DI, Argys LM (2002) The impact of government policies and neighborhood characteristics on teenage sexual activity and contraceptive use. Am J Public Health 92: 1773–1778. doi: 10.2105/ajph.92.11.1773

26. Santelli JS, Lowry R, Brener ND, Robin L (2000) The association of sexual behaviors with socioeconomic status, family structure, and race/ethnicity among US adolescents. Am J Public Health 90: 1582–1588. doi: 10.2105/ajph.90.10.1582

27. Zenilman JM, Ellish N, Fresia A, Glass G (1999) The geography of sexual partnerships in Baltimore: applications of core theory dynamics using a geographic information system. Sex Transm Dis 26: 75–81. doi: 10.1097/00007435-199902000-00002

28. Rothenberg RB, Potterat JJ, Woodhouse DE (1996) Personal risk taking and the spread of disease: beyond core groups. J Infect Dis 174 Suppl 2: S144–149. doi: 10.1093/infdis/174.supplement_2.s144

29. Lee RE, Cubbin C (2002) Neighborhood context and youth cardiovascular health behaviors. Am J Public Health 92: 428–436. doi: 10.2105/ajph.92.3.428

30. Cubbin C, Hadden WC, Winkleby MA (2001) Neighborhood context and cardiovascular disease risk factors: the contribution of material deprivation. Ethn Dis 11: 687–700.

31. Duncan SC, Duncan TE, Strycker LA (2002) A multilevel analysis of neighborhood context and youth alcohol and drug problems. Prev Sci 3: 125–133.

32. Ross CE (2000) Walking, exercising, and smoking: does neighborhood matter? Soc Sci Med 51: 265–274. doi: 10.1016/s0277-9536(99)00451-7

33. Diez Roux AV, Merkin SS, Hannan P, Jacobs DR, Kiefe CI (2003) Area characteristics, individual-level socioeconomic indicators, and smoking in young adults: the coronary artery disease risk development in young adults study. Am J Epidemiol 157: 315–326. doi: 10.1093/aje/kwf207

34. Diez-Roux AV, Kiefe CI, Jacobs DR Jr, Haan M, Jackson SA, et al. (2001) Area characteristics and individual-level socioeconomic position indicators in three population-based epidemiologic studies. Ann Epidemiol 11: 395–405. doi: 10.1016/s1047-2797(01)00221-6

35. Karvonen S, Rimpela A (1996) Socio-regional context as a determinant of adolescents' health behaviour in Finland. Soc Sci Med 43: 1467–1474. doi: 10.1016/0277-9536(96)00044-5

36. Cubbin C, Santelli J, Brindis CD, Braveman P (2005) Neighborhood context and sexual behaviors among adolescents: findings from the national longitudinal study of adolescent health. Perspect Sex Reprod Health 37: 125–134. doi: 10.1363/3712505

37. Coulton CJ, Korbin J, Chan T, Su M (2001) Mapping residents' perceptions of neighborhood boundaries: a methodological note. Am J Community Psychol 29: 371–383. doi: 10.1023/a:1010303419034

38. Orr L, Feins JD, Jacob R, Beecroft E, Abt Associates Inc, et al. (2003) Moving to Opportunity Fair Housing Demonstration Program: Interim Impacts Evaluation. US Department of Housing and Urban Development, Office of Policy Development & Research.

39. Clampet-Lundquist S, Edin K, Kling J, Duncan G (2006) Moving at-risk teenagers out of high-risk neighborhoods: Why girls fare better than boys. Working Paper #509 Princeton University.

40. Hawkins JD, Catalano RF, Miller JY (1992) Risk and protective factors for alcohol and other drug problems in adolescence and early adulthood: implications for substance abuse prevention. Psychol Bull 112: 64–105. doi: 10.1037/0033-2909.112.1.64

41. Browning SE (2012) Neighborhood, school, and family effects on the frequency of alcohol use among Toronto youth. Subst Use Misuse 47: 31–43. doi: 10.3109/10826084.2011.625070

42. Bangpan M, Operario D (2012) Understanding the role of family on sexual-risk decisions of young women: a systematic review. AIDS Care 24: 1163–1172. doi: 10.1080/09540121.2012.699667

CHAPTER 2

WHERE LIES THE RISK? AN ECOLOGICAL APPROACH TO UNDERSTANDING CHILD MENTAL HEALTH RISK AND VULNERABILITIES IN SUB-SAHARAN AFRICA

OLAYINKA ATILOLA

2.1 INTRODUCTION

The last century witnessed considerable changes in the nature and pattern of child and adolescent health problems, significant among which is the unequivocal recognition of mental disorders as a source of childhood morbidity [1]. This recognition is not unconnected with emerging evidence from multinational epidemiological surveys that mental and behavioural problems among children and adolescents are common and a worldwide phenomenon [2]. Childhood mental disorders are also associated with significant distress to the child and a major burden to the society [3–5]. Though there is yet to be any conclusive evidence that childhood mental disorders are relatively more prevalent in low-resource countries, there

Where Lies the Risk? An Ecological Approach to Understanding Child Mental Health Risk and Vulnerabilities in Sub-Saharan Africa. © Atilola O. Psychiatric Journal, **2014** (2014). http://dx.doi.org/10.1155/2014/698348. Licensed under Creative Commons Attribution 3.0 Unported License, http://creativecommons.org/licenses/by/3.0/.

are indicators to suggest that the global burden of childhood mental health problems is likely to be concentrated in low- and middle-income (LAMI) countries. In the first instance, 85% of the world's child and adolescent population live in the LAMI countries [6]. Secondly, the LAMI regions of world have poorer child-related social indicators [7], a situation which can increase the risk of childhood mental health problems [8].

Among the LAMI regions of the world, children living in sub-Saharan Africa in particular face a life of poverty, poor nutrition, and social problems which can impair their early development as well as their mental health and wellbeing [9]. Currently available epidemiological evidence shows a prevalence rate as high as 20% for childhood mental health problems in sub-Saharan Africa [10]. Perhaps inevitably, efforts at improving on the poor state of child-health and development initiatives in sub-Saharan Africa had focused on improving the physical health of children. This focus has however been on the neglect of child and adolescent mental health (CAMH) policy development as a child-health and development initiative in the region. Part of the problem is the poor understanding of CAMH issues and awareness of the consequences of child mental health problems among policy makers. As a result, CAMH service and policy development have remained low in the rungs of public-health thrust in sub-Saharan Africa [11–13]. Child and adolescent mental health policies are critical component of the healthcare delivery system of nations [12], without which preventive and restorative child mental health services cannot be hatched on an integrated platform which can ensure success. Children will therefore suffer from preventable mental health problems, while those in need of curative services may not get it. Untreated mental health problems among children constitute major social and economic burden on families and the society at large [14, 15].

Articulating a CAMH policy for any region requires a thorough and broad-based understanding of the risk and vulnerability factors for child mental health problems in such region. In fact, in other climes, such effort has been identified as a unique step towards charting a course for CAMH policy development [16–18]. Researchers working in LAMI regions have also adopted a risk and vulnerability approach to set directions for CAMH service and policy development in recent times [19]. However, there had not been any concise documentation of child mental health risk and vulnerability points in sub-Saharan Africa. This is a critical omission for a region with almost half a billion child population [20], majority of whom are also living in sundry difficult social circumstances [7]. Therefore, with a view to emphasize the appropriate target points for CAMH policy development in sub-Saharan Africa, we present a narrative on the child mental health risk and vulnerability points in the region. To ensure capturing the ramifications of risk and vulnerability points as much as possible, we adopt the Ecological Model of Childhood [21] as the descriptive framework.

2.2 ECOLOGICAL MODEL OF CHILD AND ADOLESCENT MENTAL HEALTH RISK AND VULNERABILITY FACTORS IN SUB-SAHARAN AFRICA

Bronfenbrenner's Ecological Model of Childhood [21] compartmentalized the operating milieu and the care environment of the child into 5 hierarchal but interconnected layers. These include the microsystem, mesosystem, exosystem, macrosystem, and time bound chronosystems in that order of hierarchy. The risk and vulnerability points for child mental health in the different components of the ecological care environment of the child are hereby examined.

2.3 RISK AND VULNERABILITIES WITHIN THE MICRO- AND MESOSYSTEM

In this section, peculiar risk and vulnerability points for CAMH in sub-Saharan Africa are examined starting from the family unit, being the most critical component of the ecological care environment of children [22]. Other components of the microsystem examined include the school, other childcare facilities, and the neighbourhoods where children grow up. The mesosystem of the care environment of a child is formed mainly by the quality of interaction between the agents within the microsystem. These interactions include the degree of uptake and utilisation of available childcare resources.

2.3.1 POORLY RESOURCED FAMILIES AS A RISK AND VULNERABILITY POINT

Among the key components of the microsystem of the care environment of a child is the family unit. In fact, the intricate relationship between the child and the family unit shapes all aspects of children's physical and mental development [22]. The family unit has also been described as a critical component of the care environment of children which ensures they receive the appropriate nurturance for good social and health outcomes [23]. Therefore, the presence of an appropriate, resourceful, and stable family is a key resilience factor for the mental health and wellbeing of a child. The ability of the family unit to provide optimal care for children however depends on the level of resources, including financial and social, that are available to them. Unfortunately, there are indications that a large proportion of children in sub-Saharan Africa are being nurtured under caregiving or family arrangements that may not guarantee optimal social and mental development.

To start with, about 55 million of children in sub-Saharan Africa are orphans who live in different forms of alternative care [24]. Going by the current child population of about 430 million in the region [20], this translates to about 13% of all children in the region. The sheer burden of orphans and other out-of-care children in the region is believed to have overstretched the traditional extended-family system in the region, giving rise to different forms of alternative care arrangements including child-headed households [25, 26]. Although the exact estimate is not available, many of the orphaned children in sub-Saharan Africa live in child-headed households [27, 28]. Consistent with studies from the developed countries which show that children who grew up in alternative care settings experience poorer mental health [29, 30], a study conducted in Zambia showed that children being raised in child-headed households had poorer indicators of health (including mental health) compared with their peers growing up in adult-headed households [31]. Besides the risk of being brought up in alternative care arrangements, orphans are ordinarily at risk of cumulative social disruptions and traumatic events [32] which may put them at higher risk of mental health problems. It is therefore not surprising that cross-sectional and longitudinal studies from different parts of sub-Saharan Africa have found higher prevalence rates of mental disorders among orphaned children compared with nonorphaned controls [32–34].

Moreover, a significant proportion of children in sub-Saharan Africa are born into "families" with limited childcare resources. For instance, up to 123 out of 1000 children in the region are born to children below 18 years [7]. Many of the children so born also grow up in alternative care arrangements with their attendant mental health risks. Besides this, the quality of care that can be provided by a child-mother is limited so is the likelihood of full utilisation of childcare resources. Therefore, being born to a child and being a child-mother both carry mental health risks. In a review of child mental health problems in sub-Saharan Africa, lower maternal age was an independent predictor [10].

Equally relevant is the fact that the well-known strong inclination towards a stable family life in sub-Saharan Africa is already on a fast decline [35], giving rise to an emerging generation of single-parent households in the region [36, 37]. A recent survey in South Africa, for example, found that up to 40% of children are living in single-parent households [38]. Though there are cultural differences in what constitutes the ideal family, the chances of optimal mental health and wellbeing of children are most guaranteed in a cohesive dual-parent setting [39]. Large-scale studies from the developed countries have found a higher prevalence of mental health problems among children in single-parent families [40]. Similar large-scale studies are yet to be conducted in sub-Saharan Africa but small-scale studies have established links between family-life deficits and adverse social and mental health outcomes for children [41, 42].

Furthermore, about 50% of families and household in sub-Saharan Africa live on less than USD 1.25 per day [7]. Severe limitation of financial resources can impair the ability of families to meet the social and emotional needs of children [43]. Poverty can also initiate a spiral of events that can threaten the stability of the family unit [44, 45] and as such can put the social and mental wellbeing of children at risk. A good illustration can be found in the sundry reports from many parts of sub-Saharan Africa that parental poverty is the key factor responsible for children dropping out of school, living on the street, being forced into early marriage, engaging in child labour, and living in sundry other difficult circumstances [46–49]. Therefore, by fostering family instability or putting children in precarious situations, family poverty is one of the factors within the ecological care environment that is capable of increasing the mental health risk of children. In a recent review of all the available epidemiological data on mental health problems among children in sub-Saharan Africa, most of the studies reviewed found an association between childhood psychopathology and poorer parental socioeconomic status [10]. Besides this, the highest burden of mental health problems among children in sub-Saharan Africa has been found among children living in sundry poverty-driven difficult circumstances. For instance while the prevalence of mental health problems among the general population of children in sub-Saharan Africa currently hovers around 10–30% [10], studies conducted in the region have found as high as 50–90% rate of mental health problems among children living in poverty-driven difficult circumstances like street children [50], child labourers [51], and children living on social welfare or in juvenile justice custody [52, 53].

Besides material resources, educational resources of care givers are also important in determining the quality of childcare, including the uptake of available resources for childcare. General literacy can improve awareness and uptake of newer childcare insights and practices. The adult literacy rate which is as high as 99% in some developed countries averages about 63% in sub-Saharan Africa [54, 55]. In fact, adult literacy is as low as 45% among women in the region [54, 55]. The figures for women can even be as low as 10% or less in some sub-Saharan Africa countries like Niger and Burkina Faso [55]. Without prejudice to the rich indigenous knowledge for childcare in sub-Saharan Africa which may have nothing to do with formal schooling [56], education—in terms of literacy—often serves as a proxy for knowledge and information as well as cognitive skills and societal values [57]. All these can influence good childcare choices [58]. Therefore, parental illiteracy is capable of limiting the full utilisation of available childcare resources and as such limiting the mental health reserve of their children.

2.3.2 POOR AVAILABILITY AND UPTAKE OF CHILDCARE RESOURCES AS RISK AND VULNERABILITY POINT

There is substantial evidence that the availability and uptake of Early Childhood Care and Development (ECCD) resources are key determinant of social and mental health outcomes for children [8]. In this context and thereafter, ECCD is understood as resources for health promotion, optimal nutrition, psychosocial, and cognitive stimulation, as well as other supports to strengthen the care environment of children [59]. Common ECCD resources usually include health and educational resources, maternal health services, and child nutritional support among others. Though significant effort is being made, a complex interplay of social, economic, structural, and cultural factors continues to limit availability and utilisation of ECCD resources in sub-Saharan Africa [60]. Lack or poor utilisation of ECCD resources can impair the resilience of children against physical and mental health shocks [8]. Therefore, from mental health perspectives, lack of or poor utilisation of ECCD resources in sub-Saharan Africa suggests that a large proportion of children in the region may be disadvantaged in terms of baseline resilience or mental health reserves.

Specifically, only about half of mothers in sub-Saharan Africa utilise or have access to antenatal care services or skilled birth attendance on the average [7]. The rate of antenatal-care access and utilisation is as low as 20% in some countries like Niger and Chad, while skilled birth attendance is lower than 40% in Nigeria, Chad, Ethiopia, and Niger [7]. Studies from Kenya [61] through Sudan [62] to Nigeria [63] have established a link between poor antenatal care or lack of skilled birth attendance and poor obstetric outcomes. Obstetrics complications arising from poor maternal care in sub-Saharan Africa are the key risk factor for perinatal asphyxia [64], which is very common in the region [65]. Some studies from sub-Saharan Africa had found an association between perinatal asphyxia and childhood mental disorders [66].

Similarly, up to 40% of children below 5 years in the sub-Saharan Africa are malnourished, while up to 20% do not receive complete immunisation by respective national guidelines [7]. Nutritional deficiencies and lack of full immunisation put children at a risk of childhood infectious diseases like measles, poliomyelitis, meningitis, and others which can lay a foundation for mental health problems in later childhood. On a different note, high-quality early education provided in a highly stimulating environment is expected to come with an early sense of self-esteem and confidence and a repertoire of problem-solving skills which are critical protective factors for mental health [67]. Therefore, quality early child education for instance is a fundamental mental health resilience factor. Unfortunately, access to and utilisation of early-childhood educational resources are still poor in sub-Saharan Africa. The preprimary school Gross Enrolment Rate (GER) in sub-Saharan Africa averages about 18% while the primary school Net Enrolment Ratio (NER) averages 66% [7]. Though at 86%, the rate of survival to the last grade in primary school is fair, an average secondary school NER of about 27% in the region [7] erodes this apparent gain.

Besides this, infrastructure for early education in sub-Saharan Africa is poor, and the average pupil-teacher ratio of 45:1 in the region is the highest in all the regions of the world [68]. In addition, a survey of teacher motivation and satisfaction also found that majority of elementary school teachers in sub-Saharan Africa are dissatisfied with their jobs and are poorly motivated [69]. This situation has continued to threaten the proper acquisition of early childhood foundational education and social-skill development in many parts of sub-Saharan Africa [69]. Poor pupil-teacher interaction, which can be envisaged in a situation of high pupil-teacher ratio and poor teacher motivation, reduces the chances of the child benefitting fully from the mental health benefits of school participation. It can also reduce the chances of early detection of emotional and behavioural problems [70].

Likewise, in the event that childhood mental health problem arises, availability of mental healthcare facilities is crucial. This is because untreated mental health problems among children hardly just go away; rather they are associated with social and functional impairments [4]. Therefore, availability of restorative CAMH services is a good child mental health resource. Unfortunately, resources for restorative mental health service are very limited in sub-Saharan Africa, in terms of both human and material resources [13]. Many countries in the region have an acute shortage of CAMH facilities and an abysmally low number of trained CAMH practitioners, sometimes in the ratio of 1 : 10 million child population [71]. To compound the problem, some recent studies have reported a poor utilisation of the few available mental health services for children [50].

2.3.3 RISK AND VULNERABILITIES IN THE LIVING NEIGHBOURHOOD

The neighbourhood in which children grow is also a critical component of the microsystem. The neighbourhood is part of the sources of stimulation, care, and nurturance, as well as an embodiment of values and behavioural models for children. Therefore, the neighbourhoods within which children grow up contribute significantly to children's mental health and wellbeing. Poverty, social inequalities, and poor rural development have created a situation of exodus of people to the urban areas of sub-Saharan Africa. As a result, urbanized population in sub-Saharan Africa has been on the rise. Urbanized population is as high as 50% in Nigeria and Cote d'Ivoire and over 60% in South Africa, Congo, and Cameroon [7]. In fact, with a current population of at least 10 million, Lagos (Nigeria) has acquired the status of a megacity while Nairobi (Kenya) with an annual population growth rate of 13% may soon join the league [72]. Urbanisation, especially very rapid ones, poses a lot of mental health challenges for vulnerable group of individuals, including children, in LAMI countries [73].

Many of the rapidly urbanising cities in sub-Saharan Africa lack the facilities to cater for the large influx of persons, as such, creating a situation of urban slums in many parts of the region [74]. More than 70% of urban dwellers in sub-Saharan Africa live in slums [75], expectedly with their children. This proportion is the highest for any region in the world [75]. Urban slums in low-income regions like sub-Saharan Africa are associated with lack of basic amenities, poor housing, unsafe neighbourhoods, and social exclusion [76]. These social circumstances constitute mental health risk for children. Reports from other parts of the world had found that children living in slums had poorer mental health [77, 78]. A recent study conducted among children and youth in the slums of Kampala (Uganda) found a prevalence of suicidal ideation that is very much higher than the national average [79].

2.4 RISK AND VULNERABILITIES IN THE EXOSYSTEM

The key components of the exosystem examined here include the parental workplace, community childcare facilities like social welfare and juvenile justice systems, and social-protection schemes for children.

2.4.1 POOR WORKPLACE POLICIES AS A VULNERABILITY AND RISK FACTOR

Sub-Saharan Africa is among the worst-hit regions by the shock waves of the global economic crisis [80]. The crippling effect of the global economic crisis on the economy is further complicated by the preexisting low infrastructural capacity for industrialization and job creation in the region. As a result, there is an intensive scampering for jobs in the region which creates a situation for exploitative and unhealthy working conditions [81]. Furthermore, the labour market in sub-Saharan Africa is characterized by high level of precarious forms of employment like casualised labour [82, 83] and forced labour [84]. A lot of women in sub-Saharan Africa had had to augment family income by participating in the informal and formal labour market [85]. This often comes at some cost to childcare, as women are traditionally the primary caregiver for children in the region [86].

Workplace policies in sub-Saharan Africa have not fully embraced initiatives on family-work life balance as stipulated by International Labor Organisation (ILO) Conventions [87]. For instance, none of the countries in sub-Saharan Africa make provision for parental leave which allows both parents to take paid leave to care for children [87]. Also, only a few countries in the region provide up to the recommended 14 weeks maternity leave. In fact, it is as low as 60 days in countries like Eritrea, Guinea-

Bissau, Kenya, Malawi, Mozambique, and Uganda. There is also a deficient—if not nonexistent—framework for extending paid maternity leave to workers in the informal sector in sub-Saharan Africa, which is the main employer of women in the region [88]. In the context of Bronfenbrenner's ecological model of childhood, the lack of opportunity for sharing quality time with children and the instability and unpredictability of family life that is created by precarious employment have been described as the most destructive force to child physical and mental wellbeing globally [89]. Therefore, the precarious nature of work and working in sub-Saharan Africa can be viewed as a significant potential source of risk for mental health and wellbeing of children in the region.

2.4.2 LACK OF ADEQUATE COMMUNITY AND INSTITUTIONAL CHILDCARE SYSTEMS AS A RISK FACTOR

Among the repercussions of the ongoing global economic crisis is increased incidence of child maltreatment/neglect, delinquency, and youth crime [90, 91]. In the last decade, the proportion of children coming in contact with the social welfare and juvenile justice systems in the sub-Saharan Africa as a result of neglect or delinquency had been on the rise [52, 92, 93]. The availability of a well-organized juvenile justice and social welfare system offers a good opportunity for many of these children and adolescents to receive the necessary care, guidance, mentorship, reformation, and mental health services needed for their rehabilitation and reintegration back into the society.

Unfortunately, despite a high need for juvenile justice and child social-welfare services in many parts of sub-Saharan Africa, these systems are still poorly developed in the region [42, 94, 95]. The care of children in contact with social welfare and juvenile justice institution in the region is still hinged largely on punitive incarceration or institutional seclusion without much framework for true reformation or addressing their social and mental health needs [42, 96]. The implication is that there currently exist a limited capacity and framework in the sub-Saharan Africa region for assisting children and adolescents who may be out-of-care as a result of maltreatment/neglect or in need of reformation as a result of delinquency/youth crime to regain their footing for continued mental health and wellbeing.

2.4.3 LACK OF ADEQUATE SOCIAL PROTECTION FOR VULNERABLE CHILDREN AS A RISK FACTOR

In a care environment associated with deprivation, social insecurity, and social inequalities, social protection schemes for families and children offer a unique and effective policy framework to mitigate the damaging effects on the mental health and wellbeing of children and their families. This fact is recognized by the 2005 report of the Commission for Africa [97]. Social protection schemes can mitigate the social and mental health risks of poverty and inequalities on children and their families. In spite of the modest expansion in Eastern and Southern regions of Africa in recent times [98], available data unfortunately suggests that social protection and social-welfare schemes in sub-Saharan Africa are still largely rudimentary, noncomprehensive, restrictive, or at experimental stages [99–101]. In addition, the social protection schemes in the region are still bedeviled by weak institutional framework for impactful implementation [102]. This scenario has the potential of limiting the capacity of households in sub-Saharan Africa to break the poverty cycle, provide qualitative care for children, and ensure the mental wellbeing of children.

2.5 RISK AND VULNERABILITY POINTS IN THE MACROSYSTEM

Though it is the most distant component of the care ecosystem of a child in terms of the proximity of impact, the components of the macrosystem affect the wellbeing of children through its influence on the components of the other layers of the care environment. The components of the macrosystem include cultural practices relating to children, legislative framework for the protection of children, and globalisation and its effect on children, among other things.

2.5.1 CULTURAL PRACTICES IN CHILDCARE AS A RISK FACTOR

Many of the cultures in sub-Saharan Africa place a lot of premium on childcare and have a lot of healthy practices that can enhance the mental health of children [103, 104]. In fact, some of the peculiar parenting styles in sub-Saharan Africa which promote sense of duty and responsibility, as well as subservience to culturally recognized authorities, have been speculated to promote mental wellbeing of children [103]. There are however a lot of potentially harmful traditional practices in the region that can affect the mental health of children. For instance, widespread cultural and religious beliefs in many parts of sub-Saharan Africa have entrenched corporal punishment and other forms of abusive and potentially abusive methods of child control [104]. Though the psychological effects of corporal punishment among children in sub-Saharan Africa are yet to be systematically studied [104, 105], studies from other parts of the world show that corporal punishments have deleterious effects on mental health of children [106, 107]. Similarly, linked to deep-seated and ancestrally entrenched cultural beliefs, close to 3 million girls are estimated to undergo female genital mutilation annually in sub-Saharan Africa [108]. Besides the sundry physical health implications of this traditional practice [109], harmful effects on mental health of girls and women have been documented [110].

In addition, several studies have shown that women and children are disinherited through various traditional and cultural norms in sub-Saharan African communities [111–113]. Life-course analyses have however established the importance of asset transfers in intergenerational wellbeing of persons [114, 115]. Intergenerational studies of poverty transmission in sub-Saharan Africa have found disinheritance of women and children as a perpetuating factor, with attendant adverse implications for the mental health and wellbeing of children and women [116]. Furthermore, driven by practice that is linked with strongly held cultural and religious values, sub-Saharan Africa also has one of the highest rates of child marriages in the world [117]. Child marriage can interfere with proxies of mental health like education and free socialisation and can put the child-wife in situations that increase mental health risks [118]. Other traditional practices in sub-Saharan Africa that can impact negatively on the mental health and wellbeing of children include, but not limited to, taboos against consumption of some nutritious foods by pregnant women and hierarchical or gender based distribution of food [105]. Cultural and religious beliefs are also known to contribute to delays in seeking medical care for childhood mental health problems in the region [50].

2.5.2 POOR LEGISLATIVE FRAMEWORK FOR CHILD PROTECTION AS A RISK FACTOR

The legislative framework for the protection of the wellbeing of children in a country is a component of the macrosystem of the care environment of a child. Besides a few regional charters for the protection of the rights of children, the provisions of the United Nation's Convention on the Rights of Children [119] are the framework for achieving this objective globally. The Convention on the Rights of Children (CRC) seeks to promote the physical, mental, and social wellbeing of children by conferring certain rights on children which state parties are expected to strive to protect. This legislative framework is expected to compel state parties to invest in the physical, mental, and social wellbeing of children by creating the necessary socioeconomic and legislative milieu for the protection and assurance of the rights of the child. With the exception of Somalia, all sub-Saharan African countries signed, ratified, and domesticated the CRC. However, many of these countries have not been able to fully guarantee these rights due to a combination of lack of adequate local legislative framework for operationalisation, poor political will, sociocultural barriers, and poor socioeconomic realities [120, 121]. These barriers to full implementation of child's rights continue to put children in the region at significant mental health risks. This is because most of the factors like child abuse and neglect, child labor, and lack of access to ECCD, which put children at mental health risks, are preventable within the framework of child rights.

2.5.3 GLOBALISATION AND ITS EFFECT ON CHILDHOOD AS A RISK FACTOR

The macrosystem level of the care environment of children in resource-poor regions of the world like sub-Saharan Africa is highly susceptible to disruptions arising from the globalizing influence of the world's dominant socialization. It is a well-known fact that for a long time, the spirit of "ubuntu" (one for all and all for one) has provided a strong bonding and a source of social, emotional, and material security for children and families during crisis periods in sub-Saharan African communities [122]. However, globalisation has engendered the emergence of elitist nuclear family system in sub-Saharan Africa and has created an increasing sense of individualism that undermines the spirit of ubuntu [123, 124]. In addition, economic globalisation has also widened the inequality gaps in many poor-resourced regions like sub-Saharan Africa [125] to the detriment of the mental health and wellbeing of children.

Despite the fact that cultural value and beliefs are known to influence the idioms of expression as well as manifestation of mental disorders [126], globalisation of mental healthcare has created a situation whereby childhood mental disorders in a non-Western regions like sub-Saharan Africa are increasingly being conceptualized from Western perspectives [127]. This has a potential of undermining an effective and culturally nuanced diagnosis and management of childhood mental health problems in the region. Also, some globalization-driven economic policy advice like the structural adjustment programme, deregulation and privatization policies, and currency devaluation initiatives has created disastrous economic blunders [128] which have affected the capacities of many sub-Saharan African countries to meet obligations on welfare and wellbeing of families and children [129].

2.6 IMPLICATIONS FOR CHILD AND ADOLESCENT MENTAL HEALTH POLICY DEVELOPMENT IN SUB-SAHARAN AFRICA

Though the planned focus of this paper is to be an expository on the risk and vulnerability points for child mental health for future development of CAMH policies, we will however make some general notes on the implications of the current discourse for CAMH policy development in the region. Suffice to say however that the ecological approach to CAMH risk and vulnerability points adopted in this discourse provides a broad and holistic template from which an angle to CAMH policy direction in the region can be understood. It also shows that approaches to CAMH policy development in the region must be cognizant of the fact that child mental health risks are diverse and cuts across different layers of the care environment. In line with recent recommendations for developing countries [130, 131] therefore, CAMH policy formulation in sub-Saharan Africa needs to have a multisectoral and multidisciplinary focus. This should include assigned roles for sectors including health, education, social welfare, juvenile justice, and legislative authorities. The Labor Office, environmental agencies, and community-based organizations among others will also have a role to play.

For the constraint of space we have dedicated another paper to charting a tentative course for CAMH policy in sub-Saharan Africa based on the risk and vulnerability points and using the Bronfenbrenner's ecological model of childhood as the operational framework [132]. Strategies targeted towards the micro-/mesosystem that have been recommended include but are not limited to strengthening the care capacity of the family unit through child-sensitive social-protection schemes extended to the most vulnerable families and households [132]. Significant emphasis should also be placed on providing for and removing barriers to accessing ECCD resources. There is ample evidence from sub-Saharan Africa that bridging the ECCD gap has a potential of reducing social inequalities, promoting the mental health and wellbeing of children, and breaking the intergenerational cycle of poverty [60]. Strategies to address risk and vulnerabilities in the exo- and mesosystems of the care environment of children should incorporate efforts and legislations to promote child-friendly workplace policies, strengthening the child social welfare and juvenile justice systems, ensuring further development of legislative frameworks to protect child rights, as well as community engagements on harmful traditional practices [132].

2.7 CONCLUSION

We have presented a narrative on the risk and vulnerability points for child mental health in sub-Saharan Africa, using an ecological approach. The risk and vulnerability points are broad, and cuts across many layers of the child's care environment. This underscores the need for CAMH policy development in the region to be multisectoral and multidisciplinary in design. While the social circumstance of children may differ among countries of sub-Saharan Africa, the general principles of this discourse will come in handy as each country evolves a CAMH policy.

REFERENCES

1. J. S. Palfrey, T. F. Tonniges, M. Green, and J. Richmond, "Introduction: addressing the millennial morbidity—the context of community pediatrics," Pediatrics, vol. 115, no. 4, pp. 1121–1123, 2005.

2. E. J. Costello, H. Egger, and A. Angold, "10-Year research update review: the epidemiology of child and adolescent psychiatric disorders: I. Methods and public health burden," Journal of the American Academy of Child and Adolescent Psychiatry, vol. 44, no. 10, pp. 972–986, 2005.

3. V. Patel, A. J. Flisher, S. Hetrick, and P. McGorry, "Mental health of young people: a global public-health challenge," The Lancet, vol. 369, no. 9569, pp. 1302–1313, 2007.

4. F. Smit, P. Cuijpers, J. Oostenbrink, N. Batelaan, R. de Graaf, and A. Beekman, "Costs of nine common mental disorders: implications for curative and preventive psychiatry," Journal of Mental Health Policy and Economics, vol. 9, no. 4, pp. 193–200, 2006.

5. G. A. Simpson, B. Bloom, R. A. Cohen, S. Blumberg, and K. H. Bourdon, "U.S. children with emotional and behavioral difficulties: data from the 2001, 2002, and 2003 National Health Interview Surveys," Advance Data, no. 360, pp. 1–13, 2005.

6. United Nations, "World Population Prospects: The 2008 revision," Department of Economic and Social Affairs, Population Division, Geneva, Switzerland, 2008, http://www.esa.un.org/unpd/wpp2008/index.htm.

7. Unicef, "State of World's Children, 2012 report," 2012, http://www.unicef.org/sowc/files/SOWC_2012-Main_Report_EN_21Dec2011.pdf.

8. L. J. Schweinhart, H. V. Barnes, and D. P. Weikart, Significant Benefits: The High/Scope Perry Preschool Study Through Age 27, High/Scope Press, Ypsilanti, Mich, USA, 1993.

9. S. Grantham-McGregor, Y. B. Cheung, S. Cueto, P. Glewwe, L. Richter, and B. Strupp, "Developmental potential in the first 5 years for children in developing countries," The Lancet, vol. 369, no. 9555, pp. 60–70, 2007.
10. M. A. Cortina, A. Sodha, M. Fazel, and P. G. Ramchandani, "Prevalence of child mental health problems in Sub-Saharan Africa: a systematic review," Archives of Pediatrics and Adolescent Medicine, vol. 166, no. 3, pp. 276–281, 2012.
11. O. Omigbodun, "Unifying psyche and soma for child healthcare in Africa," Journal of Child and Adolescent Mental Health, vol. 21, no. 2, pp. 7–9, 2009.
12. J. P. Shatkin and M. L. Belfer, "The global absence of child and adolescent mental health policy," Child and Adolescent Mental Health, vol. 9, no. 3, pp. 104–108, 2004.
13. S. Kleintjes, C. Lund, and A. J. Flisher, "A situational analysis of child and adolescent mental health services in Ghana, Uganda, South Africa and Zambia," African Journal of Psychiatry (South Africa), vol. 13, no. 2, pp. 132–139, 2010.
14. K. R. Merikangas, H. S. Akiskal, J. Angst et al., "Lifetime and 12-month prevalence of bipolar spectrum disorder in the national comorbidity survey replication," Archives of General Psychiatry, vol. 64, no. 5, pp. 543–552, 2007.
15. S. H. Busch and C. L. Barry, "Marketwatch-mental health disorders in childhood: assessing the burden on families," Health Affairs, vol. 26, no. 4, pp. 1088–1095, 2007.
16. H. Baker-Henningham, "Transporting evidence-based interventions across cultures: using focus groups with teachers and parents of pre-school children to inform the implementation of the Incredible Years Teacher Training Programme in Jamaica," Child: Care, Health and Development, vol. 37, no. 5, pp. 649–661, 2011.
17. Z. Wu, R. Detels, J. Zhang, V. Li, and J. Li, "Community-based trial to prevent drug use among youths in Yunnan, China," American Journal of Public Health, vol. 92, no. 12, pp. 1952–1957, 2002.
18. D. Yu and M. Seligman, "Preventing depressive symptoms in Chinese children," Prevention and Treatment, vol. 5, pp. 1–39, 2002.
19. C. Kieling, H. Baker-Henningham, M. Belfer et al., "Child and adolescent mental health worldwide: evidence for action," The Lancet, vol. 378, no. 9801, pp. 1515–1525, 2011.
20. Population Reference Bureau, "World Population Datasheet 2010," http://www.prb. org/pdf10/10wpds_eng.pdf.
21. U. Bronfenbrenner, The Ecology of Human Development: Experiments by Nature and Design, Harvard University Press, Cambridge, Mass, USA, 1979.
22. L. E. Berk, Child Development, Allyn and Bacon, Boston, Mass, USA, 5th edition, 2000.
23. Unicef, "The child in the family," 2005, http://www.unicef.org/childfamily/index_24511.html.
24. Unicef, At Home or in a Home? Formal Care and Adoption of Children in Eastern Europe And Central Asia, Unicef, Geneva, Switzerland, 2010.
25. G. Foster, "Safety nets for children affected by HIV/AIDS in Southern Africa," in A Generation at Risk: HIV/AIDS, Vulnerable Children and Security in Southern Africa, G. Foster and R. Pharoah, Eds., pp. 65–92, Institute of Security Studies, Cape Town, South Africa, 2004.

26. C. M. Miller, S. Gruskin, S. V. Subramanian, D. Rajaraman, and S. J. Heymann, "Orphan care in Botswana's working households: growing responsibilities in the absence of adequate support," American Journal of Public Health, vol. 96, no. 8, pp. 1429–1435, 2006.

27. Z. Maqoko and Y. Dreyer, "Child-headed households because of the trauma surrounding HIV/AIDS," HTS Theological Studies, vol. 63, no. 2, pp. 717–731, 2007.

28. S. Tsegaye, HIV/AIDS Orphans and Child-Headed Households in Sub-Saharan Africa, African Child Policy Reform, Johannesburg, South Africa, 2008.

29. A. F. Garland, R. L. Hough, K. M. McCabe, M. Yeh, P. A. Wood, and G. A. Aarons, "Prevalence of psychiatric disorders in youths across five sectors of care," Journal of the American Academy of Child and Adolescent Psychiatry, vol. 40, no. 4, pp. 409–418, 2001.

30. D. Bruskas, "Children in foster care: a vulnerable population at risk," Journal of Child and Adolescent Psychiatric Nursing, vol. 21, no. 2, pp. 70–77, 2008.

31. M. Chatterji, D. Leanne, V. Tom, et al., "The well-being of children affected by HIV/AIDS in Gitarama Province, Rwanda, and Lusaka, Zambia: findings from a study," Community REACH Working Paper 2, Community REACH Program Pact, Washington, DC, USA, 2005.

32. J. Sengendo and J. Nambi, "The psychological effect of orphanhood: a study of orphans in Rakai district," Health Transition Review, vol. 7, pp. 105–124, 1997.

33. B. Olley, "Health and behavioural problems of children orphaned by AIDS as reported by their caregivers in Abuja, Nigeria," Nigerian Journal of Psychiatry, vol. 6, no. 2, pp. 70–75, 2008.

34. L. D. Cluver, M. Orkin, F. Gardner, and M. E. Boyes, "Persisting mental health problems among AIDS-orphaned children in South Africa," Journal of Child Psychology and Psychiatry and Allied Disciplines, vol. 53, no. 4, pp. 363–370, 2012.

35. V. Hertrich, Nuptiality and Gender Relationships in Africa: An Overview of First Marriage Trends Over the Past 50 Years, Paper Presented at the Annual Meeting of the Population Association of America, Atlanta, Ga, USA, 2002.

36. B. Bigombe and G. M. Khadiagala, "Major trends affecting families in Sub-Saharan Africa," in Major Trends Affecting Families, United Nations, New York, NY, USA, 2003.

37. O. Wusu and U. C. Isiugo-Abanihe, "Interconnections among changing family structure, childrearing and fertility behaviour among the Ogu, Southwestern Nigeria: a qualitative study," Demographic Research, vol. 14, pp. 139–156, 2006.

38. South African Institute of Race Relations, Fast Facts, South African Institute of Race Relations, Marshalltown, South Africa, 2009.

39. K. A. Moore, S. M. Jekielek, and C. Emig, Marriage From a Child's Perspective: How Does Family Structure Affect Children, And What Can We Do About It?Child Trends Research Brief, Washington, DC, USA, 2002.

40. M. D. Bramlett and S. J. Blumberg, "Family structure and children's physical and mental health," Health Affairs, vol. 26, no. 2, pp. 549–558, 2007.

41. O. Atilola, "Can family interventions be a strategy for curtailing delinquency and neglect in Nigeria? Evidence from adolescents in custodial care," African Journal for the Psychological Study of Social Issues, vol. 15, no. 1, pp. 218–237, 2012.

42. O. Atilola, "Different points of a continuum? Cross sectional comparison of the current and pre-contact psychosocial problems among the different categories of adolescents in institutional care in Nigeria," BMC Public Health, vol. 12, p. 554, 2012.

43. L. Frame, Parent-Child Relationships in Conditions of Urban Poverty: Protection, Care and Neglect of Infants and Toddlers: Policy Brief, Center for Social Services Research, University of California, Berkeley, Calif, USA, 2001.

44. R. D. Conger and K. J. Conger, "Resilience in Midwestern families: selected findings from the first decade of a prospective, longitudinal study," Journal of Marriage and Family, vol. 64, no. 2, pp. 361–373, 2002.

45. B. R. Karney, L. Story, and T. Bradbury, "Marriages in context: interactions between chronic and acute stress among newlyweds," in Proceedings of the International Meeting on the Developmental Course of Couples Coping with Stress, pp. 12–14, Boston College, Chestnut Hill, Mass, USA, October 2002.

46. A. Assani, Etude sur les Mariages Précoces et Grossesses Précoces au Burkina-Faso, Cameroun, Gambie, Liberia, Niger et Tchad, UNICEF WCARO, Abidjan, Ivory Coast, 2000.

47. E. Osiruemu, "Poverty of parents and child labour in Benin City, Nigeria: a preliminary account of its nature and implications," Journal of Social Science, vol. 14, no. 2, pp. 115–121, 2007.

48. F. T. Nuhu and S. T. Nuhu, "Opinions and attitudes of some parents in ilorin, north-central Nigeria, towards child abuse and neglect," South African Journal of Psychiatry, vol. 16, no. 1, pp. 27–32, 2010.

49. R. R. J. Akarro and N. A. Mtweve, "Poverty and its association with child labor in Njombe District in Tanzania: the case of Igima Ward," Current Research Journal of Social Sciences, vol. 3, no. 3, pp. 199–206, 2011.

50. J. O. Abdulmalik and S. Sale, "Pathways to psychiatric care for children and adolescents at a tertiary facility in northern Nigeria," Journal of Public Health in Africa, vol. 3, no. 1, 2012.

51. P. Onyango and D. Kayongo-Male, "Child labour and health," in Proceedings of the 1st National Workshop on Child Labor and Health in Kenya, University of Nairobi, Nairobi, Kenya, 1983.

52. H. M. Maru, D. M. Kathuku, and D. M. Ndetei, "Psychiatric morbidity among children and young persons appearing in the Nairobi Juvenile Court, Kenya," East African Medical Journal, vol. 80, no. 6, pp. 282–288, 2003.

53. O. Atilola, "Prevalence and correlates of psychiatric disorders among residents of a Juvenile Remand Home in Nigeria: implications for mental health service planning," Nigerian Journal of Medicine, vol. 21, no. 4, pp. 416–426, 2012.

54. UNESCO Institute for Statistics, "Adult and Youth Literacy: Global Trends in Gender Parity," UIS Fact Sheet, no. 2, 2010, http://www.uis.unesco.org/template/pdf/Literacy/Fact_Sheet_2010_Lit_EN.pdf.

55. UNESCO, Education for All Global Monitoring Report 2010: Reaching the Marginalized, UNESCO, Paris, France, 2010.

56. A. Pence and J. Shafer, "Indigenous knowledge and early childhood development in Africa: the early childhood development virtual university," Journal for Education in International Development, vol. 2, no. 3, 2006.

57. T. P. Schultz, "Studying the impact of household economic and community variables on child mortality," Child Survival: Strategies for Research, vol. 10, pp. 215–235, 1984.

58. Y. Celik and D. R. Hotchkiss, "The socio-economic determinants of maternal health care utilization in Turkey," Social Science and Medicine, vol. 50, no. 12, pp. 1797–1806, 2000.

59. J. L. Evans, Child Rearing Practices in Sub-Saharan Africa. An Introduction to the Studies. The Consultative Group on Early Childhood Care and Development, World Bank, Washinton, DC, USA, 1994.

60. A. A. Aldoo, "Positioning ECD Nationally: trends in selected African countries," in Africa's Future, Africa's Challenge: Early Childhood Care and Development in Sub-Saharan Africa, M. Garcia, A. Pence, and J. L. Evans, Eds., World Bank, Washington, DC, USA, 2008.

61. C. A. Brown, S. B. Sohani, K. Khan, R. Lilford, and W. Mukhwana, "Antenatal care and perinatal outcomes in Kwale district, Kenya," BMC Pregnancy and Childbirth, vol. 8, p. 2, 2008.

62. E. M. Yousif and A. R. Abdul Hafeez, "The effect of antenatal care on the probability of neonatal survival at birth, Wad Medani Teaching Hospital Sudan," Sudanese Journal of Public Health, vol. 1, no. 4, pp. 293–297, 2006.

63. M. A. Okunlola, K. M. Owonikoko, A. O. Fawole, and A. O. Adekunle, "Gestational age at antenatal booking and delivery outcome," African Journal of Medicine and Medical Sciences, vol. 37, no. 2, pp. 165–169, 2008.

64. L. A. M. de Costello and D. S. Manandhar, "Perinatal asphyxia in less developed countries," Archives of Disease in Childhood, vol. 71, no. 1, pp. F1–F3, 1994.

65. Unicef/Nigeria, Federal Government of Nigeria and UNICEF Master Plan of Operations for a Country Program of Cooperation for Nigerian Children and Women—2002–2007, Unicef, Lagos, Nigeria, 2001.

66. O. O. Omigbodun, "Psychosocial issues in a child and adolescent psychiatric clinic population in Nigeria," Social Psychiatry and Psychiatric Epidemiology, vol. 39, no. 8, pp. 667–672, 2004.

67. M. Rutter, "Resilience in the face of adversity: protective factors and resistance to psychiatric disorder," British Journal of Psychiatry, vol. 147, pp. 598–611, 1985.

68. J. B. G. Tilak, "Basic education and development in Sub-Saharan Africa," Journal of International Cooperation in Education, vol. 12, no. 1, pp. 5–17, 2009.

69. P. Bennell and K. Akyeampong, "Teacher motivation in Sub-Saharan Africa and South Asia," Researching the Issues 7, 2007.

70. L. B. Liontos, At-Risk Families and Schools: Becoming Partners, ERIC Clearinghouse on Educational Management, College of Education, University of Oregon, Eugene, Ore, USA, 1992.

71. B. Robertson, O. Omigbodun, and N. Gaddour, "Child and adolescent psychiatry in Africa: luxury or necessity?" African Journal of Psychiatry (South Africa), vol. 13, no. 5, pp. 329–331, 2010.

72. UN Habitat, State of the World'S CitieS 2010/2011: Bridging the Urban Divide, UN Habitat, Nairobi, Kenya, 2012.

73. R. B. Patel and T. F. Burke, "Global health: urbanization—an emerging humanitarian disaster," New England Journal of Medicine, vol. 361, no. 8, pp. 741–743, 2009.

74. A. Daramola and E. O. Ibem, "Urban environmental problems in Nigeria: implications for sustainable development," Journal of Sustainable Development in Africa, vol. 12, no. 1, pp. 124–143, 2010.
75. United Nations Human Settlements Programme, State of the World's Cities 2006/7, Earthscan, London, UK, 2006.
76. United Nations Human Settlements Programme, The Challenge of Slums: Global Report on Human Settlements, Earthscan, London, UK, 2003.
77. R. Flournor and I. Yen, The Influence of Community Factors on Health. An Annotated Bibliography, PolicyLink, Oakland, Calif, USA, 2004.
78. S. D. Bele, T. N. Bodhare, S. Valsangkar, and A. Saraf, "An epidemiological study of emotional and behavioral disorders among children in an urban slum," Psychological Health and Medicine, vol. 18, no. 2, pp. 223–232, 2013.
79. M. H. Swahn, J. B. Palmier, R. Kasirye, and H. Yao, "Correlates of suicide ideation and attempt among youth living in the slums of Kampala," International Journal of Environmental Research and Public Health, vol. 9, no. 2, pp. 596–609, 2012.
80. International Labour Organisation, World Social Security Report 2010-2011: Providing Coverage in Times of Crisis and Beyond, International Labor Organisation, Geneva, Switzerland, 2011.
81. O. Atilola, "Partaking in the global movement for occupational mental health: what challenges and ways forward for sub-Sahara Africa?" International Journal of Mental Health Systems, vol. 6, no. 1, p. 15, 2012.
82. O. Animashaun, "Casualisation and casual employment in Nigeria: beyond contract," Labor Law Review, vol. 1, pp. 14–34, 2008.
83. O. Bodipe, The Extent and Effects of Casualisation in Southern Africa: Analysis of Lesotho, Mozambique, South Africa, Swaziland, Zambia and Zimbabwe: A Research Report for the Danish Federation of Workers, National Labor and Economic Development Institute, Johannesburg, South Africa, 2006.
84. International Labour Organisation, "A global alliance against forced labor," Report of the Director-General, International Labour Organisation, Geneva, Switzerland, 2005.
85. International Labour Organisation, Global Employment Trends, January 2010, International Labour Organisation, Geneva, Switzerland, 2010.
86. N. Cassirer and L. Addati, "Expanding women's employment opportunities: informal economy workers and the need for childcare," Conditions of Work and Employment Programme, International Labour Organisation, Geneva, Switzerland, 2007.
87. International Labour Organisation, ILO Database on Conditions of Work and Employment Laws, ILO, Geneva, 2012, http://www.ilo.org/dyn/travail.
88. ILO International Labour Organisation, African Employment Trends, ILO International Labour Organisation, Geneva, Switzerland, 2007.
89. J. T. Addison, "Urie Bronfenbrenner," Human Ecology, vol. 20, no. 2, pp. 16–20, 1992.
90. C. Harper, N. Jones, A. McKay, and J. Espey, Children in Times of Economic Crisis: Past Lessons, Future Policies, Overseas Development Institute, London, UK, 2009.
91. UN World Youth Report, Juvenile Delinquency, United Nations, Geneva, Switzerland, 2003, http://www.un.org/esa/socdev/unyin/documents/ch07.pdf.

92. Urban Management Programme, "Street children and gangs in African cities: guidelines for local authorities," Working Paper Series 18, Urban Management Programme, Nairobi, Kenya, 2000, http://www.unhabitat.org/downloads/docs/1901_41571_Streetchildren1.pdf.

93. O. Ogundipe, "Management of juvenile delinquency in Nigeria," in Proceedings of the International Conference on Special Needs Offenders, Nairobi, Kenya, October 2011.

94. C. Petty and M. Brown, "Justice for children: challenges for policy and practice in Sub-Saharan Africa," Save the Children, 1998.

95. A. Sam, Child Justice in Africa, PREDA Foundation, Olongapo City, Philippines, 2007.

96. O. Atilola, "Corrective seclusion or punitive incarceration: an overview of the state of the Nigerian juvenile justice system," European Psychiatry, vol. 25, no. 1, p. 669, 2010.

97. Commission for Africa, "Our Common Interest," Report, Commission for Africa, London, UK, 2005.

98. B. Davis, M. Gaarder, S. Handa, and Y. Yablonski, "Evaluating the impact of cash transfer programmes in sub-Saharan Africa: an introduction to the special issue," Journal of Development Effectiveness, vol. 4, no. 1, pp. 1–8, 2012.

99. A. Barrientos, "Introducing basic social protection in low-income countries: lessons from existing programmes," BWPI Working Paper 6, Brooks World Poverty Institute, Manchester, UK, 2007.

100. A. Barrientos, M. Nino-Zarazua, and M. Maitrot, Social Assistance in Developing Countries Database, Brookings World Poverty Institute and Chronic Poverty Research Centre, Manchester, UK, 2010.

101. N. Jones, Strengthening Social Protection For Children. West and Central Africa, ODI and Unicef, London, UK, 2009.

102. M. Nino-Zarazua, A. Barrientos, D. Hulme, and S. Hickey, Social Protection in Sub-Saharan Africa: Getting the Politics Right, World Poverty Institute, The University of Manchester, Manchester, UK, 2010.

103. S. Timimi, Naughty Boys: Anti-Social Behaviour, ADHD, and the Role of Culture, Palgrave Macmillan, Basingstoke, UK, 2005.

104. M. Mweru, "Why are Kenyan teachers still using corporal punishment eight years after a ban on corporal punishment?" Child Abuse Review, vol. 19, no. 4, pp. 248–258, 2010.

105. O. O. Omigbodun and M. O. Olatawura, "Child rearing practices in Nigeria: implications for Mental Health," Nigerian Journal of Psychiatry, vol. 6, no. 1, pp. 10–15, 2008.

106. K. J. Aucoin, P. J. Frick, and S. D. Bodin, "Corporal punishment and child adjustment," Journal of Applied Developmental Psychology, vol. 27, no. 6, pp. 527–541, 2006.

107. E. Durrant, "Corporal punishment: prevalence, predictors and implications for child behaviour and development," in Eliminating Corporal Punishment, S. N. Hart, Ed., pp. 49–90, UNESCO, Paris, France, 2005.

108. WHO, Eliminating Female Genital Mutilation. An Interagency Statement, World Health Organization, Geneva, Switzerland, 2008.

109. WHO Study Group, "Female genital mutilation and obstetric outcomes," The Lancet, vol. 367, no. 9525, pp. 1835–1841, 2006.

110. A. Elnashar and R. Abdelhady, "The impact of female genital cutting on health of newly married women," International Journal of Gynecology and Obstetrics, vol. 97, no. 3, pp. 238–244, 2007.

111. C. Oleke, A. Blystad, and O. B. Rekdal, "'When the obvious brother is not there': political and cultural contexts of the orphan challenge in northern Uganda," Social Science and Medicine, vol. 61, no. 12, pp. 2628–2638, 2005.

112. L. Rose, Children's Property and Inheritance Rights and their Livelihoods: The Context of HIV and AIDS in Southern and East Africa, Food and Agricultural Organization of the United Nations, Rome, Italy, 2006.

113. E. Cooper, Inheritance Practices and the Intergenerational Transmission of Poverty: A Literature Review and Annotated Bibliography, Overseas Development Institute (ODI) and Chronic Poverty Research Centre (CPRC), London, UK, 2006.

114. K. Bird and I. Shinyekwa, "Multiple shocks and downward mobility: learning from the life histories of rural Ugandans," Working Paper 36, Overseas Development Institute (ODI) and Chronic Poverty Research Centre (CPRC), London, UK, 2004.

115. M. R. Carter and C. B. Barrett, "The economics of poverty traps and persistent poverty: an asset-based approach," Journal of Development Studies, vol. 42, no. 2, pp. 178–199, 2006.

116. K. Bird, N. Pratt, T. O'Neil, and V. Bolt, "Fracture points in social policies for chronic poverty reduction," Working Paper 47, Overseas Development Institute (ODI) and Chronic Poverty Research Centre (CPRC), London, UK, 2004.

117. Unicef, Early Marriage: A Harmful Traditional Practice, Unicef, Geneva, Switzerland, 2005, http://www.unicef.org/publications/index_26024.html.

118. R. Jensen and R. Thornton, "Early female marriage in the developing world," Gender and Development, vol. 11, no. 2, pp. 9–19, 2003.

119. United Nations, Convention of the Rights of the Child, UN General Assembly, Geneva, Switzerland, 1989.

120. M. M. Mulinge, "Implementing the 1989 United Nations' Convention on the Rights of the Child in sub-Saharan Africa: the overlooked socioeconomic and political dilemmas," Child Abuse and Neglect, vol. 26, no. 11, pp. 1117–1130, 2002.

121. M. M. Mulinge, "Persistent socioeconomic and political dilemmas to the implementation of the 1989 United Nations' Convention on the Rights of the Child in sub-Saharan Africa," Child Abuse and Neglect, vol. 34, no. 1, pp. 10–17, 2010.

122. African Union, Plan of Action on the Family in Africa, African Union, Addis Ababa, Ethiopia, 2004.

123. T. Maundeni, "Residential care for children in Botswana: the past, the present, and the future," in Residential Care for Children: Comparative Perspectives, M. E. Courtney and D. Iwaniec, Eds., Oxford University Press, New York, NY, USA, 2009.

124. C. M. Miller, S. Gruskin, S. V. Subramanian, D. Rajaraman, and S. J. Heymann, "Orphan care in Botswana's working households: growing responsibilities in the absence of adequate support," American Journal of Public Health, vol. 96, no. 8, pp. 1429–1435, 2006.

125. D. Bhugra and A. Mastrogianni, "Globalisation and mental disorders: overview with relation to depression," British Journal of Psychiatry, vol. 184, pp. 10–20, 2004.

126. L. J. Kirmayer, N. Nutt, L. Lecrubier, L. Lepine, and D. Davidson, "Cultural variations in the clinical presentation of depression and anxiety: implications for diagnosis and treatment," Journal of Clinical Psychiatry, vol. 62, supplement 13, pp. 22–30, 2001.

127. S. Timimi, Pathological Child Psychiatry and the Medicalization of Childhood, Brunner-Routledge, London, UK, 2002.

128. E. Hong, Globalisation and the Impact on Health, A Third World View-Impact of SAPs in the Third World, The Peoples' Health Assembly, Savar, Bangladesh, 2000, http://www.twnside.org.sg/title/health.pdf.

129. A. O. Ong'ayo, "Political instability in Africa: where the problem lies and alternative perspectives," in Paper Presented at the Symposium: 'Afrika: een continent op drift', Stichting Nationaal Erfgoed Hotel de Wereld Wageningen, Istanbul, Turkey, September 2008, http://www.diasporacentre.org/DOCS/Political_Instabil.pdf.

130. V. Patel, A. J. Flisher, S. Hetrick, and P. McGorry, "Mental health of young people: a global public-health challenge," The Lancet, vol. 369, no. 9569, pp. 1302–1313, 2007.

131. C. Lund, S. Kleintjes, V. Campbell-Hall, et al., "Mental health policy development and implementation in South Africa: a situation analysis," Phase 1 Country Report, Mental Health and Poverty Project, Cape Town, South Africa, 2008.

132. O. Atilola, "Child mental-health policy development in sub-Saharan Africa: broadening the Perspectives using Bronfenbrenner's ecological model," Health Promotion International. In press.

PART II

THE INTERACTION OF ADOLESCENT MENTAL HEALTH WITH THE EDUCATIONAL COMMUNITY

CHAPTER 3

THE ASSOCIATION BETWEEN SCHOOL CLASS COMPOSITION AND SUICIDAL IDEATION IN LATE ADOLESCENCE: FINDINGS FROM THE YOUNG-HUNT 3 STUDY

JOAKIM D. DALEN

3.1 INTRODUCTION

Suicidal ideation can be defined as "thoughts of engaging in behaviour intended to end one's life" [1] and is an important indicator of both mental health vulnerability and the risk of engaging in suicide attempts [2,3]. It is especially common during adolescence, with prevalence increasing from age 12 and peaking by age 16, remaining elevated into the early twenties [1].

School classrooms represent an important social context for adolescents. Here, students spend a large portion of their waking hours with a group of classmates who they had no opportunity of choosing themselves and who they are required to interact with [4]. The continuous interaction among the students in each class creates unique psychosocial environ-

The Association between School Class Composition and Suicidal Ideation in Late Adolescence: Findings from the Young-HUNT 3 Study © Dalen JD. Child and Adolescent Psychiatry and Mental Health, *6,37 (2012),doi:10.1186/1753-2000-6-37. Licensed under Creative Commons Attribution 2.0 Generic License, http://creativecommons.org/licenses/by/2.0/.*

ments which vary in factors such as shared beliefs, emotions, habits and peer pressure [4,5]. These environments can influence the mental health of students in both positive and negative ways [5]. As a consequence, some school classes are likely to have more students with suicidal ideation compared to others.

It has also been suggested that suicidal ideation may cluster within schools due to suicidal behaviour transferring between individuals as a result of interpersonal interactions with other students who are suicidal [6]. That is, the probability of suicidal ideation could be higher in contexts where there are students with thoughts of taking their own lives who then communicated this ideation outward. If this is the case, then it follows that students who originally are at a low risk for experiencing suicidal ideation may be at higher risk if they have extensive contact with such at-risk individuals.

Multilevel analyses are particularly effective in examining the importance of the school class context because they enable the variation between individuals and groups to be assessed separately [7]. However, multilevel studies investigating the relationship between school context and suicidal ideation are rare [6,8,9]. In the only known study reporting between-school variation in suicidal behaviour, Young et al. [9] found that a small percentage of the variation in attempted suicide (1%), suicide risk (1.3%) and self-harm (1.6%) could be attributed to the school level. The extent to which suicidal ideation may be related to the school classroom context has not been previously examined through the use of multilevel analyses. Research on other mental health outcomes does, however, suggest that the differences between school classrooms are greater than the differences between schools [10-12].

It can be argued that the influence of the social environment on one's mental health, as well as transference of suicidal ideation, is related to the gender and socioeconomic composition within school classes. Both socioeconomic status and gender are background characteristics often found to be associated with suicidal ideation and mental health. For adolescents, a higher level of parental socioeconomic status is usually associated with fewer mental health problems [13,14], while girls tend to have a higher prevalence of suicidal ideation compared to boys [3,15-19]. If the probability of having suicidal ideation increases as a result of extensive contact with at-risk individuals, then the probability of suicidal ideation should be higher in school classes containing a greater proportion of girls or of students with low socioeconomic background.

Moreover, research has shown that a school's culture regarding academic achievement can vary greatly depending on the students' socioeconomic background [5]. Likewise, several studies have suggested that the socioeconomic composition of the school context is associated with mental health status, over and above individual socioeconomic characteristics [6,20-22]. The majority of these studies have found the level of socioeconomic status to be positively related to reports of better mental health, but as with the school context in general, studies specifically examining the relationship between socioeconomic composition of school classes and mental health are scarce. It is, however, likely that school classes, in the same way as schools themselves, will manufacture unique social environments, suggesting that there may be positive effects of a higher average level of socioeconomic background at the class level as well.

Similarly, the influence of one's psychosocial environment may also depend upon that environment's gender composition. In a review by Belfi et al. [23], the authors conclude that students in single-sex schools have higher levels of well-being compared to students in mixed schools. This is, however, a gender-specific effect because the relationship has only been documented among girls. Multilevel research analysing the association between classroom gender composition and student mental health is rare, and the few studies testing this relationship have not found significant effects [10].

In this study, suicidal ideation among a population of Norwegian adolescents is examined in relation to school class composition. Suicidal behaviour is a common problem among Norwegian adolescents, and studies on suicidal attempts and self-harm have reported prevalence rates ranging from 3.0 to 8.2 percent [24]. An additional study examining Norwegian conscripts reported a 21.7 percent prevalence rate of life-time suicidal ideation [25], while a second study of adolescents in their last year of upper secondary education (18–19 years) found the prevalence of individuals having suicidal ideation during the last week to be 10.9 percent [26].

To examine the association between suicidal ideation and school class composition, the following two research questions were formulated:

- To what degree can variation in suicidal ideation be attributed to differences between school classes?
- Is there an association between suicidal ideation and school class composition in regards to student gender and parental education?

3.2 METHODS

3.2.1 DATA

Participants were identified from the Young-HUNT 3 study, a study population composed of all adolescents attending secondary school (13–19 years old) in the Norwegian county of Nord-Trøndelag. The survey was conducted between 2006 and 2008, and data were acquired through questionnaires and a subsequent health examination. Questionnaires were completed during a school period; consequently, students that had dropped out of school were excluded. The question concerning suicidal ideation was asked only to students in upper secondary school (16–19 years). All 4357 students attending one of the 13 upper secondary schools of the county were invited to participate. Of these, 3353 responded to the questionnaire resulting in a total response rate of 77 percent. After removing cases due to missing data, the final number of students analysed was 2923 distributed across 379 school classes. Participation was voluntary, and every participant was asked to provide written informed consent. Additional information was obtained by retrieving data on parental education from the central registers of Norway. The study was approved by the Regional Committee for Medical and Health Research Ethics.

3.2.2 THE NORWEGIAN SCHOOL SYSTEM

After attending ten years of obligatory school, Norwegian adolescents have the option to continue upper secondary school, choosing between three types of general studies and nine types of vocational studies. Of all Norwegian adolescents, approximately 96 percent start upper secondary school, although a substantial number quit during the three to four years of schooling. A majority (96%) of students attend public upper secondary schools, which are administered at the county level.

3.2.3 VARIABLES

Suicidal ideation was measured by a single question aiming to capture the occurrence of suicidal ideation during one's lifetime. The question was formulated as: "Have you had thoughts about taking your own life?" Possible response categories were "Yes" and "No".

Individual explanatory variables included gender, age, socioeconomic status, living situation and parents' marital status. Parent education level was used to represent socioeconomic status, and the variable consisted of two categories: "Parents with education at college or university level" and "Parents with education lower than college or university level". When information on both parents' education was available, the higher level of education was used. If information was not available for both parents, the educational level of the remaining parent was used instead. For the living situation variable, adolescents were grouped based on whether they lived with "both parents", "one (or mainly one) parent", "away from home (either alone or with friends)" or "other possible living situations".

Descriptors of school class composition included the proportion of parents with higher education as well as the ratio of girls to boys in the class. These variables were constructed by aggregating the individual variables of parental education and gender using information on all students participating in the study. Finally, the analyses included variables indicating educational programme (general or vocational) and school grade.

3.2.4 STATISTICAL ANALYSES

To examine contextual effects on the dichotomous variable of suicidal ideation, multilevel logistic regression analysis was performed. The main advantages of this model are that it allows for the decomposition of unexplained variance between contexts and individuals, as well as effective inclusion of variables on the contextual level. In this analysis, individuals were grouped within school classes. Denoting the probability of suicidal ideation $\pi_{ij} = Pr(y_{ij} = 1)$, where i is the individual within school class j, the model can be written as

$$\log(\pi_{tj}/[1-\pi_{tj}]) = \beta_0 + \beta x_{ij} + \beta z_j + u_j$$

β_0 is the intercept, and βx_{ij} is the vector for the coefficients and values of the variables on the individual level. βz_j is the vector for the coefficients and values on the school class level. Finally, u_j denotes the random effect on the school class level. This random effect is assumed to follow a normal distribution $u_j - N(0, \sigma_u^2)$, with σ_u^2 as the variance parameter of the residual between-school class variance. Using MLwiN, all models were estimated by MCMC methods [27].

3.3 RESULTS

Table 1 presents the descriptive statistics and shows that 22.8 percent of the adolescents in the study reported suicidal ideation. Girls were more likely to report suicidal ideation compared to boys ($p<0.001$), while adolescents whose parents had a higher level of education were less likely to report suicidal ideation compared to adolescents whose parents had a lower level of education ($p<0.05$). A higher prevalence of suicidal ideation was also reported among students with divorced parents and among students who were not living with both of their parents ($p<0.001$).

The prevalence of suicidal ideation was 9.6 percent higher among students enrolled in vocational programmes than those in general programmes. Of the 379 school classes, 241 (63.6%) followed a vocational programme. However, these classes accounted for only 46.6 percent of the students, indicating that classes following a vocational program, on average, were smaller than those in a general educational programme. Finally, data from the table suggest that suicidal ideation was far less common among students in the third grade of upper secondary education.

TABLE 1: Descriptive statistics

Individual variables		N	%	(%) with suicidal ideation
Suicidal ideation				
	Yes	668	22.8	
	No	2255	77.2	
Gender				
	Boys	1404	48.0	20.2
	Girls	1519	52.0	25.3
Age				
	16	780	26.7	22.8
	17	1085	37.1	24.3
	18	879	30.1	20.7
	19	179	6.1	23.3
Parental education				
	Less than college or university	1588	54.3	24.5
	College or university	1335	45.7	20.8
School grade				
	First grade	914	31.3	25.5
	Second grade	1195	40.9	25.3
	Third grade	814	27.9	16.3
Living situation				
	Both parents	1749	59.8	18.6
	One parent	643	22.0	28.7
	Away from home	417	14.3	27.6
	Other	114	3.9	37.7
Divorced parents				
	Yes	839	28.7	29.5
	No	2084	71.3	20.2
Educational programme				
	Vocational programme	1366	46.7	28.0
	General programme	1557	53.3	18.4
	Total	2923		22.8

TABLE 1: *Cont.*

School class variables	N	%	Mean (std. dev.)
Educational programme			
Vocational programme	241	63.6	
General programme	138	36.4	
Proportion of parents with higher education			0.40 (0.27)
Proportion of girls			0.52 (0.35)
School grade			
First grade	133	35.1	
Second grade	166	43.8	
Third grade	80	21.1	
Total	379		

In multilevel models, a model with no explanatory variables can be used to estimate the intra-class correlation coefficient (ICC) [28]. The ICC is interpreted as the proportion of variance that can be attributed to the higher level in the analysis. Therefore, the ICC provides information of the degree to which suicidal ideation clusters within school classes. In the empty model (not shown) the ICC was estimated to be 0.053 indicating that 5.3 percent of the variance in suicidal ideation could be attributed to the school class level.

Model 1 in Table 2 includes explanatory variables at the individual level. After controlling for other variables, the analyses revealed that boys were less likely to disclose suicidal ideation compared to girls, while parental education and age were negligible factors. In this model, the ICC has been reduced to 2.7 percent, indicating that approximately half of the variance at the school class level could be explained by an unequal distribution of the individual level variables included in the analysis.

In Model 2, variables at the school class level were introduced. Although the proportion of parents with a high educational level had little effect on suicidal ideation, results overall suggested substantial effects of grade, educational programme and gender. Specifically, the effect of school grade indicates that third graders had the lowest probability of suicidal ideation. Regarding educational programmes, the likelihood of having suicidal ideation was substantially higher for those attending a vocational programme compared to those following a general programme. For gender composition, the results indicated that the probability of having suicidal ideation was greater in classes having a higher proportion of girls, even after taking the individual effect of gender into account. It is interesting to note that when the school class level variables were included in the analyses, the individual effect of gender decreased to the point of non-significance.

TABLE 2: Multilevel logistic regression of adolescent suicidal ideation

	Model 1	Model 2
Individual-level variables		
Gender (ref.: boys)	1.28 (1.07-1.54)**	1.10 (0.88-1.37)
Age (ref.: 16)		
17	1.05 (0.83-1.33)	1.30 (0.97-1.75)
18	0.88 (0.68-1.14)	1.77 (1.22-2.57)**
19	0.89 (0.59-1.34)	1.85 (1.13-3.05)*
Parent education (ref.: low)	0.88 (0.68-1.14)	0.99 (0.80-1.21)
Living arrangement (ref.: both parents)		
One parent	1.40 (1.01-1.91)*	1.41 (1.03-1.94)*
Away from home	1.43 (1.08-1.89)**	1.42 (1.07-1.87)*
Other	2.45 (1.61-3.72)***	2.38 (1.56-3.62)***
Divorced parents (ref.: not divorced)	1.24 (0.94-1.65)	1.20 (0.91-1.58)
School class-level variables		
Vocational subject		1.46 (1.16-1.84)**
Proportion of parents with higher education		1.07 (0.65-1.84)
Proportion of girls		1.93 (1.33-2.79)***
School grade (ref.: First grade)		
Second grade		0.77 (0.58-1.02)
Third grade		0.37 (0.25-0.54)***
Variance level 2 (Std. Error)	0.11 (0.06)	0.02 (0.030)
ICC (%)	3.2	0.6
Deviance	3088.1	3043.7

*: $P < .05$; **: $P < .01$; ***: $P < 0.001$. OR (95% CI).

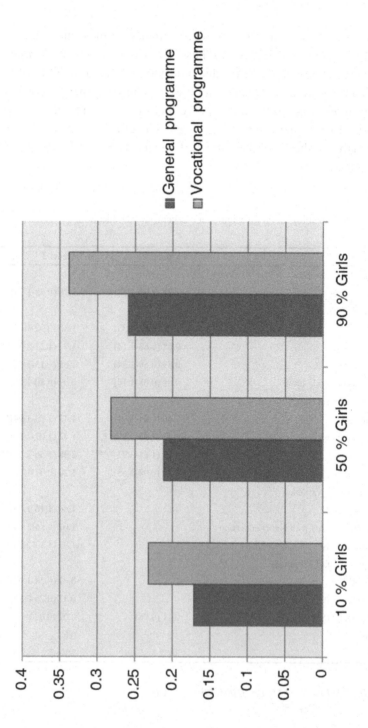

FIGURE 1: Predicted probability of suicidal ideation by gender composition and educational programme.

Figure 1 shows the predicted probabilities of suicidal ideation by gender balance and type of educational programme. The figure indicates that when all other explanatory variables were held constant, the differences in the probability of having suicidal ideation were substantial. Students in classes following a general educational programme had an approximately 6–8 percent higher probability of suicidal ideation compared to classes that followed a vocational programme. However, the difference is most clearly illustrated when comparing individuals from vocational classes having a large proportion of girls to those in general programme having mostly boys. The probability of suicidal ideation was almost twice as high for the first group compared to the latter.

It is possible that the effects of both individual and contextual variables differ between boys and girls. To examine this possibility, the same models were analysed while stratifying by gender. In this instance, the effects were similar for both genders, and differences were not significant for any of the variables.

3.4 DISCUSSION

The results of this study indicate that a significant amount of variation in suicidal ideation can be attributed to differences between school classes. However, after controlling for individual level variables, it is clear that the unequal distribution of students at risk due to individual factors explained a substantial amount of the variability. Furthermore, the results suggest that the probability of suicidal ideation is higher in classes having a greater proportion of girls as well as in classes following a vocational education programme.

The effect of gender composition on suicidal ideation is surprising as similar effects have not previously been observed. One possible explanation is that in classes with higher proportions of girls, the likelihood of having contact with others with suicidal thoughts is greater due to the overall higher risk of suicidal ideation among girls. Girls also have a tendency to prefer close emotional communication, intimacy and responsiveness in their social relationships [29]. This type of relationship may increase the chance of discussing psychological problems, such as suicidal thoughts, thus increasing the risk of transferring suicidal behaviour. Because school classes with a majority of girls will necessarily have more social relationships that include girls, it is possible that students within these classes will have more suicidal thoughts as a result.

However, the effect of gender composition could also be at least partially explained by mediating or confounding factors not included in these models. At the contextual level, one possibility is that classes with a high proportion of girls create psychosocial environments that can increase the risk for suicidal ideation in some students. On the other hand, perhaps an unequal distribution of individual level variables not included in the model also account for the gender effect. For example, school-related problems such as being bullied, social exclusion, academic stress and academic achievement have all been found to be associated with suicidal ideation [30-32]. If such problems were unequally distributed according to gender composition in our sample, the inclusion of these variables could then remove or reduce the observed effect. Finally, the individual effect of gender disappears when controlling for gender composition, suggesting that the gender differences in suicidal ideation previously observed in the literature [15-19] may partially be explained by the social context.

The absence of an association between aggregated parental education and suicidal ideation is surprising due to the regularity with which this relationship is found in the literature on mental health [13,14]. However, it is possible that the difference is due to limited variation in the population analysed. Nord-Trøndelag is one of the most homogeneous counties in Norway. Compared to other more heterogeneous populations, parental education correlates to a lesser degree with other variables related to socioeconomic status, such as income and neighbourhood disadvantage. This potential explanation is further strengthened by the fact that the vast majority of upper secondary schools are public and free to attend. Consequently, school classes in Norway are much less likely to vary in terms of socioeconomic status compared to societies where school choice is much more dependent on parental socioeconomic background.

Similar results showing that educational programme is significantly associated with suicidal ideation have been observed in the literature on other measurements of mental health [10]. It is possible that the social climates associated with vocational classes differ from classes following a general programme, and thus, may influence the probability of developing suicidal thoughts. Another plausible explanation is that there is a selection effect due to factors associated with both suicidal ideation and choice of school programme. For example, the most important factor in predicting choice of one's educational programme in Norway is one's academic achievement during the last year of lower secondary education [33]. As academic achievement has been related to the risk of suicidal ideation [34,35], it is possible that adolescents with suicidal ideation in early adolescence are more likely to choose vocational education programmes. It may also be that this selection effect extends to the gender composition effect. While general education programmes are relatively equal in regards to gender distribution, many of the vocational programmes are not. It is thus possible that the observed effect of gender composition is a result of selection into specific vocational education programmes and not specifically of the gender composition.

That third graders were found to have a lower probability of suicidal ideation was somewhat surprising due to the dependent variable being lifetime suicidal ideation. However, this effect was likely a consequence of the higher probability of suicidal ideation among students dropping out of school [36] as well as individuals having a tendency to forget they had suicidal thoughts [37]. Because the prevalence of suicidal ideation peaks by age of 16 [1], third graders may be more likely to have forgotten their previous suicidal thoughts when compared to first graders.

3.4.1 LIMITATIONS

The unclear causal relationship between school class variables and suicidal ideation is one of the major limitations of the study. This limitation was exacerbated by how the question addressing suicidal ideation was formulated. For instance, the question did not ask specifically when individuals had considered taking their own lives and could therefore have been interpreted by some students as meaning any suicidal ideation in one's lifetime. Consequently, adolescents may have reported suicidal thoughts that occurred before they began upper secondary education. Furthermore, misreporting of suicidal ideation may have occurred, whether accidental, due to recall, or purposely, due to a lack of anonymity. To minimise this problem, participants were assured that no one at their schools would see their questionnaires. However, such assurances cannot fully guarantee accurate reporting.

Another potential limitation is that the suicidal ideation variable did not take into account the severity of the suicidal thoughts. Adolescents who have thought about taking their own life do not necessarily have mental health problems or suicidal plans. The analyses may have yield different results if suicidal ideation was measured in a way that took severity into account.

Finally, variables on the individual level were restricted to background variables. Including additional individual level variables could alter the observed effects of school class variables, as well as explain unexplained variation at the school class level.

3.5 CONCLUSION

One of the main reasons for studying suicidal ideation from a school class perspective is that this context may be ideal for interventions. The results of this study indicate that adolescent suicidal ideation is associated with both gender balance and educational programme. Thus, targeting classes with these characteristics may be an effective approach as more students with suicidal ideation are likely to be included in the intervention.

REFERENCES

1. Nock MK, Borges G, Bromet EJ, Cha CB, Kessler RC, Lee S: Suicide and Suicidal Behavior. Epidemiol Rev 2008, 30:133-154.
2. Andrews JA, Lewinsohn PM: Suicidal Attempts among Older Adolescents: Prevalence and Co-occurrence with Psychiatric Disorders. J Am Acad Child Adolesc Psychiatry 1992, 31:655-662.
3. Bridge JA, Goldstein TR, Brent DA: Adolescent suicide and suicidal behavior. J Child Psychol Psychiatry 2006, 47:372-394.
4. Eccles JS, Roeser RW: Schools as Developmental Contexts During Adolescence. J Res Adolesc 2011, 21:225-241.
5. Kahlenberg RD: All together now: creating middle-class schools through public school choice. Washington, D.C.: Brookings Institution Press; 2001.

6. Bernburg JG, Thorlindsson T, Sigfusdottir ID: The spreading of suicidal behavior: The contextual effect of community household poverty on adolescent suicidal behavior and the mediating role of suicide suggestion. Soc Sci Med 2009, 68:380-389.

7. Sellström E, Bremberg S: Is there a "school effect" on pupil outcomes? A review of multilevel studies. J Epidemiol Community Health 2006, 60:149-155.

8. Thorlindsson T, Bernburg JG: Community structural instability, anomie, imitation and adolescent suicidal behavior. J Adolesc 2009, 32:233-245.

9. Young R, Sweeting H, Ellaway A: Do schools differ in suicide risk? The influence of school and neighbourhood on attempted suicide, suicidal ideation and self-harm among secondary school pupils. BMC Publ Health 2011, 11:874.

10. Andersson H, Bjørngaard J, Kaspersen S, Wang C, Skre I, Dahl T: The effects of individual factors and school environment on mental health and prejudiced attitudes among Norwegian adolescents. Soc Psychiatry Psychiatr Epidemiol 2010, 45:569-577.

11. Opdenakker M-C, Van Damme J: Effects of Schools, Teaching Staff and Classes on Achievement and Well-Being in Secondary Education: Similarities and Differences Between School Outcomes. Sch Eff Sch Improv 2000, 11:165-196.

12. Van den Oord EJCG, Rispens J: Differences between School Classes in Preschoolers' Psychosocial Adjustment: Evidence for the Importance of Children's Interpersonal Relations. J Child Psychol Psychiatry 1999, 40:417-430.

13. Fryers T, Melzer D, Jenkins R: Social inequalities and the common mental disorders. A systematic review of the evidence. Soc Psychiatry Psychiatr Epidemiol 2003, 38:229-237.

14. Yu Y, Williams DR: Socioeconomic Status and Mental Health. In Handbook of the sociology of mental health. Edited by Aneshensel CS, Phelan JC. New York: Springer; 1999:151-166.

15. Allison S, Roeger L, Martin G, Keeves J: Gender differences in the relationship between depression and suicidal ideation in young adolescents. Aust N Z J Psychiatry 2001, 35:498-503.

16. Beautrais AL: Gender issues in youth suicidal behaviour. Emerg Med 2002, 14:35-42.

17. Nock MK, Borges G, Bromet EJ, Alonso J, Angermeyer M, Beautrais A, Bruffaerts R, Chiu WT, de Girolamo G, Gluzman S, de Graaf R, Gureje O, Haro JM, Huang Y, Karam E, Kessler RC, Lepine JP, Levinson D, Medina-Mora ME, Ono Y, Pasada-Villa J, Williams D: Cross-national prevalence and risk factors for suicidal ideation, plans and attempts. Br J Psychiatry 2008, 192:98-105.

18. Ursoniu S, Putnoky S, Vlaicu B, Vladescu C: Predictors of suicidal behavior in a high school student population: a cross-sectional study. Wien Klin Wochenschr 2009, 121:564-573.

19. Wunderlich U, Bronisch T, Wittchen H-U, Carter R: Gender differences in adolescents and young adults with suicidal behaviour. Acta Psychiatr Scand 2001, 104:332-339.

20. Botticello A: A Multilevel Analysis of Gender Differences in Psychological Distress Over Time. J Res Adolesc 2009, 19:217-247.

21. Saab H, Klinger D: School differences in adolescent health and wellbeing: Findings from the Canadian Health Behaviour in School-aged Children Study. Soc Sci Med 2010, 70:850-858.

64 Adolescent Mental Health: Connections to the Community

22. Wight R, Botticello AL, Aneshensel CS: Socioeconomic Context, Social Support, and Adolescent Mental Health: A Multilevel Investigation. J Youth Adolesc 2006, 35:115-126.
23. Belfi B, Goos M, De Fraine B, Van Damme J: The effect of class composition by gender and ability on secondary school students' school well-being and academic self-concept: A literature review. Educ Res Rev 2012, 7:62-74.
24. Nrugham L, Herrestad H, Mehlum L: Suicidality among Norwegian youth: Review of research on risk factors and interventions. Nordic J Psychiatry 2010, 64:317-326.
25. Mehlum L: Suicidal ideation and sense of coherence in male conscripts. Acta Psychiatr Scand 1998, 98:487-492.
26. Halvorsen JA, Stern RS, Dalgard F, Thoresen M, Bjertness E, Lien L: Suicidal Ideation, Mental Health Problems, and Social Impairment Are Increased in Adolescents with Acne: A Population-Based Study. J Investigative Dermatol 2011, 131:363-370.
27. Browne WJ: MCMC estimation in MLwinN. Bristol: University of Bristol; 2009.
28. Hox JJ: Multilevel analysis. Techniques and Applications. Second edition. New York: Routhledge; 2010.
29. Cyranowski JM, Frank E, Young E, Shear MK: Adolescent Onset of the Gender Difference in Lifetime Rates of Major Depression: A Theoretical Model. Arch Gen Psychiatry 2000, 57:21-27.
30. Ayyash-Abdo H: Adolescent Suicide:An Ecological Approach. Psychol Schools 2002, 39:459-475.
31. Töero K, Nagy A, Sawaguchi T, Sawaguchi A, Sotonyi P: Characteristics of suicide among children and adolescents in Budapest. Pediatrics Int 2001, 43:368-371.
32. Kaltiala-Heino R, Rimpelä M, Marttunen M, Rimpelä A, Rantanen P: Bullying, depression, and suicidal ideation in Finnish adolescents: school survey. BMJ 1999, 319:348-351.
33. Markussen E: Valg og gjennomføring av videregående opplæring før Kunnskapsløftet. Acta Didactica Norge 2010, 4(17):1. 18
34. Ang R, Huan V: Relationship between Academic Stress and Suicidal Ideation: Testing for Depression as a Mediator Using Multiple Regression. Child Psychiatry Hum Dev 2006, 37:133-143.
35. Borowsky IW, Ireland M, Resnick MD: Adolescent Suicide Attempts: Risks and Protectors. Pediatrics 2001, 107:485-493.
36. Daniel S, Walsh AK, Goldston DB, Arnold EM, Reboussin BA, Wood FB: Suicidality, School Dropout, and Reading Problems Among Adolescents. J Learn Disabilities 2006, 39:507-514.
37. Klimes-Dougan B, Safer MA, Ronsaville D, Tinsley R, Harris SJ: The Value of Forgetting Suicidal Thoughts and Behaviour. Suicide Life-Threatening Behav 2007, 37:431-438.

CHAPTER 4

THE IMPACT OF PERSONAL BACKGROUND AND SCHOOL CONTEXTUAL FACTORS ON ACADEMIC COMPETENCE AND MENTAL HEALTH FUNCTIONING ACROSS THE PRIMARY-SECONDARY SCHOOL TRANSITION

SHARMILA VAZ, RICHARD PARSONS, TORBJÖRN FALKMER, ANNE ELIZABETH PASSMORE, AND MARITA FALKMER

4.1 INTRODUCTION

4.1.1 THE ISSUE: TRANSITION FROM PRIMARY TO SECONDARY SCHOOL

The transition from primary to secondary school has long been acknowledged as an important change in the lives of most students [1]–[3]. Despite contextual variations in school systems, similarities in the features of this transition exist [4]. Typically, the secondary school transition involves si-

The Impact of Personal Background and School Contextual Factors on Academic Competence and Mental Health Functioning across the Primary-Secondary School Transition. © *Vaz S, Parsons R, Falkmer T, Passmore AE, and Falkmer M.* PLoS ONE **9**,3 *(2014), doi:10.1371/journal.pone.0089874. Licensed under a Creative Commons Attribution 4.0 International License, http://creativecommons. org/licenses/by/4.0/.*

multaneous changes in school environments, relationships, and academic expectations [1], [5]–[7]. Students in Western Societies, including Australia, negotiate the school transition at a time in development when they are striving to gain independence from their parents, establish a unique identity [8], [9], and gain approval and support from peers [10]. Adjusting to the changes associated with the secondary school transition can be challenging. Unsuccessful negotiation may set some students on a trajectory of diminishing returns, not only in the short-term [11], [12], but also years thereafter [2].

4.1.2 EFFECTS OF THE SECONDARY SCHOOL TRANSITION ON TYPICALLY DEVELOPING STUDENTS' ACADEMIC COMPETENCE (AC) AND MENTAL HEALTH FUNCTIONING (MHF)

Current evidence on the effects of the secondary school transition on AC (also referred to as academic performance or academic functioning) and MHF in typically developing students is mixed. Some studies suggest mean AC scores significantly decline after an initial settling-in period [3], [13]–[15]. Not every student experiences changes to the same extent, or even in the same direction [16], [17]. For example, less academically able students have been shown to have poorer adjustment to new school regimes [1], [18]. When compared to girls, boys have been shown to be more negatively affected by self-consciousness about AC, leading to declines in self-esteem and problems with adjustment subsequent to the transition [12]. The observed variability in AC across the transition has been attributed to various reasons including: study design and measurement issues (i.e., type of study, timing of data collection, stability and specificity of measurement tools used); social reference group variance; structural and philosophical differences between schools; and differences due to gender-role identification and personality [3], [15], [16], [18]–[23]. The role that the transition itself plays in the academic attainment dip is unclear, since a causal link between the transition and subsequent attainment has yet to be established [3].

Variability in student MHF is conspicuous within the transition literature. For example in one Australian study (restricted to two primary schools and one high school), the majority (55%) of students reported stable psychological health; 20% had better functioning, and 25% reported decreased psychological functioning through the transition [24]. Variability in MHF has also been reported in the US setting, where the middle school structure is common [25]–[27]. For example, Chung and colleagues [26] found students' MHF (from years 5 to 6) followed three trajectories (average start to high; low to moderately high; consistently high). Those with worse MHF prior to transition tended to have more adaptive difficulties after the transition when compared to their peers. Other studies report students with certain mental health conditions to be at a greater disadvantage across this transition. For example, studies suggest victimization is strongly related to depression, and weakly related to anxiety [28], while others suggest students with problem behaviours (disruptive or aggressive) have greater problems adjusting to junior high school [1], [29]. Gender differences in MHF have been documented. Girls report more internalising [30] and anxiety problems [31], while boys appear to exhibit more externalising problems [24], [32]. Overall, MHF across the primary-secondary transition varies widely amongst typically developing students. While some view the transition as demanding, others thrive on the challenges that it creates [33]. Therefore, considering a student cohort to be homogenous could be misleading.

4.1.3 LIMITED FOCUS ON THE IMPACT OF PRIMARY-SECONDARY SCHOOL TRANSITION ON AC AND MHF OF STUDENTS WITH DISABILITIES

Few studies have considered the impact of transition to secondary school on AC and MHF of students with disabilities [34]. Students with learning disabilities have been reported to experience reductions in AC [35], while their typically developing counterparts show increased scores. Information on MHF of students with disabilities is variable, and depends on the construct used to define mental health. For example, when defined in terms of self-esteem, studies reported those with special educational needs (SEN) [36] and specific learning difficulties [35] to be at no greater risk than their peers. Students with special educational needs have, however, been reported to be at higher risk of bullying in secondary school (with 37% out of 110 reporting to be bullied when compared to 25% of their peers without SEN) [36]. In another study [37], while teachers reported students with specific learning difficulties to have significantly more internalising and externalising difficulties than their peers; students self-reported to have significantly fewer problems. Thus, measurement issues appear to confound the accuracy of self-reported mental health data for the disability subgroup [34].

4.1.4 EFFECT OF SCHOOL CONTEXTUAL VARIABLES ON AC AND MHF

Although not explicit to the primary-secondary transition, there is inconclusive evidence on the influence of school contextual factors on AC and MHF. Various factors such as school size; sector; organisational system; and school socio-economic status (SES), which is based on the post-code of the school, have been implicated [38]–[44]. The contribution of school contextual factors to post-transition functioning in a mainstream Australian sample remains unexplored.

4.1.5 AUSTRALIAN STUDIES ON THE PRIMARY-SECONDARY SCHOOL TRANSITION

Case studies and literature reviews dominate the Australian literature on primary-secondary school transition [23], [45]–[52]. The available deductive studies are constrained by small sample size, design (i.e., convenience sampling) or scope (i.e., predominantly focus on mental health, bullying, or the changes in the school environment) issues that limit the generalisation of their findings [24], [33], [50], [53], [54]. With too few schools involved in transition research in Australia, exploration of "school effects" on student AC and MHF across this transition is difficult (Fitz-Gibbon 1996; Smyth 1999). Similarly, for students with disabilities there are no Australian or international studies that have considered the impact of secondary school transition on perceived AC and MHF, despite inclusion of these students in the regular school system for decades [34]. The limited number and scope of studies precludes speculation on whether this subgroup may be additionally disadvantaged across the transition, even though they are at lower baseline level to their typically developing counterparts before the transition.

4.2 METHODS

4.2.1 AIMS AND OBJECTIVES

The overall aim of this study was to explore and compare perceived AC and MHF of students with and without disability, six months before and six months after transition to secondary school. The objectives were:

- determine the unique and combined effects of personal background factors (i.e., gender, disability and SES) on academic competence and mental health functioning before and after transition to secondary school;
- examine the added contribution of school contextual factors (i.e., sector, organisational structure, mean-school SES) on academic competence and mental health functioning before and after transition to secondary school, after accounting for personal background factors;
- determine the contribution of personal background factors and school contextual factors on change in academic competence and mental health functioning across the transition.

The current study is part of a larger study on the factors associated with student academic, social-emotional and participatory adjustment across the primary-secondary school transition [55].

4.2.2 DESIGN

A cohort study using a prospective, longitudinal design with two data collection points was used [Time 1 (T1) and Time 2 (T2)]. Informed written consent was obtained from school principals, parents, teachers, and written assent was obtained from students to participate in this study. In situations where the student declined to participate, even with parental consent, they were not included. All participants were made aware that they were not obliged to participate in the study, and were free to withdraw from the study at any time without justification or prejudice. At all stages, the study conformed to the National Health and Medical Research Council Ethics Guidelines [56]. Full ethics approval was obtained from Curtin University Health Research Ethics Committee, in Western Australia (WA) (Reference number HR 194/2005).

4.2.3 RECRUITMENT

The following inclusion criteria were applied to recruit students into the study:

1. Attending a regular school in the educational districts of metropolitan Perth or other major city centres of WA; and
2. Enrolled in the final year of primary school in WA (class 6 or 7) in the academic years commencing January 2006 or 2007, and due to transition to either middle or secondary school in January 2007 or 2008. Further details on the schooling system in WA are presented in Appendix A.

Students were categorised as having a disability if they were reported to have medical diagnosis or a disability or a chronic ill health condition, and were identified by their parent(s)/care-giver(s) to be attending a regular class for the majority of their weekly schooling hours (over 80% of the school hours per week), with support provided as required. Thus, a broad definition was used to define disability which entailed any addition medical health condition that had the potential of impact on an individual's daily functioning.

Several recruitment strategies were used to maximize reach and representativeness:

1. A pre-paid package (containing poster, letter of invitation, and school sector endorsement letter) was mailed out to principals from 250 primary schools listed on the Department of Education and

Training, WA website. Schools listed in the Canning, Fremantle-Peel, Swan, and West Coast educational districts of Perth and major centres of Albany, Bunbury, Mid-West, Midlands, and Esperance educational districts of WA were approached.

2. A structured procedure was followed; with principal, teacher, parent and student consent obtained in that order.

3. A poster and a letter of invitation were circulated to the Disability Services Commission (DSC), the chief government body offering services to school-children with disability in WA. The DSC also posted a link to the study on its web page.

4. A pre-paid package (containing poster, letter of invitation, school sector and DSC endorsement letters) was circulated via known service providers, consumer groups, support groups, families of students with a disability via individual providers, and to any individuals who expressed interest in the study. In order to over sample the disability subgroup, additional snowball sampling occurred via participants forwarding information to friends and family.

T1 data collection was timed to ensure that parents had a definitive letter of acceptance from the secondary school, so that the identified secondary schools could be contacted at the commencement of the following academic year. The T1 parent questionnaire requested parents to list the name of the secondary school they planned to send their child to, for follow-up purposes. Follow-up of participants was carried out using the above mentioned recruitment procedure. T2 data collection commenced 6-months after the transition (Terms 3 and 4), after students had passed through the short-lived variability in functioning due to the transition, and had time to experience the new environments which either supported or hindered their transition.

4.2.4 DATA COLLECTION

Data were collected via questionnaires, primarily paper and pencil format. T1 data collection commenced in the second semester (Terms 3 and 4) of the final year in primary school (class 6 or 7) in the academic years commencing January 2006 or 2007. At T1, data from students, a parent (or primary caregiver) and the main class teacher were collected. To ensure consistency of administration, all questionnaires were administered on site by the first author or research assistants. Administration guidelines were developed to minimize administration bias. Student questionnaires were designed to be completed within one sitting during their regularly scheduled class time (35–40 minutes). On completion of this questionnaire, students returned it to staff and were given the pre-coded parent questionnaire in a reply-paid envelope, to take home. In cases where students were absent on the date of data collection, parent and student questionnaire packages (questionnaires and administration guidelines) were mailed-out to their residence. At T1, data from 395 students from 75 primary schools were collected. There were no more than 30 (11.3%) absent students across the schools sampled, across both academic years.

Routine follow-up protocol for parent/student/teacher questionnaires included: phone call to residence within two weeks; reminder mail if questionnaires were not returned within four weeks; and at least two fortnightly reminder phone calls.

T2 questionnaire administration commenced 6-months after the transition to secondary school. Administration was undertaken in the usual class times. Given that this was the second exposure to the survey, a decision was made to mail out 40% of the parent and student questionnaires to the students' residence, with the administration guideline and reply-paid envelope enclosed in the package. At T2, data from students and the same parent (primary caregiver) were collected. A student attrition rate of 32.7% resulted in a T2 sample of 266 participants from 152 secondary schools

4.2.5 POWER CALCULATION

For the purpose of sample size estimation, it was assumed that there would be approximately 10 independent variables in the final regression model (for AC or MHF). In order to have power of .90 ($\beta = 0.1$) and with α-value of .05 (type I error), a sample size of 215 would be required to detect a small to moderate effect size of 0.1 (Sample Size Program: PASS) [57]. With an α-value of .05 and a β of .2, any between group comparisons with the smallest of groups, viz.: the 69 children with disabilities, allowed for a Cohen's d of .47 or larger to be detected.

4.2.6 DATA COLLECTION INSTRUMENTS

4.2.6.1 AC

Items from the scholastic competence domain of the Self-Perception Profile for Adolescents (SPPA) were used to measure student's perception of their AC (Harter, 1988). The SPPA has comparable internal consistency in populations of students with learning disability ($\alpha = 0.89$), and behavioural disorders ($\alpha = 0.85$) [58]. Considerate convergent, discriminant, and construct validity of the academic competence scale in an equivalent US and Australian sample has been substantiated [59]–[61]. Higher scores indicate better perceived AC.

4.2.6.2 MHF: THE STRENGTHS AND DIFFICULTIES QUESTIONNAIRE (SDQ).

The parent version of the Strengths and Difficulties Questionnaire (SDQ) was used to assess students' overall MHF [62]. The overall scores were computed by summing hyperactivity, emotional symptoms, conduct problems and peer problems subscales [62]. Moderate to high internal consistency values have been reported ($\alpha = 0.70$–0.80) [63]. Empirical studies supported the tool's discriminate and predictive validity [62], [65]. The SDQ score correlates strongly with the Child Behaviour Checklist [64] but is more sensitive in detecting hyperactivity, and equally effective in detecting internalising and externalising problems in children and adolescents [65]. Australian norms have been published for the SDQ [63]. Higher scores indicate lower MHF.

4.2.6.3 FAMILY DEMOGRAPHICS AND SCHOOL CONTEXTUAL CHARACTERISTICS.

Family demographics: Items were drawn from the Indicators of Social and Family Functioning Instrument Version-1 (ISAFF) [66] and Australian Bureau of Statistics (ABS, 2001) surveys. Parents reported details on the family demographic characteristics, residence post code, and child's disability. Information on the school sector, post code number of students enrolled in each school, and organisational structure at each school was obtained from Department of Education and Training, WA records. The school post code was used to calculate its socio-economic index (SEIFA Index), using the Commonwealth Department of Education, Employment, and Workplace Relations measure of relative socio-economic advantage and disadvantage [67]. In this study, the SEIFA decile was used as the measure of mean school-SES, with a lower decile number meaning that the school was located in an area that is relatively more disadvantaged than other areas.

4.2.7 DATA MANAGEMENT

Data were managed and analysed using Statistical Package for Social Sciences Version 20 and Statistical Analysis Software Version 9.2. Data from the 2006 and 2007 cohort were alike on all factors. Hence, for purposes of subsequent analyses, sample scores were combined. Skewness/kurtosis measures indicated reasonable symmetry. Only 1.8–2.5% of data were missing at scale levels. The estimation maximization algorithm and Little's chi-square statistic identified data to be missing completely at random, with the probability level set at 0.05 [68], [69]. Standard guidelines recommended by the SDQ developers were followed to replace missing values and sensitivity checks were undertaken to substantiate the validity of data substitution techniques employed. Dummy variables were created to represent the categorical personal background and school contextual factors (i.e., independent variables) incorporated into the regression models [68].

4.2.8 ANALYSES

The General Linear Model (GLM) procedure was used to address the study's objectives. The model was first tested with all personal background factors (i.e., gender, disability and SES) and their interactions. Since none of the interactions were statistically significant, they were removed from the model. The most parsimonious models including personal background and school contextual factors for each outcome at T1 and T2 are presented. The results from the model include the R^2 or the proportion of variance in the outcome variable that could be explained by each personal background factor; the unstandardized regression coefficients (B) and their standard errors (SE), and the Least-Square (LS) means (or estimated population marginal means), which are within-group means appropriately adjusted for the other effects in the model [70].

4.3 RESULTS

At T1, data from 395 students from 75 primary schools were collected. Mean age of the students at T1 was 11.89 years (SD = 0.45 years, median = 12 years). A student attrition rate of 32.7% resulted in a T2 sample of 266 participants from 152 secondary schools. Chi-square and paired sample t-tests demonstrated that the participants who continued to be involved in the study at T2 did not differ from those who discontinued involvement, on gender, disability, SES-level, AC and MHF. The current paper presents data of the 266 students that answered questionnaires at T1 and T2. Access to the complete data can be obtained by contacting the first author.

Tables 1 and 2 give an overview of the key demographic characteristics of the student sample. The majority of the students in the disability subgroup had asthma, auditory disability, or a learning disability. Seventy six percent (n = 203) of students were from two-parent (original or biological) families, 11% (n = 29) were from the blended/extended/combination families, while the remaining 12.8% (n = 34) were from single-parent households. English was the main language spoken in 95.5% households (n = 252). Mothers of 23% (n = 60) of the sample did not have a post-school qualification. Of those who had a post school qualification, 5% (n = 13) completed a trade/apprenticeship course, 31.5% (n = 82) completed a vocational education and training certificate from college or Training and Further Education, 20% (n = 52) had a bachelor's degree, 20.4% (n = 53) had a post graduate degree. Eighty-two percent of the mothers (n = 218) were in paid employment, and 53.5% (n = 110) of the working mothers held professional/managerial employment titles. The remaining held clerical/administrative, technical, or sales positions. T2 data were collected after 12 months. The mean age of students at T2 was 12.9 years (SD = 0.57 years, median = 13 years).

TABLE 1: Student demographic characteristics at T1: Gender, health status, and household SES-level.

Characteristics	T1	
	N = 266	%
Gender		
Boy (Mean age 11.98 years, SD = 0.44 years)	124	46.6
Girl (Mean age 11.77 years, SD = 0.46 years)	142	53.4
Health status		
No disability (Mean age 11.84 years, SD = 0.41 years)	197	74.1
Disability (Mean age 11.96 years, SD = 0.58 years)	69	25.9
Househould SES-level [66,122]		
$1–599/week (low-SES level)	23	8.7
$600–1,999/week (mid-SES level)	154	58.3
$2,000 +/week (high-SES level)	87	33.0

Of the 250 primary schools invited to participate in the study, 175 declined, resulting in a non-participation rate of 70%. Only ten (14.9% of 67) students with disability were sourced from outside the main school recruitment (through DSC and the snowball). Details on the school characteristics of the 266 students surveyed at T1 and T2 are presented in Tables 3–5.

At T1, 47% of the students (n = 125) were enrolled in the public schools, 29% (n = 77) in Catholic schools and the remaining 24% (n = 64) in independent/private schools. There was a movement out of government schools towards Catholic and Independent schools at T2, with 60% staying in the government sector while over 85% of students in other sectors at T1 remained in those sectors at T2. Almost 80% (n = 209) were in schools that followed the K7–K10/12 organisational system. The majority of the sample at both T1 and T2 (T1 = 53.0%, n = 141; T2 = 45.1%, n = 120) received their education from mid-range sized schools. Slightly more than 90% (n = 240) moved to secondary school at the completion of Year 7, and 79% (n = 211) moved to a secondary school which was not connected with their primary school. Kappa statistics was used to determine whether the agreement between school sector attendance at T1 and T2 exceeded chance levels [71]. As shown in Tables 4 and 5, a significant change in school sectors accessed by the total sample and sub-group with disability across the transition was noticed (Kappa coefficient = 0.64).

TABLE 2: Types of disabilities involved in the student sample.

Disability type	n	%
Asthma	13	18.8
Auditory diability	11	15.9
LD	8	11.6
CP	6	8.7
ADHD	6	8.7
Asperger	5	7.2
Visual disability	5	7.2
ADD	4	5.8
Juvenile diabetes	2	2.9
Osteogen imperfecta	2	2.9
ASD	1	1.4
Brachial	1	1.4
Diabetes	1	1.4
Enuresis	1	1.4
Epilepsy	1	1.4
Haemophilia	1	1.4
Hypothyroidism	1	1.4
Total	69	100

TABLE 3: School characteristics at T1 and T2. The same 266 subjects were surveyed at both time points.

	T1	T2
School Sector		
Catholic	77 (29.0%)	81 (40.5%)
Government	125 (47.0%)	79 (29.7%)
Independent private	64 (24.0%)	106 (39.9%)
School Organizational Structure		
Primary school (K–7)	209 (78.6%)	
Secondary school (Y8–10/12)		173 (65.0%)
K–12 without middle school	33 (12.4%)	52 (19.6%)
K–12 with middle school	24 (9.0%)	41 (15.4%)
Mean school SES (indexed by SEIFa[1] decile)		
1–6	45 (16.9%)	37 (13.9%)
7–8	47 (17.7%)	51 (19.2%)
9	117 (44.0%)	112 (42.1%)
10	57 (21.4%)	66 (24.8%)
Primary school size based on total number of students		
small = <375	67 (25.2%)	
mid-range = 375–975	141 (53.0%)	
large = >975	58 (21.8%)	
Secondary school size based on total number of studens		
small = <700		67 (25.2%)
mid-range = 700–1250		120 (45.1%)
large = >1250		79 (29.7%)
Year of transition		
Year 6	26 (9.8%)	
Year 7	240 (90.2%)	
Same secondary school as primary		
No		211 (79.3%)
Yes		55 (20.7%)

[1]*The SEIFA decile was used as the measure of mean school SES, with a lower decile number meaning that the school was located in an area that is relatively more disadvantaged than other areas.*

TABLE 4: Change in school sector of the total sample across the primary-secondary transition (N = 266).

T1 School sector	T2 School sector			
Sector	Government	Catholic	Independent/Private	Sum (%)
Government	75 (60.0%)	14 (11.2%)	36 (28.8%)	125 (100)
Catholic	2 (2.6%)	66 (85.7%)	9 (11.7%)	77 (100)
Independent/Private	2 (3.1%)	1 (1.6%)	61 (95.3%)	64 (100)

Numbers in each cell show the number of students and percentage of the school sector to which they belong

TABLE 5: Change in school sector of the disability subgroups across the primary-secondary transition (n = 69).

T1 School sector	T2 School sector			
Sector	Government	Catholic	Independent/Private	Sum (%)
Government	25 (69.4%)	2 (5.6%)	9 (25%)	36 (100)
Catholic	1 (5.9%)	14 (82.3%)	2 (11.8%)	17 (100)
Independent/Private	0 (0.0%)	0 (0.0%)	16 (100%)	16 (100)

4.3.1 MODEL PREDICTING AC AT T1

As shown in Table 6, personal background factors explained 14.2% of the variability in T1 AC scores. While the models included a term for gender, this appeared not to be significantly associated with either the AC scores at T1 or T2, or the change in AC scores over the transition.

Students with disability reported significantly lower AC than their typically developing counterparts. Household SES was linearly related to T1 AC; with those from higher SES households having the highest AC scores and those from socially disadvantaged households having the lowest scores.

After accounting for personal background variability, school contextual factors could explain an additional 3.1% of the variability in T1 AC. In ascending order, students from Catholic schools reported lowest AC, followed by government, and independent sector students. Students attending larger schools appeared to have lower AC scores than the other schools.

TABLE 6: Personal background and school contextual factors associated with perceived AC at T1 and T2, and across the T1–T2 transition (higher value represents better outcomes).

	Variable	B (SE)	LS-Mean	p-value
	Model predicting T1 AC			
Step 1: Personal factors	Gender			
$R^2 = 14.2\%$				
	Male	0.09 (0.08)	2.74	0.2818
	Female		2.66	
	Presence of disability			
	Yes	−0.42 (0.09)	2.49	<0.0001
	No		2.91	
	Household SES			
	low-SES = <$599	−0.67 (0.17)	2.35	<0.0001
	mid-range SES = $600–$1999	−0.30 (0.09)	2.73	
	high-SES = $2000+		3.02	
Step 2: School contextual factors	T1 School sector			
$R^2 = 17.3\%$				
	Catholic	−0.62 (0.23)	2.40	0.0236
	Government	−0.48 (0.22)	2.54	
	Independent private		3.02	
	T1 School size			
	small = <375	0.61 (0.23)	2.84	0.0215
	mid-range = 375–975	0.64 (0.24)	2.88	
	large = >975		2.23	
	Model predicing T2 AC			
Step 1: Personal factors	Gender			
$R^2 = 5.1\%$				
	Male	0.13 (0.08)	2.91	0.1021
	Female		2.78	
	Presence of disability			
	Yes	−0.18 (0.09)	2.75	0.0495
	No		2.93	
	Household SES			
	low-SES = <$599	−0.39 (0.16)	2.65	0.0226

TABLE 6: *Cont.*

	Variable	B (SE)	LS-Mean	p-value
	mid-range SES = $600–$1999	–0.19 (0.09)	2.85	
	high-SES = $2000+		3.03	
Step 2: School contextual factors	T1 school sector			
R² = 10.5%				
	Catholic	0.39 (0.38)	2.98	0.0131
	Government	0.85 (0.39)	3.44	
	Independent private		2.59	
	T1 school size			
	small = <375	0.85 (0.38)	3.27	0.0514
	mid-range = 375–975	0.92 (0.38)	3.33	
	large = >975		2.42	
	Model predicting change in AC from T1 to T2			
Step 1: Personal factors	Gender			
R² = 5.2%				
	Male	0.04 (0.07)	0.16	0.5483
	Female		0.12	
	Presence of disability			
	Yes	0.23 (0.08)	0.26	0.0046
	No		0.03	
	Household SES			
	low-SES = <$599	0.29 (0.14)	0.29	0.1168
	mid-range SES = $600–$1999	0.11 (0.08)	0.12	
	high-SES = $2000+		0.01	
Step 2: School contextual factors	T1 school structure			
R² = 9.8%				
	K-12 with middle school	–0.46	–0.28	0.0016
	K-12 without middle school	0.06	0.24	
	Primary school (K-7)		0.19	

4.3.2 MODEL PREDICTING AC AT T2

At T2, personal background factors accounted for only 5.1% of the variance in AC. The disability subgroup continued to report lower AC than their typically developing peers (p = .0495), but the magnitude of this difference was not as large as reported at T1. The linear relationship between household-SES and T2 AC continued (high-SES>mid-range SES>low-SES); but the strength of this relationship reduced significantly.

After accounting for personal background variability, T2 school contextual factors could not explain any additional variability in T2 AC scores. T1 school size and organisational type continued to account for 5.4% of the variability in T2 AC scores. Attending large schools at T1 was associated with lower prospective AC (i.e., T2 AC). Students from T1 schools that used the K-7 organisational structure reported the lowest AC scores.

4.3.3 MODEL PREDICTING CHANGE IN AC OVER THE PRIMARY-SECONDARY TRANSITION

Personal background factors explained 5.2% of the change in AC across the transition. Students with a disability showed an improvement in AC compared with other students. Those students who attended K-12 schools with middle school system appeared to show a reduced AC score across the transition compared to students from other school structure types.

4.3.4 MODEL PREDICTING MHF AT T1

At T1, personal background factors explained 21.4% of the variability in MHF (Table 7). Boys and students with a disability had lower scores than girls and students without disability respectively. An inverse relationship between MHF and household-SES was evident. In descending order, students from higher-SES households had better MHF than those from mid-range, followed by low-SES. T1 School contextual factors could not explain any additional variability in MHF than the above-mentioned personal background factors.

TABLE 7: Personal background and school contextual factors associated with MHF at T1 and T2, and across the T1–T2 transition (higher value represents worse outcomes).

	Variable	B (SE)	LS-Mean	p-value
	Model predicting T1 MHF			
Step 1: Personal factors	Gender			
$R^2 = 21.4\%$				
	Male	1.40 (0.61)	9.47	0.0229
	Female		8.06	
	Presence of disability			
	Yes	4.82 (0.70)	11.18	<0.0001
	No		6.35	
	Household SES			
	low-SES = <$599	3.82 (1.24)	10.96	0.0078
	mid-range SES = $600–$1999	1.06 (0.66)	8.20	
	high-SES = $2000+		7.14	
Step 2: School contextual factors	T1 School structure			
$R^2 = 22.8\%$				
	K-12 with middle school	0.12 (1.15)	9.05	0.0855
	K-12 without middle school	–2.13 (0.97)	6.81	
	Primary school (K-7)		8.93	
	Model predicting T2 MHF			
Step 1: Personal factors	Gender			
$R^2 = 20.1\%$				
	Male	1.09 (0.59)	9.11	0.0656
	Female		8.02	
	Presence of disability			
	Yes	4.58 (0.67)	10.86	<0.0001
	No		6.27	
	Household SES			
	low-SES = <$599	2.74 (1.23)	9.91	0.0228
	mid-range SES = $600–$1999	1.45 (0.63)	8.62	
	high-SES = $2000+		7.17	

TABLE 7: *Cont.*

	Variable	B (SE)	LS-Mean	p-value
Step 2: School contextual factors Step 2: No school variables contribute further	T1 school sector			
	Model predicting change in MHF from T1 to T2			
Step 1: Personal factors	Gender			
$R^2 = 2.1\%$				
	Male	−0.13 (0.46)	−0.43	0.7755
	Female		−0.030	
	Presence of disability			
	Yes	−0.32 (0.53)	−0.53	0.5375
	No		−0.20	
	Household SES			
	low-SES = <$599	−1.78 (0.97)	−1.61	0.1075
	mid-range SES = $600–$1999	0.18 (0.50)	0.35	
	high-SES = $2000+	·	0.17	
Step 2: School contextual factors	T1 school structure			
$R^2 = 7.0\%$				
	Catholic	−1.87 (0.64)	−0.70	0.0017
	Government	−2.10 (0.60)	−0.92	
	Independent		1.18	

4.3.5 MODEL PREDICTING MHF AT T2

At T2, personal background variability explained 20.1% of the variability in MHF. The difference in MHF between genders narrows at T2 to the point that it is not statistically significant. The students with a disability appeared to have significantly lower MHF scores at T2 (similar to T1). The inverse linear relationship between household SES and MHF persisted after the secondary school transition. Similar to the T1 model, school contextual factors could not explain any variability in MHF additional to the personal background factors discussed above.

4.3.6 MODEL PREDICTING CHANGE IN MHF OVER THE PRIMARY-SECONDARY TRANSITION

Personal background factors accounted for 2.1% of the change MHF across the transition, with none of them demonstrating statistically significant associations. An unexpected finding was the prospective impact of T1 school sector on change in MHF over the transition (explaining 5.9% of the MHF change). Students who attended independent schools at T1 reported lower MHF at T2, while those who attended other school sectors showed small improvements in their MHF.

4.4 DISCUSSION

Mixed evidence exists on the effects of this school transition on student AC and MHF. Researchers generally agree that no given student cohort is homogeneous [12], [72]. By employing a prospective longitudinal design, the current study examined the contribution of personal background factors (i.e., gender, presence of disability and household SES) and school contextual factors (i.e., size, sector, organisational model, and mean-SES) on perceived AC and overall MHF across the primary-secondary transition.

4.4.1 PERSONAL FACTORS AND AC AND MHF AT DIFFERENT TIMES ACROSS THE TRANSITION

The current study found that personal background factors explained the majority of the variability in student AC and MHF, before and after the transition. A significant reduction in the contribution of personal background factors on AC subsequent to the transition, despite AC scores staying stable across time was unexpected. This finding suggests that factors other than gender, disability and household-SES influence AC at T2 [55]. In the case of MHF, the contribution of personal background factors remained broadly constant at both times, a finding consistent with previous evidence [73].

Students with a disability had lower AC than their typically developing peers. This finding was in line with a number of previous studies [35],
[58], [74], [75]. The reduced AC in the disability subgroup could be explained by the negative social comparison processes (referred to as the
Big-fish-little-pond effect, (BFLPE) [76]. According to the BFLPE hypothesis, a student's self-concept is negatively correlated with one's peers.
Thus, a student's academic self-concept depends not only on the student's
academic accomplishments but also the accomplishments of those in the
school that the student attends. The consistently lower AC in the disability
sub-group found in the current study highlights the need for schools to
recognise and address this issue.

Of interest was an improvement in the disability subgroup's AC after the
transition. This finding could suggest that there was a less obvious BFLPE
in secondary school, or the timing of data collection which was 6-months after the transition to secondary school was not long enough for ability group-
ings among students to be obvious. Long term longitudinal studies that track
students through the secondary years of school would be beneficial in understanding the effect of regular secondary school attendance on the disability
subgroup's AC relative to their typical peers, especially in light of evidence
suggesting poorer school completion rates and employment participation
rates among youth and young adults with disability [77], [78].

The consistent poorer MHF in the disability subgroup found in the
current study could be attributed to several factors including biological
processes (e.g., deficits in cognition; language and communication, social skills); the effect of medication; the psychological burden associated
with having a disability; or the associations between mental disorders and
lifestyle risk factors [79]–[86]. Given the importance of positive mental
health in itself and the detrimental impact of mental ill health on the individual and society over time [87]–[94], the current study's findings re-
inforce the importance of comprehensive, whole-of school, mental health
prevention programs currently operational in Australian primary and secondary schools [95]–[97].

With regards to gender and AC, our study's findings support egalitarian theories of the reduced gender-stereotyped socialization over the past
decade. This could be attributed to interventions and legislation aimed at
increasing girls' motivation and participation in academic pursuits. Future

research into whether egalitarian patterns hold in subject-specific academic domains (i.e., math, computers, sciences, history) could help target specific interventions for those most in need. In the case of MHF, a significant gender bias favouring girls was evident in primary school. This finding could be a function of poorer behaviour during the last term of the school year (i.e., an effect of timing of measurement). The improvement in overall MHF in boys after the transition and the absence of any significant gender association with MHF in secondary school is a positive finding. Our findings highlight the need for primary and secondary schools to be equally sensitive and responsive to the AC and MHF needs of boys and girls.

Consistent with earlier research [1], [15], the detrimental effects of social disadvantage on AC and MHF was evident. According to the Family Investment Model (FIM), higher SES households can afford to make significant capital investments in the development of their children, while more disadvantaged families are forced to invest in more immediate needs [98], [99]. Economic deprivation affects families' well-being through an increase in family stress, which in turn decreases ability to provide stability, adequate attention, supervision, and cognitive stimulation to children [100]. The absence of any cumulative disadvantage of household-SES on AC and MHF is optimistic. Furthermore, the reduced strength of the association between social disadvantage and AC and MHF post-transition, due to the improvement in the functioning of the lower-SES group could be attributed to several factors, which include: the transition trend noted in the study (i.e., increased enrolment in independent schools); or the effect of measurement (i.e., ceiling effect of the scales used, or the small sample size of the low-SES group making the detection of significant differences difficult due to power issues); or an indication that the transition to secondary school is beneficial to the MHF and AC of students from lower-SES subgroups. Nonetheless, this sub-group needs support more than their more affluent peers.

4.4.2 SCHOOL CONTEXTUAL FACTORS AND AC AND MHF AT DIFFERENT TIMES ACROSS THE TRANSITION

Across the board, school contextual factors explained very little, if any, of the variability in MHF, but more of the change in MHF over time. These findings concur with past findings on the small contribution of school factors on student MHF [101]–[104] and relatively larger contribution on AC [105], [106] and indicate that most school contextual factors provide similar experiences [107] or that school contextual factors are less important than personal background factors on student AC and MHF. Furthermore, no secondary school contextual characteristic (i.e., size, school sector, organisational model, mean-school SES or their interactions) influenced AC and MHF in secondary school. This means that individual student factors and primary school contextual factors are more important contributors of post-transition adjustment than concurrent secondary school contextual factors. Thus, there exists a greater responsibility on primary schools to ensure that the transition needs of the disadvantaged groups are satisfactorily met.

To date, the effect of school sector (private or public) on student outcomes is uncertain. Some findings suggest that that once student-household SES is considered in the analysis, the advantage of private schooling (independent schools) disappears or becomes minimal [38], [39]. Others suggest beneficial outcomes for those in private education [40], [108], [109]. In the current study, we found that even after accounting for personal background factors, attending an independent primary school was associated with higher concurrent AC but worse prospective MHF. The benefits of independent school attendance on AC could be attributed to the better resources, more functional and supportive school climate, or fewer discipline problems noted in these schools [40]. The lower AC found amongst those who attended Catholic schools is an unexpected finding which is contrary to past studies that highlight the benefits of Catholic school attendance in terms of a steady stream of funds that permits forward planning and budgeting, and institutional autonomy [40].

A trend was noticed for the whole student sample including the disability sub-group students to move out of government schools into independent or private schools for secondary education. This has been observed in previous Australian studies [41], [42]. Despite this transition trend, the absence of any significant contribution of school SES (indexed by the SEIFA score) on AC and MHF after adjustment for personal background factors validates the applicability of whole of school mental health models across school sectors, irrespective of social stratification. This finding is positive and suggests that for our current sample, individual-household SES was more important than the mean-school SES as far as AC and MHF were concerned. Given the relative skewness of the participating schools to higher deciles, it is likely that the detection of significant differences was difficult due to power issues. Caution ought to be exercised while interpreting these findings.

4.5 LIMITATIONS

The sample of students was drawn from the Perth metropolitan area and major city centres across WA, and did not involve students from other rural and regional populations, or other major metropolitan cities in Australia. Despite extensive recruitment efforts, 70% of the schools declined to participate in the study, which may have introduced a possible bias. The study's cohort comprised 29% Catholic, 47% Government, and 24% Independent schools, which was different to the profile of all schools in Western Australia (15%, 72%, and 13% respectively) and may limit the generalizability of the findings.

The majority of the students in the disability subgroup had asthma, auditory disability, or a learning disability. The criteria for inclusion into the disability category could have resulted in the exclusion of students with more disability related physical, cognitive, social, and emotional restrictions [110]. Thus, the findings of the current study may underestimate the impact of more severe disabilities on school transition. Statistically, it is also likely that combining the reports of a heterogeneous disability subgroup, with less disability related limitations, may have reduced the sensitivity of the analyses [111]. Additionally, we did not account for the confounding effect of disability severity and comorbidity status on AC and MHF [112]. Replication of the study findings in students from other school settings, such as educational support units, separate schools that cater for students with severe disabilities or students who were home schooled and more severe disabilities is needed to extend generalizability.

In the current study, AC was evaluated by students only. Social desirability self-report bias may have exaggerated the relationship between the predictor variables and student perceived AC scores. Parents reported on their child's overall mental functioning using the SDQ, which tends to over emphasise externalising conduct features. Especially during the adolescent years, it is likely that children are more apt to have better insights into their own MHF than their parents. Additional research that involves multisource data from students, parents, teachers, and possibly clinical interviews and school records, is warranted to validate these findings [113].

Consistent with past studies [114], students from low-SES households were under-represented in our sample. Despite small numbers, the significant disadvantage found in this sub-group suggest that these students are greatly disadvantaged (i.e., the true effect size could be larger). We did not explicitly define the sub-group of individuals from Indigenous and Torres Strait communities due to ethical concerns. Further research is warranted to find out whether the findings of this study can be generalised to all sub-groups of the Australian population.

Also, the two-point longitudinal study design did not permit us study the longer-term effect of transition on AC and MHF. This is an area worthy of scrutiny.

4.6 CONCLUSIONS

The current study is one of the few studies that investigated the effects of personal background and school contextual factors on AC and MHF across the primary-secondary transition, using a student sample with and without disabilities. Our findings highlight the existence of within-group variability in student AC and MHF and the responsibility on primary schools to ensure that the needs of disadvantaged groups are satisfactorily met, as these students continue to be disadvantaged after the transition to secondary school.

It is acknowledged that risks commonly accumulate and cluster across multiple contexts of development [115], [116]. Our findings highlight the need for detailed, multi-contextual assessment of personal background and school contextual factors that influence student AC and MHF across the primary-secondary school transition. Such studies are invaluable in guiding transition-specific interventions for all students in the regular school system.

4.A1 APPENDIX A: THE SCHOOLING SYSTEM IN WA

Schooling in Western Australia (WA) is delivered under the State's Education Act (1999), the Curriculum Council Act (1997) and the Adelaide Declaration on National Goals for Schooling in the Twenty-first Century (MCEETYA, 2004). The concept of inclusion is firmly embedded within the WA Curriculum Framework [117], [118].

WA has government (public) school and non-government (private) school sectors. Government schools operate under the direct responsibility of the State Minister of Education and Training, and are represented by the Department of Education and Training (DET). The non-government sector is represented by the Catholic Education Office (CEO) and the Association of Independent Schools (AISWA). One-third of all students in Australia study in non-government schools, the majority of whom are from middle and upper socio-economic status (SES) background [119]. WA government schools are all co-educational. The privatised sector has co-educational and single-gender schools at primary and at secondary level.

Predominately, a three-stage educational structure consisting of pre-primary, primary, and secondary operates in most government and non-government schools. Schools organisational structures range from traditional primary-secondary school configurations (Kindergarten – Year 7, and Years 8–12), through separate structures within larger frameworks from Kindergarten - Year 12 (K-12), to specially designated middle schools (Year 6/7- Year 8 or 10/12) [120]. There are relatively few designated middle schools in WA when compared to the US and the rest of Australia [120]. During the time of data collection for this study, primary-secondary secondary school transition in WA occurred at the completion of Year seven (i.e., the year in which students turned 13). Post 2009, as part of a state-wide planning framework, a phased relocation of Year 7 students into the secondary settings is being undertaken on case-by-case [121].

Additionally, the models of inclusion for students with disabilities adopted in schools across WA vary widely with regard to student contact time in the regular classroom. In some inclusive instances, students with disabilities who are based in regular classrooms spend some time in specialised units or classes designed to cater to their needs. Students with a chronic illness also spend time out in hospital/home, or require assistance from nurses at school. The term regular schools in this paper is used to refer to a mainstreamed situation, in which students attend a regular class for almost 80% of the school hours per week, with support from specialised service providers offered as required.

REFERENCES

1. Anderson LH, Jacobs J, Schramm S, Splittgerber F (2000) School transitions: Beginning of the end or a new beginning? International Journal of Educational Research 33. doi: 10.1016/s0883-0355(00)00020-3
2. Seidman E, French S (2004) Developmental trajectories and ecological transitions: A two-step procedure to aid in choice of prevention and promotion interventions. Development and Psychopathology 16: 1141–1159. doi: 10.1017/s0954579404040179
3. West P, Sweeting J, Young R (2010) Transition matters: pupils' experiences of the primary–secondary school transition in the West of Scotland and consequences for well-being and attainment. Research Papers in Education 25: 21–50. doi: 10.1080/02671520802308677
4. Humphrey N, Ainscow M (2006) Transition Club: Facilitating Learning, Participation and Psychological Adjustment during the Transition to Secondary School. European Journal of Psychology of Education 21: 319–331. doi: 10.1007/bf03173419
5. Hargreaves A (1986) Two cultures of schooling: The case of middle schools. London: Falmer Press.
6. Juvonen J, Vi-Nhuan L, Kaganoff T, Augustine C, Constant L (2004) Focus on the wonder years: Challenges facing the American middle school. Santa Monica: Rand Corporation.
7. Eccles JS, Midgley C, Wigfield A, Buchanan CM, Reuman D, et al. (1993) Development during adolescence: The impact of stage-environment fit on adolescents' experiences in school and in families. American Psychologist 48: 90–101. doi: 10.1037/0003-066x.48.2.90
8. Erikson EH (1968) Identity:Youth and crisis. New York: Norton.
9. Weiss RS (1973) Loneliness: The experience of emotional and social isolation. Cambridge, MA: MIT Press.
10. Larson RW, Verma S (1999) How children and adolescents spend time across the world: Work, play, and developmental opportunities. Psychological Bulletin 125: 701–736. doi: 10.1037//0033-2909.125.6.701
11. Roeser RW, Strobel K, Quihuis G (2002) Studying early adolescents' academic motivation, social-emotional functioning, and engagement in learning: Variable and person-centered approaches. Anxiety, Stress and Coping 15: 345–368. doi: 10.1080/10615800021000056519

12. Lord S, Eccles JS, McCarthy K (1994) Surviving the junior high school transition: Family processes and self-perceptions as protective risk factors. Journal of Early Adolescence 14: 162–199. doi: 10.1177/027243169401400205

13. Wigfield A, Eccles JS (1994) Children's Competence Beliefs, Achievement Values, and General Self-Esteem: Change Across Elementary and Middle School. Journal of Early Adolescence 14: 107–138. doi: 10.1177/027243169401400203

14. Watt HMG (2004) Development of adolescents' self perceptions, values and task perceptions according to gender and domain in 7th through 11th grade Australian students. Child Development 75: 1556–1574. doi: 10.1111/j.1467-8624.2004.00757.x

15. McGee CR, Ward J, Gibbons J, Harlow A (2003) Transition to secondary school: A literature review. A Report to the Ministry of Education. Hamilton, University of Waikato, New Zealand

16. Block J, Robins RW (1993) A longitudinal study of consistency and change in self-esteem from early adolescence to early adulthood. Child Development 64: 909–923. doi: 10.1111/j.1467-8624.1993.tb02951.x

17. Harter S (1999) The construction of self: A developmental perspective. New York: Guilford.

18. Galton M, Morrison I, Pell T (2000) Transfer and transition in English schools: reviewing the evidence. International Journal of Educational Research 33: 341–363. doi: 10.1016/s0883-0355(00)00021-5

19. Marsh HW (1989) Age and sex effects in multiple dimensions of self-concept: Preadolescence to early adulthood. Journal of Educational Psychology 81: 417–430. doi: 10.1037/0022-0663.81.3.417

20. Nottlemann E (1987) Competence and self-esteem during the transition from childhood to adolescence. Developmental Psychology 23: 441–450. doi: 10.1037/0012-1649.23.3.441

21. Simmons R, Blyth D (1987) Moving into adolescence: The impact of pubertal change and school context. Hawthorn, NJ: Aldine de Gruyter.

22. Eccles JS, Midgley C (1989) Stage-environment fit: Developmentally appropriate classrooms for young adolescents. In: Ames R, Ames C, editors. Research on motivation in education. New York: Academic Press. pp. 139–181.

23. Luke A, Elkins J, Weir K, Land R, Carrington V, et al. (2003) Beyond the middle: A report about literacy and numeracy development of target group students in the middle years of schooling, Volume 1. In: Commonwealth Department of Education SaTatUoQ, editor.

24. Wallis J, Barrett PM (1998) Adolescent adjustment and the transition into high school. Journal of Child and Family Studies 7: 43–58. doi: 10.1023/a:1022908029272

25. Barber BK, Olsen JA (2004) Assessing the transitions to middle and high school. Journal of Adolesent Research 19: 3–30. doi: 10.1177/0743558403258113

26. Chung H, Elias M, Schneider K (1998) Patterns of individual adjustment change during middle school transition. The Journal of School Psychology 92: 20–25. doi: 10.1016/s0022-4405(97)00051-4

27. Lohaus A, Elben C, Ball J, Klein-Hessling J (2004) School transition from elementary to secondary school: changes in psychological adjustment. Educational Psychology 24: 161–173. doi: 10.1080/0144341032000160128

28. Hawker DSJ, Boulton MJ (2000) Twenty Years' Research on Peer Victimization and Psychosocial Maladjustment: A Meta-analytic Review of Cross-sectional Studies. Journal of Child Psychology and Psychiatry 41: 441–455. doi: 10.1111/1469-7610.00629

29. Berndt TJ, Mekos D (1995) Adolescents' perceptions of the stressful and desirable aspects the transition to junior high school. Journal of Research on Adolescence 5: 123–142. doi: 10.1207/s15327795jra0501_6

30. Anderman EM (2002) School effects on psychological outcomes during adolescence. Journal of Educational Psychology 94: 795–808. doi: 10.1037/0022-0663.94.4.795

31. Benner AD, Graham S (2009) The transition to high school as a developmental process among multi-ethnic urban youth. Child Development 80: 356–376. doi: 10.1111/j.1467-8624.2009.01265.x

32. Roderick M (2003) What's happening to the boys? Early high school experiences and school outcomes among African American male adolescents in Chicago. Urban Education 38: 538–607. doi: 10.1177/0042085903256221

33. Bahr N, Pendergast D (2007) The millennial adolescent. Canberra: Australian Council for Educational Research.

34. Hughes LA, Banks P, Terras MM (2013) Secondary school transition for children with special educational needs: a literature review. Support for Learning 28: 24–34. doi: 10.1111/1467-9604.12012

35. Forgan JW, Vaughn S (2000) Adolescents With and Without LD Make the Transition to Middle School. Journal of Learning Disabilities 33: 33–43. doi: 10.1177/002221940003300107

36. Evangelous M, Vangelous M, Taggart B, Sylva K, Melhuish E, et al. (2008) Effective Preschool, Primary and Secondary Education 3–14 Project (EPPSE 3–14): What Makes a Successful Transition from Primary to Secondary School ? Nottingham: DCSF Publications.

37. Tur-Kaspa H (2002) The socioemotional adjustment of adolescents with LD in the kibbutz during high school transition periods. Journal of Learning Disabilities 35: 87–96. doi: 10.1177/002221940203500107

38. Organisation for Economic Co-operation and Development [OECD] (2003) School factors related to quality and equity: Results from PISA 2000. Paris: OECD.

39. Gorard S (2006) The true impact of school diversity? In: Hewlett M, Pring R, Tulloch M, editors. Comprehensive education: evolution, achievement and new directions. Northampton: University of Northampton Press.

40. Perry LB (2007) School composition and student outcomes: A review of emerging areas of research 2007; Fremantle, WA. Murdoch University

41. Lamb S (2007) School reform and inequality in urban Australia: A case of residualising the poor. In: Teese R, Lamb S, Duru-Belat M, editors. Education and Inequality Dordrecht: Springer. pp. 1–38.

42. Lamb S, Long M, Baldwin G (2004) Performance of the Australian education and training system. Melbourne: Centre for Post compulsory Education and Lifelong Learning, University of Melbourne.

43. Lamb S, Walstab A, Teese R, Vickers M, Rumberger R (2004) Staying on at school: Improving student retention in Australia. Brisbane: Queensland Department of Education and the Arts.

44. Bonell C, Parry W, Wells H, Jamal F, Fletcher A, et al. (2012) The effects of the school environment on student health: A systematic review of multi-level studies. Health & Place doi: 10.1016/j.healthplace.2012.12.001

45. Edgar D (2001) The patchwork nation: Re-thinking government – re-building community. Pymble, N.S.W.: HarperCollins.

46. Lo Bianco J, Freebody P (1997) Australian literacies: Informing national policies on literacy education. Melbourne: Language Australia.

47. Luke A, Land R, Christie P, Kolatsis A, Noblett G (2002) Standard Australian english and languages for Queensland Aboriginal and Torres Strait Islander students. Brisbane: Indigenous Education Consultative Body.

48. Hanewald R (2013) Transition Between Primary and Secondary School: Why it is Important and How it can be Supported. Australian Journal of Teacher Education 38. doi: 10.14221/ajte.2013v38n1.7

49. Howard S, Johnson B (2004)Transition from primary to secondary school: Possibilities and paradoxes.

50. Kirkpatrick D (1993) Student perceptions of the transition from primary to secondary school. Australian Association for Research in Education Conference. Geelong.

51. Kirkpatrick D (1997) Making the Change. The transition from primary to secondary school. Education Australia 36: 17–19.

52. Marston J (2008) Perceptions of students and parents involved in primary to secondary school tranistion programs. Australian Association for Research in Education. Brisbane: Australian Association for Research in Education.

53. Chadbourne R (2001) Middle schooling for the middle years. What might the jury be considering?. Southbank, Victoria: Australian Education Union.

54. Carrington V, Pendergast D, Bahr N, Kapitzke C, Mayer D, et al. (2002) Education futures: Transforming teacher education (Re-framing teacher education for the middle years). Proceedings of the 2001 National Biennial Conference of the Australian Curriculum Studies Association

55. Vaz S (2010) Factors affecting student adjustment as they transition from primary to secondary school: A longitudinal investigation. Perth: Curtin University.

56. National Health and Medical Research Centre [NHMRC] (2005) Human research ethics handbook: A research law collection.

57. NCSS (1996) PASS 6.0 user's guide. Kaysville, UT: NCSS.

58. Harter S, Whitesell N, Junkin L (1998) Similarities and differences in domain-specific and global self-evaluations of learning disabled, behaviorally disordered, and normally achieving adolescents. American Educational Research Journal 35: 653–680. doi: 10.3102/00028312035004653

59. Zubrick S, Silburn SR, Garton A (1993) Field instrument development for the Western Australian child health study. Perth, WA: Western Australian Research Institute for Child Health.

60. Passmore A (1998) The relationship between leisure and mental health in adolescents. Perth University of Western Australia.

61. Harter S (1982) The perceived competence scale for children. Child Development 53: 87–97. doi: 10.2307/1129640

62. Goodman R (1997) The strengths and difficulties questionnaire: A research note. Journal of Child Psychology and Psychiatry 38: 581–586. doi: 10.1111/j.1469-7610.1997.tb01545.x

63. Mellor D (2005) Normative data for the strengths and difficulties questionnaire in Australia. Australian Psychologist 40: 215–222. doi: 10.1080/00050060500243475

64. Achenbach TM (1991) Manual for the youth self-report and 1991 profile. Burlington, VT: University of Vermont Department of Psychiatry

65. Goodman R, Scott S (1999) Comparing the Strengths and Difficulties Questionnaire and the Child Behaviour Checklist: Is small beautiful? Journal of Abnormal Child Psychology 1.

66. Zubrick S, Williams A, Silburn SR, Vimpani G (2000) Indicators of social and family functioning. Canberra: Commonwealth of Australia.

67. Australian Bureau of Statistics [ABS] (2011) 2033.0.55.001 - Census of Population and Housing: Socio-Economic Indexes for Areas (SEIFA). Canberra: ABS.

68. Meyers LS, Gamst G, Guarino AJ (2006) Applied multivariate research: Design and implication. CA: Sage Publications, Inc.

69. Tabachnick B, Fidell L (2007) Using multivariate statistics. Boston, MA: Pearson Education Inc. and Allyn & Bacon.

70. Tabachnick B, Fidell L (2001) Using multivariate statistics Boston, MA: Allyn and Bacon.

71. Cohen JM (1960) A coefficient of agreement for nominal scales. Educational and Psychological Measurement 20: 37–46. doi: 10.1177/001316446002000104

72. Bahr N (2005) The middle years learner. In: Pendergast D, Bahr N, editors. Teaching middle years: Rethinking curriculum, pedagogy and assessment Crows Nest, NSW: National Middle School Association pp. 49–64.

73. Davis C, Martin G, Kosky R, O'Hanlon A (2000) Early Intervention in the Mental Health of Young People: A Literature Review. Monograph published by The Australian Early Intervention Network for Mental Health in Young People.

74. Snowling M, Muter V, Carroll J (2007) Outcomes in adolescence of children at family-risk of dyslexia. Journal of Child Psychology & Psychiatry 48: 609–618. doi: 10.1111/j.1469-7610.2006.01725.x

75. Zeleke S (2004) Self-concepts of students with learning disabilities and their normally achieving peers: a review. European Journal of Special Needs Education 19: 145–170. doi: 10.1080/08856250410001678469

76. Marsh HW, Hau KT (2004) Big fish, little pond effect. On academic self-concept. Self Concept Research, Driving International Research Agendas. Manly.

77. Howlin P, Moss P (2012) Adults with autism spectrum disorders. The Canadian Journal of Psychiatry 57: 275–283.

78. AVECO (2012) Youth unemployment: The crisis we cannot afford. London: AVECO.

79. Haager D, Vaughn S (1995) Parent, teacher, and self-reports of the social competence of students with learning disabilities. Journal of Learning Disabilities 28: 205–215. doi: 10.1177/002221949502800403

80. Newman L (2004) Family involvement in the educational development of youth with disabilities: A special topic report of findings from the national longitudinal transition study-2 (NLTS-2). Menlo Park, CA: SRI International.

81. Prince M, Patel V, Saxena S, Maj M, Maselko J, et al. (2007) No health without mental health. The Lancet 370: 859–877. doi: 10.1016/s0140-6736(07)61238-0

82. Lucas RE (2007) Long-term disability is associated with lasting changes in subjective well-being: evidence from two nationally representative longitudinal studies. J Person Soc Psychol 92: 717–730. doi: 10.1037/0022-3514.92.4.717

83. Emerson E, Honey A, Llewellyn G, Madden R (2009) The Well-being of Australian Adolescents and Young Adults with Self-reported Long-term Health Conditions, Impairments or Disabilities: 2001 and 2006. Australian Journal of Social Issues 44: 39–54.

84. Gallo LC, Matthews KA (2003) Understanding the association between socioeconomic status and physical health: do negative emotions play a role? Psychol Bull 129: 10–51. doi: 10.1037/0033-2909.129.1.10

85. Sawyer MG, Arney FM, Baghurst PA, Clark JJ, Graetz BW, et al. (2000) The mental health of young people in Australia: Child and adolescent component of the National Survey of Mental Health and Wellbeing. Canberra, Australia: Department of Health and Aged Care, Mental Health and Special Programs Branch.

86. Wight RG, Botticello AL, Aneshensel CS (2006) Socioeconomic context, social support, and adolescent mental health: A multilevel investigation. Journal of Youth and Adolescence 35: 115–126. doi: 10.1007/s10964-005-9009-2

87. Zubrick S, Silburn SR, Gurrin L, Teoh H, Shepherd C, et al. (1997) The Western Australian Child Health Survey: Education, health and competence. Perth, WA: Australian Bureau of Statistics and the Institute for Child Health Research.

88. Zubrick S, Silburn SR, Burton P, Blair EM (2000) Mental health disorders in children and young people: Scope, cause and prevention. Australian and New Zealand Journal of Psychiatry 34: 570–578. doi: 10.1046/j.1440-1614.2000.00703.x

89. Rutter M (1995) Relationships between mental disorders in childhood and adulthood. Acta Psychiatrica Scandinavica 91: 73–85. doi: 10.1111/j.1600-0447.1995.tb09745.x

90. Petticrew M, Chisholm D, Thomson H, Jane-LLlopis E (2005) Generating evidence on determinants, effectiveness and cost effectiveness. In: Herrman I, Saxena H, Moodie R, editors. Promoting Mental Health: Concepts, Emerging Evidence, Practice. Geneva: World Health Organisation.

91. Geller B, Zimerman B, Williams M, Bolhofner K, Craney JL (2001) Bipolar disorder at prospective follow-up of adults who had prepubertal major depressive disorder. American Journal of Psychiatry 158: 125–127. doi: 10.1176/appi.ajp.158.1.125

92. Geller B, Zimerman B, Williams M, Bolhofner K, Craney JL (2001) Adult Psychosocial Outcome of Prepubertal Major Depressive Disorder. Journal of the American Academy of Child and Adolescent Psychiatry 40: 673–677. doi: 10.1097/00004583-200106000-00012

93. Orvaschel H, Lewinsohn PM, Seeley JR (1995) Continuity of Psychopathology in a Community Sample of Adolescents. Journal of the American Academy of Child and Adolescent Psychiatry 34: 1525–1535. doi: 10.1097/00004583-199511000-00020

94. Cicchetti D, Rogosch FA (1999) Psychopathology as Risk for Adolescent Substance Use Disorders: A Developmental Psychopathology Perspective. Journal of Clinical Child Psychology 28: 355–365. doi: 10.1207/s15374424jccp280308

95. Roberts C, Ballantyne F, Van der Klift P (2002) Aussie Optimism: Social life skills program. Teacher resource. Perth, WA: Curtin University of Technology.

96. Cross D, Erceg E (2002) Friendly schools and families. Perth: Edith Cowan University.

97. World Health Organisation [WHO] (1996) Promoting health through schools - The World Health Organisation's global school health initiative. Geneva: World Health Organisation.

98. Becker GS, Thomes N (1986) Human capital and the rise and fall of families. Journal of Labor Economics 4: 1–139. doi: 10.1086/298118

99. Bradley RH, Corwyn RF (2002) Socio-economic status and child development. Annual Review of Psychology 53: 371–399.

100. Hauser RM, Brown BV, Prosser WR (1997) Indicators of children's wellbeing New York Russell Sage Foundation

101. Saab H, Klinger D (2010) School differences in adolescent health and wellbeing: Findings from the Canadian Health Behaviour in School-aged Children Study. Social Science & Medicine 70: 850–858. doi: 10.1016/j.socscimed.2009.11.012

102. Andersson H, Bjørngaard J, Kaspersen S, Wang CA, Skre I, et al. (2010) The effects of individual factors and school environment on mental health and prejudiced attitudes among Norwegian adolescents. Social Psychiatry and Psychiatric Epidemiology 45: 569–577. doi: 10.1007/s00127-009-0099-0

103. Roeger L, Allison S, Martin G, Dadds V, Keeves J (2001) Adolescent depressive symptomatology. Australian Journal of Psychology 53: 134–139. doi: 10.1080/00049530108255135

104. Konu AI, Lintonen TP, Autio VJ (2002) Evaluation of Well-Being in Schools - A Multilevel Analysis of General Subjective Well-Being. School Effectiveness and School Improvement 13: 187–200. doi: 10.1076/sesi.13.2.187.3432

105. Hattie J (1999) Influences on student learning. University of Auckland

106. Hattie J (2003) Teachers make a difference: What is the research evidence? Council for Educational Research Annual Conference on Building Teacher Quality. Melbourne.

107. Rutter M, Maughan B (2002) School Effectiveness Findings 1979–2002. Journal of School Psychology 40: 451–475. doi: 10.1016/s0022-4405(02)00124-3

108. Waters SK, Cross D, Shaw T (2010) Does the nature of schools matter? An exploration of selected school ecology factors on adolescent perceptions of school connectedness. British Journal of Educational Psychology 80: 381–402. doi: 10.1348/000709909x484479

109. Waters SK, Cross D, Shaw T (2010) How important are school and interpersonal student characteristics in determining later adolescent school connectedness, by school sector? Australian Journal of Education 54: 6. doi: 10.1177/000494411005400207

110. Bell M, Dempsey I (2001) Enrolment and placement practices for students with special needs in NSW government schools: A critical analysis of current policy. Special Education Perspectives 10: 3–14.

111. Portney LG, Watkins MP (2000) Foundations of clinical research: Applications to practice. Upper Saddle River, New Jersey: Prentice- Hall.

112. Yeo M, Sawyer S (2005) Chronic illness and disability. British Medical Journal 330: 721–723. doi: 10.1136/bmj.330.7493.721

113. Stone LL, Otten R, Engels RC, Vermulst AA, Janssens JM (2010) Psychometric properties of the parent and teacher versions of the strengths and difficulties questionnaire for 4- to 12-year-olds: a review. Clinical child and family psychology review 13: 254–274. doi: 10.1007/s10567-010-0071-2

114. Kipke RC (2008) Culture in rvaluation #6: Low socio-economic status populations in California. UC Davis: Tobacco Control Evaluation Center.

115. Gutman LM, Sameroff AJ, Cole R (2003) Academic growth curve trajectories from 1st grade to 12th grade: effects of multiple social risk factors and preschool child factors. Dev Psychol 39: 777–790. doi: 10.1037/0012-1649.39.4.777

116. Jimerson S, Egeland B, Sroufe LA, Carlson B (2000) A Prospective Longitudinal Study of High School Dropouts Examining Multiple Predictors Across Development. Journal of School Psychology 38: 525–549. doi: 10.1016/s0022-4405(00)00051-0

117. Council Curriculum (1998) Curriculum framework for kindergarten to year 12 education in Western Australia. Perth. Western Australia.

118. Department of Education and Training [DET] (2004) Pathways to the Future: A Report of the Review of Educational Services for Students with Disabilities in Government Schools. East Perth, W.A.

119. Ryan C, Watson L (2004) The drift to private schools in Australia: Understanding its features (No. Discussion Paper No. 479). Australian National University.

120. Council of Government School Organisations [COGSA] (2005) Middle schooling concepts and approaches: A council of government school organisations' discussion paper. Northern Territory: The Northern Territory Council of Government School Organisations.

121. Department of Education and Training [DET] (2007) The future placement of year 7 students in WA public schools: A study. Perth Government of Western Australia.

122. Australian Bureau of Statistics [ABS] (2001) ABS 2001 Census Dictionary (Cat. No. 2901.0).

CHAPTER 5

MENTAL HEALTH PROBLEMS AND EDUCATIONAL ATTAINMENT IN ADOLESCENCE: 9-YEAR FOLLOW-UP OF THE TRAILS STUDY

KARIN VELDMAN, UTE BÜLTMANN, ROY E. STEWART, JOHAN ORMEL, FRANK C. VERHULST, AND SIJMEN A. REIJNEVELD

5.1 INTRODUCTION

Successful educational attainment (e.g., achievement of at least upper secondary education) is associated with many favorable later-life social economic outcomes, including occupational achievement, financial security, or positive lifestyle behaviors. Mental health problems may negatively affect educational attainment and thus have adverse consequences during the entire life course [1]. The economic costs of childhood mental health problems are enormous. Smith and Smith [2] calculated that childhood mental health problems in the US cause a reduction in family income of about $10,400 per year. Mental health problems cover a broad range of emotional and behavioral problems, like externalizing problems (i.e. aggressive and

Mental Health Problems and Educational Attainment in Adolescence: 9-Year Follow-Up of the TRAILS Study. © *Veldman K, Bültmann U, Stewart RE, Ormel J, Verhulst FC, and Reijneveld SA. PLoS ONE, 9,7 (2014), doi:10.1371/journal.pone.0101751. Licensed under a Creative Commons Attribution 4.0 International License, http://creativecommons.org/licenses/by/4.0/.*

rule-breaking behavior), internalizing problems (i.e. depressive and anxiety problems, withdrawn behavior, and somatic complaints) and attention problems.

Lee and colleagues [3], [4] found that mental disorders were associated with low educational attainment in nine high-income countries and seven middle- and low-income countries. For externalizing problems, consistent negative associations with educational attainment were demonstrated, e.g., negative associations have been found for conduct disorder and oppositional defiant disorder [5]–[8].

For the association of internalizing problems with educational attainment mixed results have been reported. While several studies reported that internalizing problems were not associated with educational attainment [6], [8]–[11], others showed associations with high school dropout, high school graduation failure and failure to enter college [7], [12]–[15]. For attention problems, several studies reported a statistically significant association with low educational attainment [5], [6], [8], [16].

To date, the evidence regarding the effects of mental health problems on educational attainment is inconclusive, probably due to methodological problems. First, although most studies use longitudinal data [5], [8], [11], [13]–[15], changes over time in mental health problems are seldom addressed [12], [16]. Second, measurement error may be relatively large due to reliance on just one informant. Even though it is known that use of multiple informants increases the reliability of the given information [17], [18], to our knowledge none of the aforementioned studies employed more than one informant, i.e. either the adolescent [8], [10] or a parent [9], [12]. Finally, most studies concern the US-setting and studies in the European setting are sparse [3], [4], [11]. When interpreting results from the US, differences between welfare systems have to be considered, i.e. results based on a liberal system cannot directly be translated to a social democratic system.

Thus, the aims of this study were to examine the prospective associations of mental health problems at age 11 and changes over time in mental health problems between age 11 and 16 on educational attainment at age 19. For both aims multiple informants were used, i.e. adolescents and their parents, and analyses were stratified by gender.

5.2 METHODS

5.2.1 ETHICS STATEMENT

The Dutch Central Committee on Research Involving Human Subjects approved all the TRAILS study protocols. All children and their parents provided written informed consent to participate.

5.2.2 STUDY DESIGN AND SAMPLE

TRAILS (TRacking Adolescents' Individual Lives Survey) is a prospective cohort study of Dutch adolescents, aiming to study the etiology and course of psychopathology [19], [20]. The study started in March 2001. Five municipalities in the Northern part of the Netherlands, both urban and rural areas, were asked to provide the name and address of all children born between October 1, 1989 and September 30, 1990 (first 2 municipalities) or October 1, 1990 and September 30, 1991 (last 3 municipalities). Of all children approached for participation (N = 3145), 6.7% were excluded because of mental or physical incapability or language problems. Of the participating group (N = 2934), N = 2230 children and one or both of their parents provided informed consent to participate (76%, mean age 11.09, SD 0.55). At baseline, no differences in psychopathology between responders and non-responders were observed [20]. Of the baseline participants (N = 2230), N = 2149 children participated in the second wave (96.4% of baseline, mean age 13.5, SD 0.53), N = 1816 in the third wave (81.4% of baseline, mean age 16.25, SD 0.69) and N = 1881 in the fourth wave (84.3% of baseline, mean age 19.05, SD 0.58). A more detailed description of the design, sample, procedures and non-response analysis can be found elsewhere [19]–[21]. The present study used data of 1711 (76.8% of baseline) TRAILS participants, from whom educational or occupational status was known at age 19.

5.2.3 MEASURES

Educational attainment was measured at age 19 with two questions on the highest diploma obtained or on the current educational level if still at school. Educational attainment was categorized into: low (primary, lower vocational and lower secondary education), medium (intermediate vocational and intermediate secondary), and high (higher secondary, higher vocational and university) (see figure 1).

5.2.4 THE DUTCH EDUCATIONAL SYSTEM

The Dutch educational system is presented in Figure 1. Children go to primary school from age 4 to 12. Admission to secondary school is based on the teachers' advice in primary school in combination with the outcome of a national test (CITO). Secondary education consists of a differentiated, multi-track system: schools that provide vocational education or job training and preparatory schools for entrance to tertiary education.

Mental health problems were measured using the Youth Self Report (YSR) and the Child Behavior Checklist (CBCL) at age 11 and 16 [22]. The YSR and CBCL contain a list of behavioral and emotional problems, scored as 0 = not true, 1 = somewhat or sometimes true, or 2 = very or often true in the past 6 months. Standardized YSR and CBCL scores were combined into one measure, as multi-informant information provides a better prediction of mental health problems [17], [18]. The subscales aggressive behavior and delinquent behavior together form the scale externalizing problems ($\alpha = 0.85$). Scale scores for externalizing problems range from 0 to 64, with higher scores indicating more externalizing problems. The scale internalizing problems contains the subscales anxious/depressed behavior, somatic complaints and withdrawn/depressed behavior ($\alpha = 0.87$).). Scale scores range from 0 to 62, with higher scores indicating more internalizing problems. The subscale attention problems contains items regarding difficulties with concentrating, paying attention for a long time, daydreaming or getting lost in his/her thoughts. ($\alpha = 0.68$). Scale scores range from 0 to 18, with higher scores indicating more attention problems.

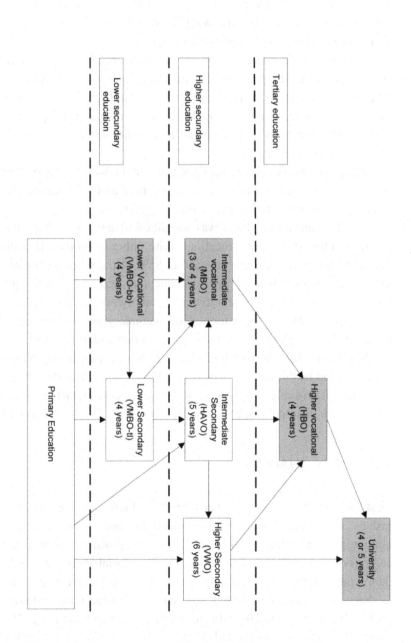

FIGURE 1: The Dutch educational system.

Intelligence was determined at age 11 with the Vocabulary and Block Design subtests of the Revised Wechsler Intelligence Scales for Children (WISC-R) [23] leading to IQ-scores [24], [25].

Academic performance at age 11 was measured by asking the teacher five questions about the effort and achievement of their pupils, like "the pupil has a good work pace" and "the pupil performs beneath his standards". Teachers rated the academic performance on a 5-point Likert scale. Some questions were recoded, and higher scores indicated better academic performance.

Family composition was measured at age 11 with two questions regarding the number of parents in the household and if biological parents were divorced in the period from birth to age 11.

Parental educational level was measured at age 11 with a question about the highest level of education of the father or mother. If both levels were known (which was the case in 85% of the parents), the highest level of education was used. Level of education was categorized into: low (primary, lower vocational and lower secondary education), medium (intermediate vocational and intermediate secondary and higher secondary education) and high (higher vocational education and university).

Physical health was measured at age 11 with the question: "How was your physical health the last two years?" Participants rated their health on a 5-point Likert-scale (1 = very poor, 5 = very good), which was recoded into 1 = poor health (1, 2), 2 = quite healthy (3) and 3 = good health (4, 5).

5.2.5 DATA ANALYSES

First, to test differences between low, medium and high educational groups, chi-quadrat-tests were performed for categorical variables (i.e. gender, parental educational level, family composition, physical health) and one-way ANOVA analyses for continuous variables (i.e. age, IQ, academic performance, externalizing, internalizing and attention problems).

Second, to examine whether externalizing, internalizing and attention problems at age 11 and 16 predicted educational attainment at age 19 multinomial logistic regression analyses were conducted. Multinomial logistic regression instead of ordinal logistic regression was performed because the test of parallel lines showed that the relationship between attention problems and the log-odds was not the same for all log-odds ($X^2 = 5.62$, p-value = 0.02). Crude associations were calculated (model 1), followed by adjustments for age, gender, IQ, parental educational level and physical health (model 2). Model 3 was additionally adjusted for internalizing, externalizing and attention problems. Model 4 was additionally adjusted for academic performance (data not shown).

Third, to examine the relationship between changes over time in mental health problems and educational attainment, difference scores between age 11 and 16 were computed for externalizing, internalizing and attention problems. To test if the difference scores in externalizing, internalizing and attention problems between age 11 and 16 were associated with educational attainment at age 19, multinomial logistic regression analyses were performed. Model 1 was adjusted for baseline mental health problems, model 2 was additionally adjusted for age, gender, IQ, parental educational level and physical health. Model 3 was additionally adjusted for internalizing, externalizing and attention problems, and model 4 was additionally adjusted for academic performance (data of model 4 not shown).

Multiple imputation was performed because complete-case analyses could be conducted on only 1142 adolescents (66.7% of total sample). Data for internalizing, externalizing and attention problems were missing for 6.8% to 24.8% of respondents. Multiple imputation of missing data was performed on item level and thirty times to minimize the risk of bias and the loss of statistical power [26]. It was assumed that data are missing at random (MAR) or missing completely at random (MCAR) [27].

All analyses were conducted for the total sample and for boys and girls separately, using SPSS version 20.

5.3 RESULTS

5.3.1 SAMPLE CHARACTERISTICS

Of the total sample (N = 1711), 107 (6.2%) adolescents had a low level of educational attainment, 1211 (70.7%) a medium level of educational attainment, and 394 (23.0%) had a high level of educational attainment.

Significant differences between educational groups were found for age, parental educational level, family composition, IQ, academic performance, physical health, externalizing problems (self- and parents' report), attention problems (self- and parents' report), difference score externalizing problems (self- and parents' report) and difference score internalizing problems (parents' report). Table 1 shows the sample characteristics per level of educational attainment.

TABLE 1: Descriptive information of the dependent, independent and confounding variables.

Variables	Age	Educational Attainment Low	Medium	High	P-value
Gender (N, %)	11				0.18
Boys		55 (51.4)	650 (53.7)	8.6)	
Girls		52 (48.6)	561 (46.3)	163 (41.4)	
Age (mean, SD)	19	19.2 (0.66)	19.0 (0.58)	19.1 (0.56)	0.01
Parental educational level (N, %)	11				<0.001
Low		47 (44.3)	279 (23.2)	6.4)	
Medium		45 (42.5)	486 (40.4)	17.6)	
High		14 (13.2)	438 (36.4)	392 (76)	
Family Composition (N,%)	11				<0.001
1 parent		37 (34.6)	262 (21.6)	60 (15.2)	
2 parents		70 (65.4)	949 (78.4)	334 (84.8)	
IQ (mean, SD)	11	87.9 (13.8)	96.5 (13.1)	110.8 (12.3)	<0.001
Academic Performance (mean, SD)	11	3.0 (0.8)	3.6 (0.8)	4.4 (0.5)	<0.001
Physical Health (N, %)	11				0.01
Poor		3 (2.8)	18 (1.5)	8 (2.0)	
Medium		11 (10.3)	106 (8.8)	23 (5.8)	
Good		93 (86.9)	1087 (89.8)	363 (92.1)	
Externalizing Problems (mean, SD)	11				
Self-report (YSR)		10.2 (7.6)	8.9 (6.4)	7.8 (5.3)	<0.001
Parents' report (CBCL)		9.5 (6.9)	7.8 (6.4)	5.3 (4.6)	<0.001
Internalizing problems (mean, SD)	11				
Self-report (YSR)		13.0 (8.7)	11.7 (7.5)	11.2 (7.1)	0.09
Parents' report (CBCL)		8.3 (6.6)	7.9 (6.1)	7.3 (5.9)	0.15

TABLE 1: *Cont.*

| Variables | Age | Educational Attainment | | | P-value |
		Low	Medium	High	
Attention problems (mean, SD)	11				
Self-report (YSR)		4.9 (2.8)	4.5 (2.8)	3.9 (2.4)	<0.001
Parents' report (CBCL)		5.8 (3.8)	4.5 (3.3)	2.3 (2.1)	<0.001
Externalizing problems (mean change since 11, SD)	16				
Self-report (YSR)		3.0 (8.9)	1.5 (7.7)	0.3 (6.3)	<0.001
Parents' report (CBCL)		1.3 (7.2)	−1.6 (6.1)	−1.7 (4.4)	<0.001
Internalizing problems (mean change since 11, SD)	16				
Self-report (YSR)		1.1 (10.9)	−1.8 (8.3)	−2.0 (7.8)	0.71
Parents' report (CBCL)		0.3 (6.2)	−1.6 (6.0)	−2.2 (5.9)	0.01
Attention problem (mean change since 11, SD)	16				
Self-report (YSR)		1.2 (3.7)	0.9 (3.3)	0.8 (3.1)	0.52
Parents' report (CBCL)		−0.9 (3.1)	−0.9 (3.1)	−0.5 (2.1)	0.05

Chi-square tests are performed for categorical variables and one-way ANOVA analyses for continuous variables.

5.3.2 MENTAL HEALTH AT AGE 11 AND EDUCATIONAL ATTAINMENT AT AGE 19

For externalizing, internalizing and attention problems a significant association was found (model 1). After adjustment for age, gender, IQ, parental educational level and physical health, the association between internalizing problems and low educational attainment was no longer significant (model 2). Model 3 shows that after adjustment for the other mental health problems, only the association for attention problems at age 11 and low educational attainment remained statistically significant. When adjusted for academic performance, the association of attention problems at age 11 with low educational attainment at age 19 attenuated and was no longer significant (data not shown).

Results were the same for boys and girls (see Table 2).

TABLE 2. Multinomial logistic regression analysis of educational attainment at age 19 and externalizing, internalizing and attention problems at age 11.

	Model 1		Model 2		Model 3	
	OR	95% CI	OR	95% CI	OR	95% CI
Low vs. high educational attainment						
Externalizing problems	2.33***	1.78–3.06	1.70**	1.18–2.46	1.41	0.94–2.11
Internalizing problems	1.36*	1.04–1.77	1.32	0.93–1.88	0.70	0.48–1.02
Attention problems	3.48***	2.60–4.66	1.78**	1.20–2.64	3.19***	2.11–4.83
Middle vs. high educational attainment						
Externalizing problems	1.71***	1.44–2.03	1.56**	1.21–2.01	1.34*	1.03–1.74
Internalizing problems	1.14	0.98–1.32	1.25	1.00–1.56	0.75*	0.60–0.94
Attention problems	2.35***	1.97–2.81	1.53**	1.19–1.96	2.28***	1.77–2.95

*P<0.05, **p<0.01, ***P<0.001. Model 1: Crude model, Model 2: Adjusted for age, gender, IQ, parental educational level, and physical health, Model 3: Adjusted for age, gender, IQ, parental educational level, physical health, internalizing and/or externalizing and/or attention problems.

TABLE 3: Multinomial logistic regression analysis of educational attainment at age 19 and difference scores of externalizing, internalizing and attention problems between age 11 and 16.

	Model 1		Model 2		Model 3	
	OR	95% CI	OR	95% CI	OR	95% CI
Low vs. high educational attainment						
Externalizing problems	3.12***	2.20–4.44	3.34***	2.12–5.28	3.12***	1.83–5.32
Internalizing problems	1.72**	1.20–2.46	1.52	0.92–2.52	0.71	0.42–1.19
Attention problems	2.30***	1.55–3.41	2.34**	1.42–3.86	1.51	0.85–2.68
Middle vs. high educational attainment						
Externalizing problems	1.70***	1.38–2.10	1.92***	1.42–2.58	1.63**	1.18–2.23
Internalizing problems	1.21*	1.00–1.45	1.37*	1.04–1.80	0.74*	0.57–0.96
Attention problems	1.64***	1.34–2.02	1.95***	1.47–2.59	1.66**	1.22–2.24

*P<0.05, **p<0.01, ***P<0.001. Model 1: Crude model, Model 2: Adjusted for age, gender, IQ, parental educational level, and physical health, Model 3: Adjusted for age, gender, IQ, parental educational level, physical health, internalizing and/or externalizing and/or attention problems.

5.3.3 CHANGES IN MENTAL HEALTH PROBLEMS BETWEEN AGE 11 AND 16 AND EDUCATIONAL ATTAINMENT AT AGE 19

Table 3 shows that for increasing externalizing, internalizing and attention problems a significant association was found for the total sample, crude and adjusted for age, gender, IQ, parental educational level and physical health (model 1 and 2). When stratified by gender, the association between increasing internalizing problems and low educational attainment was statistically significant for girls only (OR 2.21, 1.25–3.94).

After adjustment for the other mental health problems, no differences between boys and girls were found for the association between increasing externalizing, internalizing and attention problems and low educational attainment. For the total sample, only the association for increasing externalizing problems between age 11 and 16 and low educational attainment remained statistically significant (model 3).

5.4 DISCUSSION

The study examined the prospective associations of mental health problems and changes of mental health problems measured at age 11 and 16 with educational attainment of adolescents at age 19. We found that externalizing and attention problems at age 11 predicted low educational attainment at age 19. Moreover, increasing externalizing and internalizing (only for girls) between age 11 and 16 predicted low educational attainment at age 19.

Our finding of the prospective associations of externalizing and attention problems with low educational attainment is in line with previous US-based studies [5], [6], [8]. This indicates that externalizing and attention problems negatively affect school attainment, not only in a liberal welfare system, but also in a social-democratic welfare system as the Netherlands. It is possible that the underlying mechanism is similar for both contexts. One of the most likely mechanisms is social selection, i.e. that mental health problems cause low socioeconomic status. With the current data we were not able to address the social causation hypothesis, i.e. that low socioeconomic status cause mental health problems, but with future data of the TRAILS study it will be possible. Our finding of negative associations of externalizing and attention problems with low educational attainment might be due to the influence of externalizing and attention problems on other persons, such as teachers. Children and adolescents showing externalizing and attention problems are at greater risk to get involved with delinquent peers, to be dismissed from class and to receive negative feedback and therefore might have an increased risk of lower educational attainment [28].

After adjustment for internalizing and attention problems, the association between externalizing problems at age 11 and low educational attainment at age 19 was no longer significant. This might be explained by the fact that children with attention problems are at risk of having externalizing problems [29]. When looking at changes over time, McLeod and Fettes analyzed trajectories of externalizing and internalizing problems with educational attainment [12]. The findings of McLeod and Fettes regarding externalizing problems were similar with ours, i.e. increasing externalizing problems were significantly associated with low educational attainment.

For internalizing problems at age 11, the association with low educational attainment at age 19 attenuated and was no longer significant after adjustment for externalizing and attention problems. Prior research showed mixed findings, an explanation might be that the earlier reported associations were due to co-occurrence of internalizing problems with externalizing and attention problems. This is supported by the observation that studies which adjusted for psychiatric comorbidity, did not find significant associations [5], [6], [11], whereas studies which did not adjust for comorbidity found significant associations [7], [12]. In contrast, we found a significant associations of increasing internalizing problems between age 11 and 16 and low educational attainment at age 19. Girls with increasing internalizing problems have to be viewed as a high-risk group for low educational attainment, which needs specific attention. It can be speculated that girls enter a downward spiral, in which internalizing problems cause more problems at school, which in turn may lead to more internalizing problems.

The association between attention problems and low educational attainment was no longer significant after adjustment of academic performance. Probably both attention problems and academic performance are associated with educational attainment. Furthermore, attention problems and academic performance are related as well, i.e. children with attention problems are more likely to show poor academic performance. In the present study, the outcome was measured with a behavioral questionnaire. The scale attention problems contains mainly questions about attention problems and only a few questions about hyperactivity. Therefore, it was not possible to derive the diagnosis ADHD from this scale. However, several studies showed that childhood attention problems rather than hyperactivity predict educational attainment [16], [30], [31].

This study has several strengths and limitations. Data was used from a large, longitudinal representative population sample with 9-year follow up. With using repeated measurements we were able to examine mental health problems and their course over time from a life-course perspective. Another strength was the high retention rate at the different measurement waves, ranging from 81.4% to 96.4%. Moreover, we obtained information on adolescents' mental health problems from multiple informants, limiting the likelihood of information bias [17], [18]. We acknowledge that differences between the self- and parent-report of mental health problems disappeared, while these differences could have been informative as well. The level of mental health problems is based on self-report and parent-report and not on a diagnostic interview, the gold standard. However, in this study we were not only interested in the negative effects of severe mental health problems, but in the effects of mild mental health problems as well. In addition, reliable and valid measures were used to assess mental health problems (i.e. YSR and CBCL) [22].

Limitations concern results which are based on an imputed data set with the assumption that data was missing at random. If this assumption is not correct (e.g., that adolescents did not participate due to their mental health problems), it might have biased the results. We compared the imputed data with complete cases, but no differences were observed. Another point of attention is the calculation of difference scores of mental health problems between age 16 and 11. Therefore we were not able to examine if stable high mental health problems would have a negative effect on educational attainment. It would have been interesting to look at these problems as well, but due to the low number of adolescents with stable high mental health problems this was not possible [32].

Our study clearly showed that pre-adolescents' mental health problems and changes over time in mental health problems, are strongly associated with low educational attainment. This emphasizes the need for early detection, e.g., via well-child assessments and school monitoring [33]. Especially children whose mental health problems increase over time deserve attention, as they seem to be at greater risk of low educational attainment.

Early detection is of no use without early interventions, e.g., a better training of teachers and other school personnel to offer those children and their parents appropriate help, i.e. help that is tailored to meet the needs of children in their specific context. Behavioral problems and healthy behaviors are not separate entities, but are strongly related [34]. Therefore, interventions should focus on clusters of deviant behavior of children and adolescents at risk and require an integrated approach to improve the chances of these adolescents towards a successful entry of the labor market.

REFERENCES

1. Ettner SL, Frank RG, Kessler RC (1997) The impact of psychiatric disorders on labor market outcomes. Ind Labor Relat Rev 51: 64–81. doi: 10.2307/2525035
2. Smith JP, Smith GC (2010) Long-term economic costs of psychological problems during childhood. Soc Sci Med 71: 110–115. doi: 10.1016/j.socscimed.2010.02.046
3. Lee S, Tsang A, Breslau J, Aguilar-Gaxiola S, Angermeyer M, et al. (2009) Mental disorders and termination of education in high-income and low- and middle-income countries: Epidemiological study. Br J Psychiatry 194: 411–417. doi: 10.1192/bjp. bp.108.054841
4. Lee S, Tsang A, Breslau J, Aguilar-Gaxiola S, Angermeyer M, et al. (2011) Mental disorders and termination of education education in high-income and low- and middle-income coutnries: Epidemiological study: Correction. Br J Psychiatry 198: 327. doi: 10.1192/bjp.bp.108.054841
5. Breslau J, Lane M, Sampson N, Kessler RC (2008) Mental disorders and subsequent educational attainment in a US national sample. J Psychiatr Res 42: 708–716. doi: 10.1016/j.jpsychires.2008.01.016
6. Breslau J, Miller E, Joanie Chung W-J, Schweitzer JB (2011) Childhood and adolescent onset psychiatric disorders, substance use, and failure to graduate high school on time. J Psychiatr Res 45: 295–301. doi: 10.1016/j.jpsychires.2010.06.014
7. Kessler RC, Foster CL, Saunders WB, Stang PE (1995) Social consequences of psychiatric disorders, I: Educational attainment. Am J Psychiatry 152: 1026–1032.

8. Miech RA, Caspi A, Moffitt TE, Wright BRE, Silva PA (1999) Low Socioeconomic Status and Mental Disorders: A Longitudinal Study during Young Adulthood. Am J Sociol 104: 1096–1131. doi: 10.1086/210137

9. Duchesne S, Vitaro F, Larose S, Tremblay RE (2007) Trajectories of Anxiety During Elementary-school Years and the Prediction of High School Noncompletion. J Youth Adolesc 37: 1134–1146. doi: 10.1007/s10964-007-9224-0

10. Woodward LJ, Fergusson DM (2001) Life course outcomes of young people with anxiety disorders in adolescence. J Am Acad Child Adolesc Psychiatry 40: 1086–1093. doi: 10.1097/00004583-200109000-00018

11. Jonsson U, Bohman H, Hjern A, von Knorring L, Olsson G, et al. (2010) Subsequent higher education after adolescent depression: a 15-year follow-up register study. Eur Psychiatry 25: 396–401. doi: 10.1016/j.eurpsy.2010.01.016

12. McLeod JD, Fettes DL (2007) Trajectories of Failure: The Educational Careers of Children with Mental Health Problems. Am J Sociol 113: 653–701. doi: 10.1086/521849

13. Needham BL (2009) Adolescent Depressive Symptomatology and Young Adult Educational Attainment: An Examination of Gender Differences. J Adolesc Heal 45: 179–186. doi: 10.1016/j.jadohealth.2008.12.015

14. Fletcher JM (2008) Adolescent depression: diagnosis, treatment, and educational attainment. Health Econ 17: 1215–1235. doi: 10.1002/hec.1319

15. Fletcher JM (2010) Adolescent depression and educational attainment: results using sibling fixed effects. Health Econ 19: 855–871. doi: 10.1002/hec.1526

16. Pingault J-B, Tremblay RE, Vitaro F, Carbonneau R, Genolini C, et al. (2011) Childhood Trajectories of Inattention and Hyperactivity and Prediction of Educational Attainment in Early Adulthood: A 16-Year Longitudinal Population-Based Study. Am J Psychiatry 168: 1164–1170. doi: 10.1176/appi.ajp.2011.10121732

17. Achenbach TM, McConaughy SH, Howell CT (1987) Child/adolescent behavioral and emotional problems: implications of cross-informant correlations for situational specificity. Psychol Bull 101: 213–232. doi: 10.1037/0033-2909.101.2.213

18. Verhulst FC, van der Ende J (1992) Agreement between parents' reports and adolescents' self-reports of problem behavior. J Child Psychol Psychiatry 33: 1011–1023. doi: 10.1111/j.1469-7610.1992.tb00922.x

19. Huisman M, Oldehinkel AJ, de Winter A, Minderaa RB, de Bildt A, et al. (2008) Cohort profile: the Dutch "TRacking Adolescents' Individual Lives' Survey'; TRAILS. Int J Epidemiol 37: 1227–1235. doi: 10.1093/ije/dym273

20. De Winter AF, Oldehinkel AJ, Veenstra R, Brunnekreef JA, Verhulst FC, et al. (2005) Evaluation of non-response bias in mental health determinants and outcomes in a large sample of pre-adolescents. Eur J Epidemiol 20: 173–181. doi: 10.1007/s10654-004-4948-6

21. Ormel J, Oldehinkel AJ, Sijtsema J, van Oort F, Raven D, et al. (2012) The TRacking Adolescents' Individual Lives Survey (TRAILS): design, current status, and selected findings. J Am Acad Child Adolesc Psychiatry 51: 1020–1036. doi: 10.1016/j.jaac.2012.08.004

22. Achenbach T, Rescorla L (2001) Manual for the ASEBA School-Age Forms & Profiles. Burlington VT: University of Vermont, Research Center for Children, Youth, & Families.

23. Wechsler D (1974) Wechsler Intelligence Scale for Children - Revised. New York: Psychological Corporation.

24. Sattler J (1992) Assessment of Children. San Diego: Author.

25. Silverstein AB (1967) Validity of WISC short forms at three age levels. J Consult Psychol 31: 635–636. doi: 10.1037/h0025110

26. White IR, Royston P, Wood AM (2011) Multiple imputation using chained equations: Issues and guidance for practice. Stat Med 30: 377–399. doi: 10.1002/sim.4067

27. Graham JW (2009) Missing data analysis: making it work in the real world. Annu Rev Psychol 60: 549–576. doi: 10.1146/annurev.psych.58.110405.085530

28. Henry KL, Huizinga DH (2007) School-related risk and protective factors associated with truancy among urban youth placed at risk. J Prim Prev 28: 505–519. doi: 10.1007/s10935-007-0115-7

29. Monuteaux MC, Biederman J, Doyle AE, Mick E, Faraone S V (2009) Genetic risk for conduct disorder symptom subtypes in an ADHD sample: specificity to aggressive symptoms. J Am Acad Child Adolesc Psychiatry 48: 757–764. doi: 10.1097/chi.0b013e3181a5661b

30. Massetti GM, Lahey BB, Pelham WE, Loney J, Ehrhardt A, et al. (2008) Academic achievement over 8 years among children who met modified criteria for attention-deficit/hyperactivity disorder at 4–6 years of age. J Abnorm Child Psychol 36: 399–410. doi: 10.1007/s10802-007-9186-4

31. Lee SS, Hinshaw SP (2010) Predictors of Adolescent Functioning in Girls With Attention Deficit Hyperactivity Disorder (ADHD): The Role of Childhood ADHD, Conduct Problems, and Peer Status. J Clin Child Adolesc Psychol: 37–41.

32. Jaspers M, de Winter AF, Veenstra R, Ormel J, Verhulst FC, et al. (2012) Preventive child health care findings on early childhood predict peer-group social status in early adolescence. J Adolesc Health 51: 637–642. doi: 10.1016/j.jadohealth.2012.03.017

33. Jaspers M, de Winter AF, de Meer G, Stewart RE, Verhulst FC, et al. (2010) Early findings of preventive child healthcare professionals predict psychosocial problems in preadolescence: the TRAILS study. J Pediatr 157: 316–321. doi: 10.1016/j.jpeds.2010.02.015

34. Van Nieuwenhuijzen M, Junger M, Velderman MK, Wiefferink KH, Paulussen TWGM, et al. (2009) Clustering of health-compromising behavior and delinquency in adolescents and adults in the Dutch population. Prev Med (Baltim) 48: 572–578. doi: 10.1016/j.ypmed.2009.04.008

SCHOOL MENTAL HEALTH SERVICES: SIGNPOST FOR OUT-OF-SCHOOL SERVICE UTILIZATION IN ADOLESCENTS WITH MENTAL DISORDERS? A NATIONALLY REPRESENTATIVE UNITED STATES COHORT

MARION TEGETHOFF, ESTHER STALUJANIS, ANGELO BELARDI, AND GUNTHER MEINLSCHMIDT

6.1 INTRODUCTION

Mental disorders place a great challenge on the health care system. They are highly prevalent not only in adults [1] but also in adolescents and children [2], [3], [4], [5], [6], [7], with enormous implications for health-related quality of life [8] and health economy [9]. The urgent need to integrate mental health into all aspects of health research and health-care delivery has been realized by major health institutions and scientific journals, as documented for example in The Lancet series on Global Mental Health

School Mental Health Services: Signpost for Out-of-School Service Utilization in Adolescents with Mental Disorders? A Nationally Representative United States Cohort. © Tegethoff M, Stalujanis E, Belardi A, and Meinlschmidt G. PLoS ONE, *9*,6 (20134), doi:10.1371/journal.pone.0099675. Licensed under Creative Commons Attribution 4.0 International License, http://creativecommons.org/licenses/by/4.0/.

and strategic research goals and health action plans by the Grand Challenges in Global Mental Health initiative and the American Academy of Pediatrics [10], [11], [12].

Many children and adolescents with mental disorders do not receive adequate care [13], [14], even though effective treatment approaches for mental disorders exist [15]. The median interval between the first onset of a mental disorder and first contact with the treatment sector is nearly a decade [16], although early intervention offers the hope to prevent long-term mental health problems and increase wellbeing and productivity [17].

The school sector has been reported to be a major contact point for children and adolescents with emotional or behavioral problems [13], [18], [19], [20], and the further development of school-based mental health promotion programs for children and adolescents ranks among the top ten challenges identified by the Grand Challenges in Global Mental Health initiative [10]. Results of the International School Psychology Survey reveal that the number of students per school psychologist is alarmingly high, counting from 470 students per school psychologist in Italy to more than 26000 students per school psychologist in parts of Germany [21]. Besides this low ratio of school psychologists to students, the function of school psychologists is rather complex and involves a wide range of tasks among which only one is intervention supply [22], suggesting that sound and comprehensive treatment of children and adolescents with mental disorders remains hardly feasible in the school setting to date. Instead, the school sector has unrivaled access to children and adolescents and, with this unique feature, is exceptionally situated to link children and adolescents with mental disorders to out-of-school services addressing mental health problems and to high-quality care at early disorder stages. However, the role of the school sector as a guide to such out-of-school services remains poorly understood [18], [23]. To improve our understanding of common trajectories of service use in children and adolescents, it has been claimed that it is important to clarify the sequence of health care sector utilization and to move beyond studying single sectors to the study of the potentially more relevant patterns of sector use [13], [24].

The main objective of this study was to estimate in a nationally representative United States cohort, focusing on adolescents with a lifetime mental disorder, the role of school mental health services as guide to care in out-of-school service sectors for the treatment of mental disorders.

6.2 MATERIALS AND METHODS

6.2.1 STUDY SAMPLE

This study was conducted using data from the National Comorbidity Survey Replication Adolescent Supplement (NCS-A). The NCS-A, a nationally representative face-to-face survey of 10148 United States adolescents (ages 13–18 years) that was carried out in a dual-frame design between February 2001 and January 2004 [25], [26], [27], has previously been described in detail [25], [26], [28]. Further information on the NCS-A is available at http://www.icpsr.umich.edu/icpsrweb/ICPSR/studies/28581/version/2. Our analyses are based on a subsample of 6483 out of 10123 adolescents who were in school at the time of survey and for whom interviews as well as parent questionnaires (long versions) were available.

6.2.2 ETHICS STATEMENT

Adolescents and parents provided written informed consent, and the Human Subjects Committees of both Harvard Medical School and the University of Michigan approved the NCS-A.

6.2.3 ASSESSMENT OF MENTAL DISORDERS

To examine lifetime mental disorders in adolescents, trained interviewers used the WHO Composite International Diagnostic Interview (CIDI) Version 3.0, a structured clinical interview assessing major classes of Diagnostic and Statistical Manual of Mental Disorders (DSM)-IV disorders, including affective disorders (i.e. major depressive disorder, dysthymia, bipolar disorder I, bipolar disorder II), anxiety disorders (i.e. agoraphobia, generalized anxiety disorder, social phobia, specific phobia, panic disorder, post-traumatic stress disorder, separation anxiety disorder), behavior disorders (i.e. attention deficit hyperactivity disorder, oppositional defiant disorder, conduct disorder), substance use disorders (i.e. alcohol abuse/dependence, drug abuse/dependence), and eating disorders (i.e. anorexia nervosa, bulimia nervosa, binge eating disorder). The applied version of the CIDI was computer-assisted and has been adjusted for adolescents, with ensured interview quality and concordance with a clinical reappraisal subsample [25], [27], [28], [29]. In addition to the CIDI interview in the adolescents, parents or parent deputy were inquired to respond to a self-administered questionnaire (SAQ) assessing whether their offspring was suffering from attention-deficit/hyperactivity disorder, conduct disorder, oppositional defiant disorder, major depressive disorder, and dysthymic disorder, as for these disorders parental reports have been shown to be of additional diagnostic value [30], [31], [32]. Information from adolescents and parents was integrated whenever it was available from both, and we defined mental disorder as present if DSM-IV criteria were fulfilled either based on adolescent or parent report. Age of onset was specified as the age at which a certain mental disorder developed for the first time. If more than one mental disorder was present within a mental disorder class, age of onset of the first mental disorder in this class was taken as age of onset of this class. Accordingly, if analyses were performed in the subsample of children and adolescents with "any mental disorder", age of onset of the very first mental disorder was used as age of onset.

6.2.4 ASSESSMENT OF SERVICE USE

Adolescents and parents provided information on child/adolescent mental health service use across multiple sectors, based on the Service Assessment for Children and Adolescents [33]. Levels of agreement between parent and adolescent reports were acceptable [13], [33]. Respondents were asked whether the adolescents ever in their lifetime had gone to see any professionals or facilities for problems with their emotions, behavior, or use of alcohol and drugs, including in- and outpatient care. According to a previous study, service use was classified into the following categories [13]: i) school services, including individual or group psychological counseling/therapy, and ii) out-of-school services, including a) the mental health specialty sector, including community mental health centers or outpatient mental health clinics, mental health professionals, partial hospitalization or day treatment programs, drug or alcohol treatment units/clinics, hospitals and residential treatment centers, b) the medical specialty sector, including emergency rooms, pediatricians or family doctors, and c) other services, including telephone hotlines, self help groups, counselors or family preservation workers, probation or juvenile justice corrections officers or court counselors, spiritual advisors, respite care providers, any other kind of healer, group homes, foster homes, detention centers, prisons/jails, or emergency shelters. Moreover, respondents were asked how old they had been when they first used the reported type of service.

6.2.5 STATISTICAL ANALYSES

All statistical analyses are based on post-stratification weighted data, which allowed for the correction of minor discrepancies in distributions of school and/or sociodemographic characteristics between the sample and the population [25]. We performed the descriptive analyses of service utilization in different sectors and of the sample's sociodemograhic characteristics by calculating frequencies and percentages of these discrete variables. We computed separate discrete-time proportional hazard models with a non-parametric baseline hazard function, using complementary log-log regression to estimate temporal relationships between school and out-of-school service use for mental disorders, with school service use (versus no school service use) defined as time-varying predictor and mental health specialty service use, medical specialty service use, other service use, and any out-of-school service use defined as outcomes [34]. Analyses were performed in the subsamples of children and adolescents with any i) affective disorder, ii) anxiety disorder, iii) behavior disorder, iv) substance use disorder, v) eating disorder, and vi) mental disorder. We present hazard ratios (HR) and their 95% confidence intervals (CI). To account for the complex structure of the survey data, we used the Taylor series linearization method.

TABLE 1: Information on mental health service utilization in different sectors and on sociodemographic characteristics of the study sample (N = 3656*).

Service utilization			
Service sector		n	Weighted %
School mental health service sector		842	25.24
Any out-of-school service sector		1908	55.87
Mental health specialty sector		1129	32.70
Medical specialty sector		350	10.01
Other out-of-school service sector		552	16.73
Sociodemographic characteristics			
Sociodemographic factor	Category	n	Weighted %
Sex	Female	1907	49.58
	Male	1749	50.42
Age	13–14 y	1364	34.28
	15–16 y	1428	41.36
	17–18 y	864	24.36
Race	Hispanic	475	15.52
	Black	667	15.95
	Other	227	5.10
	White	2287	63.44
Parental education (highest level of either parent)	Less than high school	470	14.10
	High school	1092	29.42
	Some college	826	23.22
	College grad	1268	33.27
Poverty index ratio	≤1.5	560	15.82
	≤3	711	20.26
	≤6	1209	32.47
	>6	1176	31.46
Region	Northeast	674	16.93
	Midwest	1187	23.93
	South	1152	34.28
	West	643	24.86
Urbanicity	Metro	1506	46.45
	Other urban	1306	39.31
	Rural	844	14.24

TABLE 1: *Cont.*

Service utilization			
Service sector		n	Weighted %
Number of biological parents living with the adolescent	0	381	11.03
	1	1517	42.21
	2	1758	46.77
Birth order	Oldest	1235	36.71
	Youngest	1047	26.54
	Others	1374	36.75
Number of siblings	0	161	4.10
	1	939	25.80
	2	963	27.92
	3 or more	1593	42.19

*Abbreviations: y, years. *Subsample of the National Comorbidity Survey-Adolescent Supplement (NCS-A) including all participants providing self- and parent-reported information on mental disorders, with at least one mental disorder.*

We re-evaluated the results after adjusting p values of the 24 main tests for multiple comparisons using the Holm formula [35], [36], [37], thereby accounting for the number of tests.

To validate our results, we conducted the following secondary analyses: To control for potential confounding, we repeated the analyses after adjusting for several sociodemographic factors, as sociodemographic factors have previously been shown to influence mental health service utilization in children and adolescents [13], [38], [39], [40]. We used those sociodemographic factors that have been included in previous epidemiological studies of child and adolescent mental health as predictors of mental disorder prevalence [7], and simultaneously included them in the analyses, with the categories indicated in Table 1.

Moreover, we repeated the analyses three times, controlling for either i) number of categories in which a mental disorder was present (1/2/> = 3), ii) age of onset of the type of mental disorder characterizing the subsample in which the analysis was performed (affective disorders:

1–10 years/11–12 years/13–14 years/15–18 years; anxiety disorders: 1–4 years/5–6 years/7–10 years/11–18 years; behavior disorders: 1–4 years/5–7 years/8–12 years/13–18 years; substance use disorders: 1–13 years/14 years/15 years/16–18 years; eating disorders: 1–12 years/13 years/14 years/15–18 years; any mental disorder: 1–4 years/5–6 years/7–11 years/12–18 years; limits between the categories were defined by cutoffs as close as possible to the quartiles of the respective age distributions), or iii) presence of further types of mental disorders not characterizing the subsample in which the analysis was performed (yes/no).

We interpreted with caution all results that were statistically significant in the main analyses but not stable after Holm correction or secondary analyses.

There were a low percentage of subjects with missing information on service use and we dealt with missing data by restricting each analysis to subjects with complete data (see Table 2). We evaluated the results using two-sided tests of significance set at a level of 0.05. Statistical analyses were performed using STATA/MP 13 (Stata Corporation, College Station, Texas).

6.3 RESULTS

6.3.1 STUDY COHORT DESCRIPTIVES

Out of 6483 adolescents, 3656 adolescents (56.4%) were diagnosed with a lifetime mental disorder. Information on utilization of service sectors addressing mental health problems and on sociodemographic characteristics of the study cohort including these mentally disordered adolescents are presented in Table 1.

6.3.2 PREDICTION OF OUT-OF-SCHOOL MENTAL HEALTH SERVICE UTILIZATION BY SCHOOL MENTAL HEALTH SERVICE USE

Table 2 presents results of the discrete-time proportional hazard analyses of the associations between school and subsequent out-of-school service utilization for mental problems in children and adolescents with lifetime mental disorders. School service use predicted subsequent service utilization in the medical specialty sector in children and adolescents with affective disorders, anxiety disorders, behavior disorders, substance use disorders, and eating disorders, and any mental disorder, subsequent service utilization in other service sectors in children and adolescents with anxiety disorders, behavior disorders, and substance use disorders, and any mental disorder, subsequent service utilization in the mental health specialty sector in children and adolescents with any mental disorder, and subsequent service utilization in any out-of-school service sector in children and adolescents with anxiety disorders and any mental disorder.

After adjusting for multiple testing, all but the predictions for subsequent service utilization in the mental health specialty sector and in any out-of-school service sector in children and adolescents with any mental disorder remained statistically significant.

6.3.3 SECONDARY ANALYSES

When we repeated the analyses after adjusting for either sociodemographic factors, number of categories in which a mental disorder was present, age of onset of the type of mental disorder characterizing the subsample in which the analysis was performed, or further types of mental disorders not characterizing the subsample in which the analysis was performed, levels of significance were mostly comparable to those presented in Table 2. However, the temporal prediction of mental health specialty service use by antecedent school service use was no longer significant in the subsample of children and adolescents with any mental disorder in the secondary analyses adjusting for sociodemographic factors (HR = 1.36, 95% CI = 0.85–2.19, p = 0.20), and number of disorder categories (HR = 1.50, 95% CI = 0.94–2.39, p = 0.08), and the temporal prediction of any out-of-school service use by antecedent school service use was no longer significant in the subsample of children and adolescents with any mental disorder in the secondary analyses adjusting for sociodemographic factors (HR = 1.48, 95% CI = 0.99–2.22, p = 0.06). Instead, the temporal prediction of other service use by antecedent school service use reached marginal significance in the subsample of children and adolescents with any affective disorder in the secondary analyses adjusting for number of disorder categories (HR = 1.81, 95% CI = 1.04–3.13, p = 0.04) and further types of mental disorder (HR = 1.79, 95% CI = 1.05–3.04, p = 0.03). Detailed results of the secondary analyses are available on request.

6.4 DISCUSSION

This study, conducted with 6483 adolescents of a nationally representative United States cohort, provides as yet missing association estimates of school and subsequent out-of-school service utilization for mental problems in children and adolescents with a lifetime mental disorder. Results indicate that school services may serve as guide to certain out-of-school service sectors addressing mental disorders, especially the medical specialty sector, but not the mental health specialty sector.

Our results complement previous descriptive evidence regarding service use patterns in adolescents with mental disorders [13], [18], [23] by elucidating the role of the school service sector in the trajectory of child and adolescent service utilization for mental disorders, and suggest that the school sector plays a central role as guide to the medical specialty sector.

The roles of the medical and the mental health specialty sectors in mental health care have been addressed previously. Several studies have confirmed the prominent position of the medical specialty sector in providing services for mental disorders [41], even though the mental health specialty sector has been reported to be the major service sector for children and adolescents with mental disorders [13] and the most common subsequent service sector in adolescents entering the service system through the school mental health sector [18]. While mental health care in the medical specialty sector has improved over the past decade through a better understanding of mental disorders, the availability of practicable screening tools, provision of psychotherapy in these settings, and further development and promotion of psychotropic medications that are mostly prescribed by primary care physicians [24], [42], [43], [44], most primary care pediatricians and child and adolescent psychiatrists believe that pediatricians should identify and refer, but not treat, their patients' mental health problems [45]. Indeed, the appropriateness of treatment of mental disorders in the medical specialty sector as compared to the mental specialty sector remains a matter of debate [46], [47], [48], [49], [50], which should be kept in mind when evaluating the referral patterns observed in the present study.

There is considerable evidence that sociodemographic characteristics of children and adolescents with mental disorders influence whether or not services for mental disorders are utilized; such sociodemographic characteristics include, amongst others, ethnicity, family income, different patient, parental and familial factors, health insurance coverage, and service availability [13], [38], [39], [40], [51], [52], [53]. Much less is known about what influences, in those making use of mental health care, the sequence of sector utilization on their pathway through the service system; for example what influences whether children/adolescents with mental disorders are seeking care in the medical sector or the mental health sector. Therefore, it has been claimed that it is important to clarify the role of potential factors, including referral patterns by professionals, service availability, child and family preferences, professional competencies, and financial considerations, in order to better understand what determines the service paths of children and adolescents seeking help for mental disorders [13].

Our study has several strengths, including the large nationally representative sample [25], a fully structured diagnostic interview covering a wide range of adolescent mental disorders, with good quality criteria [25], [29], and the integration of adolescent and parent information on adolescent mental disorders, as previously suggested [32]. Given the good response rate and the small amount of missing data, it is unlikely that loss of subjects has introduced relevant selection bias.

The study also has several limitations to be considered, including amongst others the cross-sectional design of the study, as previously discussed [28], [54].

Moreover, first, service utilization has been assessed by self-report, but the validity and reliability of such data has been challenged, especially in terms of non-response and recall bias, which is no issue in large health care utilization databases [55], [56]. However, the NCS-A has not been linked with health care utilization databases, but instead provides self-reported information on service utilization for mental disorders based on a well-established instrument [13], [33]. In adults, concordance between self-reported health care and mental health care utilization and registration data has been shown to be fair [57], [58], [59], and the rather low magnitude of bias in estimates of health care utilization due to non-response in health surveys has previously encouraged the continued use of interview health surveys [60]. A study on the reliability of children's and adolescents' responses on the Child and Adolescent Services Assessment, the groundwork of the Service Assessment for Children and Adolescents [33], revealed that reports of lifetime service use were as reliable as were reports of service use in the preceding three months, even though it should be acknowledged that respondents reported inpatient, other overnight and juvenile justice services more reliably than outpatient and school services [61]. It should also be noted that relying on health care utilization databases faces other limitations, including the exclusion of services provided outside the health care system [56], and the advantages of checklists over routine data sources have been previously documented [62].

Second, even though we controlled for several potential confounders, we cannot exclude confounding by unconsidered factors, including disorder severity. However, we did not reveal a relationship between school mental health service use and subsequent utilization of the mental health specialty sector, and controlling for number of disorder categories did not change the results remarkably, both of which suggests that disorder severity did not confound the presented results in a relevant manner.

Third, the observed associations do not inform about causal but about temporal relationships, and even though the study of causality is wanted, it remains challenging in such a large representative cohort. Until such studies are available, the elucidation of the position of the school sector in the trajectory of service use for mental disorders allows for a better understanding of common service paths of children and adolescents, as has previously been claimed [13].

Fourth, the aim of our analyses was to estimate whether school mental health service use serves as a guide to the use of any out-of-school service sectors; however, we did not compare school service use with use of a specific out-of-school service sector regarding their prediction of service use in further sectors. Therefore, it may be interesting to scrutinize in future studies whether the here observed referral patterns are specific for school mental health services.

TABLE 2: Discrete-time proportional hazard models for school mental health service utilization (time-varying) predicting out-of-school service use in different sectors.

	Mental health specialty sector			Medical specialty sector			Other out-of-school service sector			Any out-of-school service sector		
	HR	(95% CI)	p-value	HR	(95% CI)	p-value	HR	(95% CI)	p-value	HR	(95% CI)	p-value
Any affective disorder	1.17	(0.84–1.63)	0.353	3.01	(1.77–5.12)	<0.001	1.67	(0.95–2.91)	0.071	1.16	(0.86–1.57)	0.335
Any anxiety disorder	1.55	(0.85–2.84)	0.147	3.87	(1.97–7.64)	<0.001	3.15	(2.17–4.56)	<0.001	1.99	(1.41–2.82)	<0.001
Any behavior disorder	1.29	(0.85–1.95)	0.230	2.49	(1.62–3.82)	<0.001	1.99	(1.29–3.06)	0.003	1.50	(0.92–2.45)	0.103
Any substance use disorder	1.16	(0.70–1.91)	0.553	4.12	(1.87–9.04)	<0.001	2.48	(1.57–3.94)	<0.001	1.47	(0.92–2.34)	0.102
Any eating disorder	0.19	(0.02–1.79)	0.144	10.72	(2.31–49.70)	0.003	0.85	(0.15–4.95)	0.857	0.48	(0.13–1.83)	0.276
Any mental disorder	1.76	(1.11–2.77)	0.017	2.97	(1.94–4.54)	<0.001	2.33	(1.54–3.53)	<0.001	1.71	(1.17–2.49)	0.007

Abbreviations: CI, confidence interval; HR, hazard ratio.

Note: All analyses are based on samples for which information on mental disorders was available from both self and parent report (N = 6483). Due to missing information on service utilization, sizes of the completer samples are as follows: Mental health specialty secotr: n = 6358. Medical specialty sector: n = 6326. Other out-of-school service sector: n = 6322. Any out-of-school service secotr: n = 6307). To calculate the hazard ratios, periods without any event were dropped.

The clinical and public health relevance of the role of the school sector in the trajectory of service use for mental disorders in children and adolescents becomes evident against the background of the urgent need to reduce unmet mental disorder treatment demands and improve access to mental health care [13], [16], together with the limited ability of school mental health services to provide comprehensive treatment on-site on the one hand and their unique position in accessing children and adolescents with mental disorders and linking them to out-of-school services on the other hand [21], [63]. It has previously been criticized that the coordination of the different health care sectors is often insufficient, thus representing a barrier for the patients and impairing the supply with appropriate treatments [64]. By raising the awareness of unidirectional referral patterns of school mental health services, our results may pave the way to improve the school mental health service system and multilateral collaborations between sectors where required, which is in line with current strategic research goals and task forces [10], [63]. Notably, our findings raise the question as to whether the school mental health sector sufficiently takes advantage of its unique position in linking mentally disordered students with the out-of-school service system beyond the medical specialty sector.

The supply of mental health services in places where children and adolescents are easily accessible is only one among several action steps that have been proposed to increase access to mental health care for children and adolescents with mental disorders. Further suggestions include the improvement of access to information on available mental health care options, inclusion of children and adolescents in treatment planning, and offering assistance in finding one's way through the rather complicated service system [65]. The bottom line is that, to be most effective in increasing access to child mental health care, strategies should target not only at structural barriers to care, such as inadequate insurance coverage, but also at barriers related to the understanding of mental health problems and services; for example, public education campaigns may help to increase the awareness and knowledge of mental disorders and mental health care services [66], [67].

Whether the here presented role of school mental health services as a guide to out-of-school services for mental disorders in the United States is generalizable to other countries remains to be elucidated, as not only the school mental health system but also insurance and health care systems, including access to mental health care systems, vary considerably worldwide [64], [68]. Future studies should focus on the role of school mental health services in the trajectory of mental health service use in other countries. Moreover, future research should include prospective data and the integration of self-report of service utilization and service utilization databases. It will also be important to evaluate the appropriateness of the mental health service use trajectory emanating from the school mental health sector and to learn about modifiable factors influencing referral patterns of school mental health services, in order to be able to take action and guide or optimize such referral patterns, if necessary.

To the best of our knowledge, this is the first comprehensive study of the role of the school mental health sector as a guide to mental health care in out-of-school sectors, using data of mentally disordered adolescents of a nationally representative United States cohort. Results indicate that school mental health services may serve as a guide to certain out-of-school service sectors for children and adolescents with various mental disorders, especially the medical specialty sector, but not the mental health specialty sector. While highlighting the relevance of school mental health services in the trajectory of mental care, our findings also suggest to further investigate into a stronger collaboration between school mental health services and mental health specialty services in order to improve and guarantee adequate mental care at early life stages.

REFERENCES

1. Wittchen HU, Jacobi F, Rehm J, Gustavsson A, Svensson M, et al. (2011) The size and burden of mental disorders and other disorders of the brain in Europe 2010. European neuropsychopharmacology: the journal of the European College of Neuropsychopharmacology 21: 655–679. doi: 10.1016/j.euroneuro.2011.07.018

2. Essau CA, Conradt J, Petermann F (2000) Frequency, comorbidity, and psychosocial impairment of depressive disorders in adolescents. Journal of adolescent research 15: 470–481. doi: 10.1177/0743558400154003

3. Essau CA, Conradt J, Petermann F (2000) Frequency, comorbidity, and psychosocial impairment of anxiety disorders in German adolescents. Journal of anxiety disorders 14: 263–279. doi: 10.1016/s0887-6185(99)00039-0

4. Brauner CB, Stephens CB (2006) Estimating the prevalence of early childhood serious emotional/behavioral disorders: challenges and recommendations. Public Health Rep 121: 303–310.

5. Costello EJ, Egger H, Angold A (2005) 10-year research update review: the epidemiology of child and adolescent psychiatric disorders: I. Methods and public health burden. J Am Acad Child Adolesc Psychiatry 44: 972–986. doi: 10.1097/01. chi.0000172552.41596.6f

6. Roberts RE, Attkisson CC, Rosenblatt A (1998) Prevalence of psychopathology among children and adolescents. Am J Psychiatry 155: 715–725.

7. Kessler RC, Avenevoli S, Costello EJ, Georgiades K, Green JG, et al. (2012) Prevalence, persistence, and sociodemographic correlates of DSM-IV disorders in the National Comorbidity Survey Replication Adolescent Supplement. Arch Gen Psychiatry 69: 372–380. doi: 10.1001/archgenpsychiatry.2011.160

8. Sawyer MG, Whaites L, Rey JM, Hazell PL, Graetz BW, et al. (2002) Health-related quality of life of children and adolescents with mental disorders. Journal of the American Academy of Child and Adolescent Psychiatry 41: 530–537. doi: 10.1097/00004583-200205000-00010

9. Guevara JP, Mandell DS, Rostain AL, Zhao H, Hadley TR (2003) National estimates of health services expenditures for children with behavioral disorders: an analysis of the medical expenditure panel survey. Pediatrics 112: e440. doi: 10.1542/peds.112.6.e440

10. Collins PY, Patel V, Joestl SS, March D, Insel TR, et al. (2011) Grand challenges in global mental health. Nature 475: 27–30. doi: 10.1038/475027a

11. Prince M, Patel V, Saxena S, Maj M, Maselko J, et al. (2007) No health without mental health. Lancet 370: 859–877. doi: 10.1016/s0140-6736(07)61238-0

12. Foy JM (2010) Enhancing pediatric mental health care: report from the American Academy of Pediatrics Task Force on Mental Health. Introduction. Pediatrics 125 Suppl 3S69–74. doi: 10.1542/peds.2010-0788c

13. Merikangas KR, He JP, Burstein M, Swendsen J, Avenevoli S, et al. (2011) Service utilization for lifetime mental disorders in U.S. adolescents: results of the National Comorbidity Survey-Adolescent Supplement (NCS-A). Journal of the American Academy of Child and Adolescent Psychiatry 50: 32–45. doi: 10.1016/j. jaac.2010.10.006

14. Offord DR, Boyle MH, Szatmari P, Rae-Grant NI, Links PS, et al. (1987) Ontario Child Health Study. II. Six-month prevalence of disorder and rates of service utilization. Archives of general psychiatry 44: 832–836. doi: 10.1001/archpsyc.1987.01800210084013

15. Weisz JR, Jensen-Doss A, Hawley KM (2006) Evidence-based youth psychotherapies versus usual clinical care: a meta-analysis of direct comparisons. The American psychologist 61: 671–689. doi: 10.1037/0003-066x.61.7.671

16. Wang PS, Berglund P, Olfson M, Pincus HA, Wells KB, et al. (2005) Failure and delay in initial treatment contact after first onset of mental disorders in the National Comorbidity Survey Replication. Archives of general psychiatry 62: 603–613. doi: 10.1001/archpsyc.62.6.603

17. Kieling C, Baker-Henningham H, Belfer M, Conti G, Ertem I, et al. (2011) Child and adolescent mental health worldwide: evidence for action. Lancet 378: 1515–1525. doi: 10.1016/s0140-6736(11)60827-1

18. Farmer EM, Burns BJ, Phillips SD, Angold A, Costello EJ (2003) Pathways into and through mental health services for children and adolescents. Psychiatric services 54: 60–66. doi: 10.1176/appi.ps.54.1.60

19. Burns BJ, Costello EJ, Angold A, Tweed D, Stangl D, et al. (1995) Children's mental health service use across service sectors. Health affairs 14: 147–159. doi: 10.1377/hlthaff.14.3.147

20. Farmer EM, Stangl DK, Burns BJ, Costello EJ, Angold A (1999) Use, persistence, and intensity: patterns of care for children's mental health across one year. Community mental health journal 35: 31–46. doi: 10.1023/a:1018743908617

21. Jimerson SR, Graydon K, Curtis MJ, Staskal R, Oakland TD, et al. (2007) The International School Psychology Survey: Insights From School Psychologists Around the World. The Handbook of International School Psychology. Thousand Oaks, CA, USA: Sage Publications, Inc.

22. Watkins MW, Crosby EG, Pearsson JL (2001) Role of the School Psychologist. School Psychology International 22: 64–73. doi: 10.1177/01430343010221005

23. Wood PA, Yeh M, Pan D, Lambros KM, McCabe KM, et al. (2005) Exploring the relationship between race/ethnicity, age of first school-based services utilization, and age of first specialty mental health care for at-risk youth. Mental health services research 7: 185–196. doi: 10.1007/s11020-005-5787-0

24. Wang PS, Demler O, Olfson M, Pincus HA, Wells KB, et al. (2006) Changing profiles of service sectors used for mental health care in the United States. The American journal of psychiatry 163: 1187–1198. doi: 10.1176/appi.ajp.163.7.1187

25. Kessler RC, Avenevoli S, Costello EJ, Green JG, Gruber MJ, et al. (2009) National comorbidity survey replication adolescent supplement (NCS-A): II. Overview and design. J Am Acad Child Adolesc Psychiatry 48: 380–385. doi: 10.1097/chi.0b013e3181999705

26. Kessler RC, Avenevoli S, Costello EJ, Green JG, Gruber MJ, et al. (2009) Design and field procedures in the US National Comorbidity Survey Replication Adolescent Supplement (NCS-A). Int J Methods Psychiatr Res 18: 69–83. doi: 10.1002/mpr.279

27. Kessler RC, Merikangas KR (2004) The National Comorbidity Survey Replication (NCS-R): background and aims. Int J Methods Psychiatr Res 13: 60–68. doi: 10.1002/mpr.166

28. Merikangas K, Avenevoli S, Costello J, Koretz D, Kessler RC (2009) National comorbidity survey replication adolescent supplement (NCS-A): I. Background and measures. J Am Acad Child Adolesc Psychiatry 48: 367–369. doi: 10.1097/chi.0b013e31819996f1

29. Kessler RC, Avenevoli S, Green J, Gruber MJ, Guyer M, et al. (2009) National comorbidity survey replication adolescent supplement (NCS-A): III. Concordance of DSM-IV/CIDI diagnoses with clinical reassessments. J Am Acad Child Adolesc Psychiatry 48: 386–399. doi: 10.1097/chi.0b013e31819a1cbc

30. Cantwell DP, Lewinsohn PM, Rohde P, Seeley JR (1997) Correspondence between adolescent report and parent report of psychiatric diagnostic data. Journal

of the American Academy of Child and Adolescent Psychiatry 36: 610–619. doi: 10.1097/00004583-199705000-00011

31.   De Los Reyes A, Kazdin AE (2005) Informant discrepancies in the assessment of childhood psychopathology: a critical review, theoretical framework, and recommendations for further study. Psychological bulletin 131: 483–509. doi: 10.1037/0033-2909.131.4.483

32.   Grills AE, Ollendick TH (2002) Issues in parent-child agreement: the case of structured diagnostic interviews. Clin Child Fam Psychol Rev 5: 57–83.

33.   Stiffman AR, Horwitz SM, Hoagwood K, Compton W 3rd, Cottler L, et al. (2000) The Service Assessment for Children and Adolescents (SACA): adult and child reports. Journal of the American Academy of Child and Adolescent Psychiatry 39: 1032–1039. doi: 10.1097/00004583-200008000-00019

34.   Willett JB, Singer JD (2004) Discrete-time survival analysis. In: Kaplan D, editor. The SAGE Handbook of Quantitative Methodology for the Social Sciences. Thousand Oaks, London, New Delhi: Sage Publications, Inc.

35.   Aickin M, Gensler H (1996) Adjusting for multiple testing when reporting research results: the Bonferroni vs Holm methods. American journal of public health 86: 726–728. doi: 10.2105/ajph.86.5.726

36.   Holm S (1979) A Simple Sequentially Rejective Multiple Test Procedure. Scandinavian journal of statistics 6: 65–70.

37.   Newson RB (2010) Frequentist q-values for multiple-test procedures. The Stata Journal 10: 568–584.

38.   Zahner GE, Daskalakis C (1997) Factors associated with mental health, general health, and school-based service use for child psychopathology. American journal of public health 87: 1440–1448. doi: 10.2105/ajph.87.9.1440

39.   Cunningham PJ, Freiman MP (1996) Determinants of ambulatory mental health services use for school-age children and adolescents. Health services research 31: 409–427.

40.   Costello EJ, Janiszewski S (1990) Who gets treated? Factors associated with referral in children with psychiatric disorders. Acta psychiatrica Scandinavica 81: 523–529. doi: 10.1111/j.1600-0447.1990.tb05492.x

41.   Marino S, Gallo JJ, Ford D, Anthony JC (1995) Filters on the pathway to mental health care, I. Incident mental disorders. Psychological medicine 25: 1135–1148. doi: 10.1017/s0033291700033110

42.   Zito JM, Safer DJ, dosReis S, Gardner JF, Boles M, et al. (2000) Trends in the prescribing of psychotropic medications to preschoolers. JAMA: the journal of the American Medical Association 283: 1025–1030. doi: 10.1001/jama.283.8.1025

43.   Olfson M, Marcus SC, Druss B, Pincus HA (2002) National trends in the use of outpatient psychotherapy. The American journal of psychiatry 159: 1914–1920. doi: 10.1176/appi.ajp.159.11.1914

44.   Spitzer RL, Kroenke K, Williams JB (1999) Validation and utility of a self-report version of PRIME-MD: the PHQ primary care study. Primary Care Evaluation of Mental Disorders. Patient Health Questionnaire. JAMA: the journal of the American Medical Association 282: 1737–1744. doi: 10.1001/jama.282.18.1737

45.   Heneghan A, Garner AS, Storfer-Isser A, Kortepeter K, Stein RE, et al. (2008) Pediatricians' role in providing mental health care for children and adolescents: do

pediatricians and child and adolescent psychiatrists agree? Journal of developmental and behavioral pediatrics: JDBP 29: 262–269. doi: 10.1097/dbp.0b013e31817dbd97

46. Wang PS, Lane M, Olfson M, Pincus HA, Wells KB, et al. (2005) Twelve-month use of mental health services in the United States: results from the National Comorbidity Survey Replication. Archives of general psychiatry 62: 629–640. doi: 10.1001/archpsyc.62.6.629

47. Wells KB, Kataoka SH, Asarnow JR (2001) Affective disorders in children and adolescents: addressing unmet need in primary care settings. Biological psychiatry 49: 1111–1120. doi: 10.1016/s0006-3223(01)01113-1

48. Wang PS, Berglund P, Kessler RC (2000) Recent care of common mental disorders in the United States: prevalence and conformance with evidence-based recommendations. Journal of general internal medicine 15: 284–292. doi: 10.1046/j.1525-1497.2000.9908044.x

49. Wang PS, Demler O, Kessler RC (2002) Adequacy of treatment for serious mental illness in the United States. American journal of public health 92: 92–98. doi: 10.2105/ajph.92.1.92

50. Young AS, Klap R, Sherbourne CD, Wells KB (2001) The quality of care for depressive and anxiety disorders in the United States. Archives of general psychiatry 58: 55–61. doi: 10.1001/archpsyc.58.1.55

51. Burns BJ, Costello EJ, Erkanli A, tweed D, Farmer EMZ, et al. (1997) Insurance coverage and mental health service use by adolescents with serious emotional disturbances. Journal of Child and Family Studies 6: 89–111.

52. Verhulst FC, van der Ende J (1997) Factors associated with child mental health service use in the community. Journal of the American Academy of Child and Adolescent Psychiatry 36: 901–909. doi: 10.1097/00004583-199707000-00011

53. Saxena S, Thornicroft G, Knapp M, Whiteford H (2007) Resources for mental health: scarcity, inequity, and inefficiency. Lancet 370: 878–889. doi: 10.1016/s0140-6736(07)61239-2

54. Kessler RC, Avenevoli S, McLaughlin KA, Green JG, Lakoma MD, et al. (2012) Lifetime co-morbidity of DSM-IV disorders in the US National Comorbidity Survey Replication Adolescent Supplement (NCS-A). Psychological medicine 42: 1997–2010. doi: 10.1017/s0033291712000025

55. Bhandari A, Wagner T (2006) Self-reported utilization of health care services: improving measurement and accuracy. Medical care research and review: MCRR 63: 217–235. doi: 10.1177/1077558705285298

56. Schneeweiss S, Avorn J (2005) A review of uses of health care utilization databases for epidemiologic research on therapeutics. Journal of clinical epidemiology 58: 323–337. doi: 10.1016/j.jclinepi.2004.10.012

57. Reijneveld SA, Stronks K (2001) The validity of self-reported use of health care across socioeconomic strata: a comparison of survey and registration data. International journal of epidemiology 30: 1407–1414. doi: 10.1093/ije/30.6.1407

58. Reijneveld SA (2000) The cross-cultural validity of self-reported use of health care: a comparison of survey and registration data. Journal of clinical epidemiology 53: 267–272. doi: 10.1016/s0895-4356(99)00138-9

59. Killeen TK, Brady KT, Gold PB, Tyson C, Simpson KN (2004) Comparison of self-report versus agency records of service utilization in a community sample of indi-

viduals with alcohol use disorders. Drug and alcohol dependence 73: 141–147. doi: 10.1016/j.drugalcdep.2003.09.006

60. Gundgaard J, Ekholm O, Hansen EH, Rasmussen NK (2008) The effect of non-response on estimates of health care utilisation: linking health surveys and registers. European journal of public health 18: 189–194. doi: 10.1093/eurpub/ckm103

61. Farmer EMZ, Angold A, Burn BJ, Costello EJ (1994) Reliability of Self-Reported Service Use: Test-Retest Consistency of Children's Responses to the Child and Adolescent Services Assessment (CASA). Journal of Child and Family Studies 3: 307–325. doi: 10.1007/bf02234688

62. Knight M, Stewart-Brown S, Fletcher L (2001) Estimating health needs: the impact of a checklist of conditions and quality of life measurement on health information derived from community surveys. J Public Health Med 23: 179–186. doi: 10.1093/pubmed/23.3.179

63. Hogan MF (2003) New Freedom Commission Report: The President's New Freedom Commission: Recommendations to Transform Mental Health Care in America. Psychiatric Services 54.

64. Remschmidt H, Belfer M (2005) Mental health care for children and adolescents worldwide: a review. World psychiatry: official journal of the World Psychiatric Association 4: 147–153.

65. Report of the Surgeon Generals Conference on Children's Mental Health: A National Action Agenda. American Journal of Health Education 32: 179–182. doi: 10.1080/19325037.2001.10603461

66. Jorm AF (2000) Mental health literacy. Public knowledge and beliefs about mental disorders. The British journal of psychiatry: the journal of mental science 177: 396–401. doi: 10.1192/bjp.177.5.396

67. Owens PL, Hoagwood K, Horwitz SM, Leaf PJ, Poduska JM, et al. (2002) Barriers to children's mental health services. Journal of the American Academy of Child and Adolescent Psychiatry 41: 731–738. doi: 10.1097/00004583-200206000-00013

68. Jacob KS, Sharan P, Mirza I, Garrido-Cumbrera M, Seedat S, et al. (2007) Mental health systems in countries: where are we now? Lancet 370: 1061–1077. doi: 10.1016/s0140-6736(07)61241-0

CHAPTER 7

A TWO-YEAR PERSPECTIVE: WHO MAY EASE THE BURDEN OF GIRLS' LONELINESS IN SCHOOL?

AUDHILD LØHRE, MARIANNE N. KVANDE, ODIN HJEMDAL, AND MONICA LILLEFJELL

7.1 BACKGROUND

Loneliness is a threat to students' wellbeing and health. Perceived loneliness at school has shown negative associations with both emotional and somatic symptoms, especially among girls [1]. Furthermore, loneliness in girls has demonstrated longitudinal associations with lower levels of perceived school wellbeing [2]. Thus, research on loneliness indicates an urgent need to search for factors that may reduce the burden of girls' loneliness. Other adversities related to loneliness are victimisation, caused by bullying, and the perception of having academic problems. It has been shown that students with low levels of academic achievement or learning disabilities are lonelier, have poorer social adjustment and more emotional problems than students with average or high levels of academic achievement [3-6].

The subjective experience of being victimised by bullying has often been measured by the frequency of verbal and/or physical harassment

A Two-Year Perspective: Who May Ease the Burden of Girls' Loneliness in School? © Løhre A, Kvande MN, Hjemdal O, and Lillefjell M. Child and Adolescent Psychiatry and Mental Health, *8,10 (2014), doi:10.1186/1753-2000-8-10. Licensed under Creative Commons Attribution 2.0 Generic License, http://creativecommons.org/licenses/by/2.0/.*

and also by the frequency of social exclusion [7]. Definitions of bullying usually include imbalance of power; aggressive behaviour; and repetitive negative acts [8,9]. The prevalence of victimisation has been shown to vary considerably between countries, even when the same measurements have been applied [10,11]. There seems, however, to be a consensus that victimisation is related both to mental health problems [12]; poor psychosocial adjustment [13-15]; and to a higher risk of psychosomatic problems [16,17]. The association between victimisation and ill health has been found to be fairly similar between countries [18]. Further, a dose–response relation between victimisation and ill health has been reported, in that an increased frequency of victimisation was related to higher levels of ill health symptoms [10,19,20].

Loneliness is less studied than victimisation and has received far less public attention during the last decades. As summarised by Peplau and Perlman [21], definitions on loneliness typically comprise an unpleasant or distressing subjective experience of deficiencies in a person's social relationships. The distinction between loneliness and aloneness is crucial [22]; aloneness may give time for reflection and rest, whereas loneliness is a negative and hurtful feeling [23,24]. In line with the findings in research on victimisation, it has been shown that loneliness is related to mental health and adjustment problems [25]. There is strong evidence that loneliness is related to anxiety [26-28] and depression [29-31], but few studies have reported associations between loneliness and somatic symptoms [1]. Loneliness among children and adolescents has been studied mainly in the school setting, and few researchers have tested initiatives to buffer feelings of loneliness [32-34]. Furthermore, as far as we are aware, no studies have reported on relational trust as a potential to reduce harmful effects of loneliness in school.

Resilience is a research approach that focuses on factors and processes buffering the effects of adversity and stressful life events. Consistently across studies, growing up with at least one trusted person has been identified as a very important protective factor. This could be a parent or another person, such as a teacher, coach, or neighbour [35-37]. It has also been found consistently throughout the resilience research that growing up with an early established and secure attachment to the caregiver is important for the development of a capacity to trust, and for the stimulation of emotional regulation and mentalising capacities (e.g. self-reflection) [35,38]. Having one adult who can be trusted, such as a parent, neighbour, trainer or a teacher may be an especially important protective factor in buffering adversity.

7.1.1 AIMS OF THE STUDY

The first aim was to investigate the association of perceived loneliness with female students' self-reported school wellbeing two years later in a model adjusting for perceived academic problems and victimisation caused by bullying. The second aim addressed the relationship between loneliness and later school wellbeing and assessed the influence of having a range of people whom the girls trusted sufficiently to contact if hurtful or difficult situations arose.

7.2 METHODS

7.2.1 PARTICIPANTS AND PROCEDURE

In this study, 119 girls from five convenience sampled public schools in Mid-Norway provided information two years apart; May-June 2002 (T1) and May-June 2004 (T2). At T1 the girls were in grades 1–8 (age 7–14) and at T2 in grades 3–10 (age 9–16). The total population of girls and boys at baseline and the transmission of students to other schools in the project period are described in detail elsewhere [2]. The rate of participation at the two-year follow-up was 99%.

Data were collected by using the School Wellbeing Questionnaire (SWQ) [39]. School nurses and headmasters administered the data collection. The younger students were interviewed by trained school nurses who used the questionnaire as a guide, whereas the older students completed the questionnaires themselves under the instruction of a trained teacher or the school nurse during a lesson allocated to this task. More information about the instrument and methods are available in other publications [1,39].

7.2.2 MEASURES

The SWQ contained items on three potential areas of adversity: perceived academic problems; victimisation (being bullied); and loneliness. Furthermore, the students' comments on having someone to turn to in difficult situations were included in the SWQ in addition to measures of the outcome of perceived school wellbeing.

7.2.2.1 SCHOOL WELLBEING AT T1 AND T2

One global question: "How do you like it at school?" with four response options; very bad (1), not so good, good, and very good (4).

7.2.2.2 ACADEMIC PROBLEMS AT T1

Four questions each linked to a certain subject: "Do you have problems with: "reading"; "writing"; "mathematics"; or "foreign language (English)?" Each had four response options: no problems (1), some problems, quite a few problems, and lots of problems (4). In the analysis, we used the question(s) with the highest response score of the four questions (the maximum score, i.e. one score only).

7.2.2.3 VICTIMISATION AT T1

Three questions each prefaced by: "During recess, are you bothered in some way that makes you feel bad?" and the following then were specified: being "teased"; being "hit, kicked or pushed"; and being "left out, excluded". Each of the three questions had five response options; never

(1), seldom, sometimes, about every week, and about every day (5). The maximum score of the three questions was used in the analysis.

7.2.2.4 LONELINESS AT T1

One question: "Do you ever feel lonely at school?" with five response options; never (1), seldom, sometimes, about every week, and about every day (5).

7.2.2.5 TRUSTED OTHERS AT T1 AND T2

Five questions each linked to identified groups of people: "Who can you talk to if something hurtful or difficult happens to you: class advisor"; "other teachers"; "other students"; "your parents"; "other adults"? Each question had four response options; no-never (1), maybe, probably, and certainly (4).

7.2.3 STATISTICS

The distribution of the population of 119 girls was described by the dispersion, median, and interquartile range (IQR) of the outcome (school wellbeing T2) and the independent variables. Correlations between trusted others at T1 and T2 were assessed by Spearman's rho. For use in logistic regression analyses, the outcome was dichotomised into the categories of bad (very bad/not so good) and good (good/very good) school wellbeing. Associations between the potential adversities and the dichotomised outcomes were tested in a multivariable analysis, adjusting for grades and earlier school wellbeing. Next, 10 multivariable adjusted models were constructed by including each of the five groups of trusted people separately; firstly, using the scores at T1 and secondly, using the scores at both T1 and T2. The multivariable models were also calculated with adjustments made for schools. All tests were two-sided, and p-values <0.05 were considered significant. The statistical analyses were performed in SPSS for Windows (version 20.0 SPSS, Chicago, Illinois).

7.2.4 ETHICS AND PROCEDURES

The surveys were approved by the statutory School Collaborative Committees, and the collection of data was approved by The Norwegian Data Inspectorate. Information letters signed by the headmaster and by the principal investigator (AL) were sent to all parents, describing the aims of the surveys, and emphasising that participation was voluntary, and that the collected information was confidential. In addition, parents were informed about the surveys in school meetings and, in each class, teachers informed in greater details. Students/parents who did not want to participate were asked to notify their main teacher or headmaster; however, no parent or student refused to take part.

7.3 RESULTS

Self-reported school wellbeing levels were high with more than 90% reporting good or very good (Table 1). Fewer than 10% reported quite a few or lots of academic problems; about 6% reported weekly or daily victimisation; and just over 3% experienced loneliness weekly or daily. Parents were the most trusted group of people with approximately 80% of the girls at T1 and 89% at T2 saying they would probably or certainly turn to them in difficult situations. Class advisors formed the second most trusted group of people at T1 and the third most trusted at T2, competing the group comprising other students. The greatest increase in trust was seen in the group consisting of other students: the percentage of girls reporting that they trusted other students increased from 58% at T1 to 74% at T2.

Correlations were calculated to assess any changes, between T1 and T2, in the degree of trust felt for specified groups of trusted others (Table 2). For class advisor, students, and parents, the correlations between T1 and T2 were statistically significant, but below rho 0.40. Other teachers and other adults showed non-significant correlations between the two points in time.

TABLE 1: Distribution of response options for the outcome and the independent variables

Variables	Response options					Total	Median	IQR[#]
	1	2	3	4	5			
	%	%	%	%	%			
School wellbeing T2[a]	3.4	3.4	42.4	50.8		118	4	3–4
School wellbeing T1[a]	0	6.8	47.0	46.2		117	3	3–4
Academic problems T1[b]	34.5	56.3	7.6	1.7		119	2	1–2
Victimisations T1[c]	50.4	24.4	19.3	3.4	2.5	119	1	1–3
Loneliness T1[c]	52.1	24.4	20.2	1.7	1.7	119	1	1–2
Class advisor T1[a]	16.0	17.9	16.0	50.0		106	3.5	2–4
Other teachers T1[a]	21.1	22.1	18.9	37.9		95	3	2–4
Students T1[a]	15.1	26.4	13.2	45.3		106	3	2–4
Parents T1[a]	3.6	16.2	8.1	72.1		111	4	3–4
Other adults T1[a]	26.7	36.0	17.4	19.8		86	2	1–3
Class advisor T2[a]	11.1	21.4	13.7	53.8		117	4	2–4
Other teachers T2[a]	17.5	28.1	21.9	32.5		114	3	2–4
Students T2[a]	0.9	25.0	21.6	52.6		116	4	2–4
Parents T2[a]	3.4	7.6	10.2	78.8		118	4	4–4
Other adults T2[a]	25.9	33.3	18.5	22.2		108	2	1–3

[#]*25-75th percentile.* [a]*From 1 (worst) to 4 (best).* [b]*From 1 (best) to 4 (worst).* [c]*From 1 (best) to 5 (worst).*

Note: Loneliness at T1 was the variable of special interest with School wellbeing at T2 as the outcome. Adjustments included School wellbeing, Academic problems, and Victimisation; all at T1. People, whom the girls trusted to contact at T1, were assessed to see if any of those groups of persons modified the association of loneliness with later school wellbeing. Corresponding groups of persons at T2 were included as adjustment.

TABLE 2: Spearman's rho correlations: trusted others

	Class advisor T2	Other teachers T2	Students T2	Parents T2	Other adults T2
Class advisor T1	0.39**	0.21*	0.01	0.08	-0.02
Other teachers T1	0.37**	0.19	0.05	0.29**	0.16
Students T1	0.17	0.08	0.37**	-0.03	0.14
Parents T1	0.22*	0.27**	0.07	0.25**	0.27**
Other adults T1	0.38**	0.19	0.12	0.16	0.13

*$p < 0.05$. **$p < 0.01$. Note: Correlations between T1 and T2 for the same groups of trusted others are marked with bold numbers.*

TABLE 3: Associations of potential adversities (T1) with school wellbeing (T2)[a]

Adverse factors	Odds ratio (95% CI)	p-value
Academic problems	0.89 (0.24 to 3.32)	0. 862
Victimisation	1.91 (0.68 to 5.40)	0. 223
Loneliness	0.35 (0.13 to 0.92)*	0. 033

[a]*adjusted for grades and school wellbeing (T1) in a multivariable logistic regression analysis. *Note: The longitudinal association of loneliness with later school wellbeing was strongly negative, with p-value < 0.05.*

Associations between the potential adversities at T1 and school wellbeing at T2 were explored by mean of a multivariable regression analysis, adjusted for grades and school wellbeing at T1 (Table 3). For lonely girls, the odds of reporting high levels of school wellbeing two years later were reduced by 65% compared to other girls (odds ratio, 0.35, 95% CI 0.13 to 0.92). Loneliness was the only variable demonstrating a strong and negative independent contribution.

Next, the influence was explored of each of the trusted others upon the relationship between loneliness at T1 and school wellbeing at T2. In Table 4, each of the five groups of trusted others was added separately (a-e) in the multivariable analyses, adjusted for grades and school wellbeing at T1. The question to be answered was whether any of the trusted others modified the negative association of loneliness with later school wellbeing. In Model 1a-e, the scores of trusted others at T1 were included, one by one. Further, to assess a possible influence of trusted others at T2, the scores of trusted others at T1 and T2 were included simultaneously in Model 2a-e. In Model 1a, the influence of loneliness on later school wellbeing was fully attenuated by having a trusted class advisor at T1. By adding class advisor at T2 (Model 2a), the association was even weaker, and additionally, class advisor at T2 demonstrated a strong and positive independent contribution (odds ratio, 3.68, 95% CI 1.06 to 12.79). Other adults at T1 showed a corresponding modifying influence on the association between loneliness and later school wellbeing (Model 1e), but this influence was somewhat reduced when other adults at T2 was added (Model 2e). None of the other groups of trusted persons (other teachers, students, or parents in Models b-d) affected the strongly negative association between loneliness and later school wellbeing, except other teachers at T1 and T2 when they were included simultaneously (Model 2b).

TABLE 4: Influence of trusted others on the relation between loneliness (T1) and school wellbeing (T2)

	Model 1 (a-e)¤		Model 2 (a-e)¤	
	Odds ratio (95% CI)	p-value	Odds ratio (95% CI)	p-value
a. Class advisor				
Loneliness	0.48 (0.16 to 1.41)§	0. 181	0.52 (0.16 to 1.68)§	0. 272
Class advisor T1	1.99 (0.79 to 5.01)	0. 145	1.51 (0.60 to 3.79)	0. 382
Class advisor T2			3.68 (1.06 to 12.79)	0. 040
b. Other teachers				
Loneliness	0.30 (0.10 to 0.88)	0. 029	0.35 (0.12 to 1.05)§	0.060
Other teachers T1	1.02 (0.46 to 2.25)	0. 963	1.10 (0.49 to 2.47)	0. 813
Other teachers T2			1.64 (0.67 to 3.99)	0. 279
c. Students				
Loneliness	0.35 (0.12 to 0.97)	0.043	0.25 (0.06 to 0.96)	0. 043
Students T1	1.66 (0.72 to 3.83)	0.239	1.20 (0.45 to 3.16)	0. 720
Students T2			2.79 (0.78 to 9.95)	0. 115
d. Parents				
Loneliness	0.26 (0.08 to 0.81)	0. 021	0.24 (0.07 to 0.78)	0. 017
Parents T1	0.54 (0.15 to 1.91)	0. 339	0.58 (0.17 to 2.03)	0. 396
Parents T2			0.74 (0.24 to 2.24)	0. 589
e. Other adults				
Loneliness	0.50 (0.17 to 1.49)§	0. 212	0.38 (0.12 to 1.27)§	0.117
Other adults T1	1.13 (0.41 to 3.09)	0. 813	1.29 (0.46 to 3.61)	0. 629
Other adults T2			0.62 (0.25 to 1.55)	0. 307

¤*adjusted for academic problems, victimisation, school wellbeing and grades (T1) in multivariable logistic regression models. §the influence of loneliness turns to be non-significant (p-value ≥0.05). Note: In Model 1 (a-e), the scores of each group of trusted others at T1 were included separately in Model 1a to Model 1e. In the right part of the table (Model 2 (a-e)), the scores of each group of the trusted others at T1 and T2 were included simultaneously.*

Participants in this study were recruited from five schools, and it could be asked whether "school" should have been included as a covariate in the adjustments, together with grade and school wellbeing at T1. Because of the relatively low number of participants, the covariates were kept to a minimum; therefore, school was not included in the results presented above. However, we ran corresponding analyses to those in Tables 3 and 4, also adjusting for school. When school was included, the negative association between loneliness and school wellbeing was even stronger (odds ratio, 0.27, 95% CI 0.09 to 0.76) compared to the corresponding association in Table 3. The influence of teachers was generally weaker when school was included but, in line with the tabulated results, class advisor still fully attenuated the association of loneliness with later school wellbeing. The influence of other teachers, and also other adults, disappeared compared to Models 2b and 2e, respectively. For students and parents, there were no substantial changes.

7.4 DISCUSSION

This longitudinal study assessed the influence of different groups of trusted people on the relationship between girls' perceived loneliness at school and their self-reported school wellbeing two years later. Among the 119 girls in grades 1–8, loneliness at school was strongly related to low levels of school wellbeing. However, having class advisors whom they trusted sufficiently to turn to in difficult or hurtful situations fully attenuated the negative association of loneliness with later school wellbeing. Also, other non-specified adults fully attenuated the longitudinal association between loneliness and school wellbeing. On the other hand, trusted people such as parents, peers at school, or other teachers did not substantially affect the relationship between girls' loneliness and later school wellbeing. For parents, this is especially surprising since 80-90% of the girls reported, two years apart, that they probably or certainly would talk to their parents if something bad or difficult happened.

7.4.1 THE INFLUENCE OF POTENTIAL ADVERSITIES

Of the three potential adversities; academic problems, victimisation and loneliness, the latter was the only adversity showing a strong relationship with later school wellbeing. It has been shown previously in cross-sectional studies that loneliness may be more damaging to wellbeing at school than both victimisation caused by bullying and students' perceptions of academic problems [39-41]; however, this relationship has been inadequately explored in longitudinal studies [2].

7.4.2 STABILITY OF TRUST OVER THE TWO YEARS

For each group of trusted persons, the correlations between T1 and T2 were unexpectedly low. For parents especially a higher stability was expected between the two points in time as parents constituted by far the most trusted group at both data collection points. We did not find theoretical or empirical support for this low correlation of rho 0.25. The girls reported the highest stability of trust in the class advisor, a finding that might be ascribed to the important role of main teachers in Norwegian schools. Contrary to this, other teachers and other adults showed no significant stability. This may reflect that other teachers and other adults, such as coaches, change during a few school years.

7.4.3 THE IMPORTANCE OF TRUSTED TEACHERS

Our results highlight the great importance of teachers to girls who feel lonely at school. Among lonely girls, who trusted their class advisor sufficiently to contact her in difficult or hurtful situations, statistical analysis showed that reported loneliness did not significantly affect their later wellbeing at school. This indicates that lonely girls were just as likely to experience good school wellbeing as non-lonely girls.

One possible explanation of the class advisor's impact on the relationship between loneliness and wellbeing at school may be that these three measures are all related to the school setting. This cannot be the only explanation, however, as our data demonstrated a notable difference between the impact of the class teacher and that of other teachers. This difference may be related to the Norwegian school system where the class advisor represents stability by teaching most of the lessons, typically over 3–4 years, whereas other teachers meet the students less frequently. Besides being a buffer for the harmful influence of loneliness over the two year perspective, reports on trusted class advisor at T2 also showed a concurrent and strong association directly with the girls' school wellbeing.

The results indicate that trust in other teachers was less important to the girls' school wellbeing; other teachers had no influence on the negative association of loneliness with school wellbeing two years later and, by adding trust in other teachers at T2, the association was only modestly changed. In line with the resilience literature [42,43], there are reasons to suggest that stable and long-lasting relationships with main teachers are valuable to most students, and especially to those who feel lonely.

7.4.4 THE ROLE OF OTHERS

Our results demonstrated that parents were the most trusted group of people, and this corresponds to findings illustrating the importance of children and adolescents being closely attached to their parents [44]. The results revealed in the multivariable analyses therefore were surprising; having trust in parents did not ease the burden of loneliness; in fact, the negative association between loneliness and later school wellbeing was enforced by adding 'trusted parents'. One explanation of this finding may be that parents are usually separated from the school setting, only occasionally taking part in school activities with their children and the teachers. The "setting" argument is, however, questionable seen in light of the minimal influence of other teachers who, by definition, are inside the school setting. Another explanation could be a weak attachment [45] between the lonely girl and her parents; it is possible that lonely girls tend not to trust their parents. However, our study was not designed to answer that possibility. A third explanation may be that the lonely girls hid their hurtful feelings related to perceived loneliness at school and never told their parents, corresponding to hidden feelings of shame and inferiority linked to invisible symptoms of depression and anxiety [46,47]. Nevertheless, the suggestions above leave the question open: why do we not see any positive influence of trusted parents on the association of loneliness with later school wellbeing?

Positive peer relationships, such as having friends, being accepted by peers and the quality of friendship are shown to protect against loneliness [48,49]. We are not aware of any study that discusses the role of peers in buffering the harmful effects of loneliness. In our study, reporting trust in other students had no influence on the relationship between loneliness and later school wellbeing. Cassidy and Berlin suggested that adequate peer relations mediate a link between weak parent attachments and loneliness in children [45]. To our knowledge, no studies have addressed this hypothesis.

In accordance with findings in the resilience research [35,37], our results showed that other trusted adults may mitigate the bad influence of adversity, in this case loneliness. Those adults were probably outside the school setting, but are not identified in our data. They might have been a relative, a trainer, or someone else who was trusted—and maybe the only one [50,51].

7.4.5 STRENGTHS AND LIMITATIONS

The longitudinal population based design and the very high rate of participation are the strengths of this study. The schools were all public and ranged from inland to costal environments in rural communities. A weakness of the study is that students from urban settings were not included, and it is difficult to anticipate to what degree the results from this convenience sampling of schools may be generalised. Furthermore, it is possible that psychiatric co-morbidity (not included in the study) may have affected the results by influencing perceptions of loneliness; placing trust in other people; and perceptions of school wellbeing. Later studies should consider including measures of emotional symptoms or diseases. All students answered the same set of questions and were guided by school nurses or teachers, all of whom were trained and knew the purpose of the study. The younger students were interviewed by the nurses, whereas the older students completed their questionnaires in a lesson allocated to this task, guided by a teachers or a nurse. These different procedures could have introduced systematic errors between the younger and older student groups. Nevertheless, the congruence in the influence of trusted others between T1 and T2 indicate that the findings are robust and can withstand variations in methods, as well as in age, in this student population. It will, however, be of great value to replicate this study using larger samples or populations.

7.5 CONCLUSIONS

Loneliness in girls strongly predicted school wellbeing two years later. Among three potential adversities, loneliness was the only variable showing a strong and negative longitudinal association with school wellbeing. The perception of having academic problems, or being victimised by bullying, did not contribute individually to school wellbeing. However, having a class advisor at T1 whom the girl trusted sufficiently to contact in stressful situations clearly reduced the burden of loneliness. Also, having another trusted adult (not identified) at T1 eased the burden of loneliness. In contrast, other trusted people at T1 such as trusted parents, students, or other teachers did not affect the relationship between loneliness and later school wellbeing. Furthermore, adjusting for the same groups of trusted others at T2 in the respective analyses showed no substantial changes in the results. This demonstrated the consistency in the results; the longitudinal associations were fairly similar to the cross-sectional associations. The influence of other adults should be recognised but, as they were not identified as individuals, they cannot guide interventions. On the contrary, the impact of the main teacher—the class advisor—calls for attention in schools, health services and public health in general. This finding highlights the great clinical importance of the stability and trust that main teachers may represent for their students, and especially for lonely and vulnerable girls.

7.5.1 CONSENT

Data in this publication was drawn from surveys in a school project. All students and parents were given oral as well as written information about the surveys and the project. They were told that participation in the surveys was voluntary, and that the collected information was confidential. Students/parents who did not want to participate were to inform the headmaster or their class advisor. No parents or students denied participating, and informed consent was given by participating and completing questionnaires.

REFERENCES

1. Løhre A, Lydersen S, Vatten LJ: Factors associated with internalizing or somatic symptoms in a cross-sectional study of school children in grades 1–10. Child Adolesc Psychiatry Ment Health 2010, 4(1):33.
2. Løhre A, Moksnes UK, Lillefjell M: Gender differences in predictors of school well-being? Health Educ J 2014, 73(1):90-100.
3. Kemp C, Carter M: The social skills and social status of mainstreamed students with intellectual disabilities. Educ Psychol 2002, 22(4):391-411.
4. Nowicki EA: A meta-analysis of the social competence of children with learning disabilities compared to classmates of low and average to high achievement. Learn Disabil Q 2003, 26(3):171-188.
5. Valås H: Students with learning disabilities and low-achieving students: peer acceptance, loneliness, self-esteem, and depression. Soc Psychol Educ 1999, 3(3):173-192.
6. Williams GA, Asher SR: Assessment of loneliness at school among children with mild mental retardation. Am J Ment Retard 1992, 96(4):373-385.
7. Olweus D: Bullying at School: What we Know and What we can do. Oxford: Blackwell Publishing; 1993.
8. Smith PK: Bullying: Recent Developments. Child Adolesc Ment Health 2004, 9(3):98-103.
9. Smith PK, Brain P: Bullying in schools: lessons from two decades of research. Aggress Behav 2000, 26(1):1-9.
10. Due P, Holstein BE, Lynch J, Diderichsen F, Gabhain SN, Scheidt P, Currie C: Bullying and symptoms among school-aged children: international comparative cross sectional study in 28 countries. Eur J Public Health 2005, 15(2):128-132.
11. Eslea M, Menesini E, Morita Y, O'Moore M, Mora-Merchán JA, Pereira B, Smith PK: Friendship and loneliness among bullies and victims: data from seven countries. Aggress Behav 2004, 30(1):71-83.

12. Arseneault L, Bowes L, Shakoor S: Bullying victimization in youths and mental health problems: much ado about nothing? Psychol Med 2010, 40(05):717-729.

13. Gini G, Albiero P, Benelli B, Altoè G: Does empathy predict adolescents' bullying and defending behavior? Aggress Behav 2007, 33(5):467-476.

14. Nansel TR, Overpeck M, Pilla RS, Ruan WJ, Simons-Morton B, Scheidt P: Bullying behaviors among US youth: prevalence and association with psychosocial adjustment. JAMA 2001, 285(16):2094-2100.

15. Rigby K: Consequences of bullying in schools. Can J Psychiatry 2003, 48(9):583-590.

16. Gini G, Pozzoli T: Association between bullying and psychosomatic problems: a meta-analysis. Pediatrics 2009, 123(3):1059-1065.

17. Gini G, Pozzoli T: Bullied children and psychosomatic problems: a meta-analysis. Pediatrics 2013, 132(4):720-729.

18. Nansel TR, Craig W, Overpeck MD, Saluja G, Ruan WJ: Cross-national consistency in the relationship between bullying behaviors and psychosocial adjustment. Arch Pediatr Adolesc Med 2004, 158(8):730-736.

19. Løhre A, Lydersen S, Paulsen B, Maehle M, Vatten LJ: Peer victimization as reported by children, teachers, and parents in relation to children's health symptoms. BMC Public Health 2011, 11:278.

20. Stickley A, Koyanagi A, Koposov R, McKee M, Roberts B, Ruchkin V: Peer victimisation and its association with psychological and somatic health problems among adolescents in northern Russia. Child Adolesc Psychiatry Ment Health 2013, 7(1):15.

21. Peplau LA, Perlman D: Perspectives on loneliness. In Loneliness: A Sourcebook of Current Theory, Research and Therapy. Edited by Peplau LA, Perlman D. New York: Wiley; 1982:1-18.

22. Galanaki E: Are children able to distinguish among the concepts of aloneness, loneliness, and solitude? Int J Behav Dev 2004, 28(5):435-443.

23. Buchholz ES, Catton R: Adolescents' perceptions of aloneness and loneliness. Adolescence 1999, 34(133):203-213.

24. Larson RW: The uses of loneliness in adolescence. In Loneliness in Childhood and Adolescence. Edited by Rotenberg KJ, Hymel S. Cambridge: Cambridge University Press; 1999:244-262.

25. Rotenberg KJ, Hymel S: Loneliness in Childhood and Adolescence. Cambridge: Cambridge University Press; 1999.

26. Coplan RJ, Closson LM, Arbeau KA: Gender differences in the behavioral associates of loneliness and social dissatisfaction in kindergarten. J Child Psychol Psychiatry 2007, 48(10):988-995.

27. Goossens L, Marcoen A: Adolescent loneliness, self-reflection, and identity: from individual differences to developmental processes. In Loneliness in Childhood and Adolescence. Edited by Rotenberg KJ, Hymel S. Cambridge: Cambridge University Press; 1999:225-243.

28. Inderbitzen-Pisaruk H, Clark ML, Solano CH: Correlates of loneliness in midadolescence. J Youth Adolesc 1992, 21(2):151-167.

29. Galanaki E, Polychronopoulou S, Babalis T: Loneliness and social dissatisfaction among behaviourally at-risk children. Sch Psychol Int 2008, 29(2):214-229.

30. Koenig LJ, Abrams RF: Adolescent loneliness and adjustment: a focus on gender differences. In Loneliness in Childhood and Adolescence. Edited by Rotenberg KJ, Hymel S. Cambridge: Cambridge University Press; 1999:296-322.

31. Qualter P, Brown S, Munn P, Rotenberg K: Childhood loneliness as a predictor of adolescent depressive symptoms: an 8-year longitudinal study. Eur Child Adolesc Psychiatry 2010, 19(6):493-501.

32. Baskin TW, Wampold BE, Quintana SM, Enright RD: Belongingness as a protective factor against loneliness and potential depression in a multicultural middle school. Couns Psychol 2010, 38(5):626-651.

33. Kvarme LG, Helseth S, Sørum R, Luth-Hansen V, Haugland S, Natvig GK: The effect of a solution-focused approach to improve self-efficacy in socially withdrawn school children: a non-randomized controlled trial. Int J Nurs Stud 2010, 47(11):1389-1396.

34. Besevegis E, Galanaki EP: Coping with loneliness in childhood. Eur J Dev Psychol 2010, 7(6):653-673.

35. Fonagy P, Target M: Attachment and reflective function: their role in self-organization. Dev Psychopathol 1997, 9(04):679-700.

36. Masten AS, Coatsworth JD: The development of competence in favorable and unfavorable environments: lessons from research on successful children. Am Psychol 1998, 53(2):205-220.

37. Werner EE, Smith RS: Journeys from Childhood to Midlife: Risk, Resilience, and Recovery. Ithaca, New York: Cornell University Press; 2001.

38. Werner EE, Smith RS: Overcoming the Odds. High Risk Children from Birth to Adulthood. Ithaca & London: Cornell University Press; 1992.

39. Løhre A, Lydersen S, Vatten LJ: School wellbeing among children in grades 1–10. BMC Public Health 2010, 10:526.

40. Løhre A: The impact of loneliness on self-rated health symptoms among victimized school children. Child Adolesc Psychiatry Ment Health 2012, 6:20.

41. Samdal O, Nutbeam D, Wold B, Kannas L: Achieving health and educational goals through schools - a study of the importance of the school climate and the students' satisfaction with school. Health Educ Res 1998, 13(3):383-397.

42. Masten AS: Ordinary magic: resilience processes in development. Am Psychol 2001, 56(3):227-238.

43. Werner EE: What can we learn about resilience from large-scale longitudinal studies? In Handbook of Resilience in Children. Edited by Goldstein S, Brooks RB. New York: Springer; 2013:87-102.

44. Bowlby J: A Secure Base: Parent–Child Attachment and Healthy Human Development. New York, NY, US: Basic Books; 1988.

45. Cassidy J, Berlin LJ: Understanding the origins og childhood loneliness: contributions of attachment theory. In Loneliness in Childhood and Adolescence. Edited by Rotenberg KJ, Hymel S. Cambridge: Cambridge University Press; 1999:34-55.

46. Gilbert P: The relationship of shame, social anxiety and depression: the role of the evaluation of social rank. Clin Psychol Psychother 2000, 7:174-189.

47. Lewis HB: The Role of Shame in Symptom Formation. Lawrence Erlbaum Associates, Inc: Hillsdale, NJ, England; 1987.

48. Asher SR, Paquette JA: Loneliness and peer relations in childhood. Curr Dir Psychol Sci 2003, 12(3):75-78.
49. Parker JG, Saxon JL, Asher SR, Kovacs DM: Dimensions of children's friendship adjustment: implications for understanding loneliness. In Loneliness in Childhood and Adolescence. Edited by Rotenberg KJ, Hymel S. Cambridge: Cambridge University Press; 1999:201-224.
50. Resnick MD, Bearman PS, Blum RW, Bauman KE, Harris KM, Jones J, Tabor J, Beuhring T, Sieving RE, Shew M, Ireland M, Bearinger LH, Udry JR: Protecting adolescents from harm. Findings from the National Longitudinal Study on Adolescent Health. JAMA 1997, 278(10):823-832.
51. Resnick MD, Harris LJ, Blum RW: The impact of caring and connectedness on adolescent health and well-being. J Paediatr Child Health 1993, 29(s1):S3-S9.

PART III

THE INTERACTION OF ADOLESCENT MENTAL HEALTH WITH PEER AND FAMILY RELATIONSHIPS

CHAPTER 8

CYBER AND TRADITIONAL BULLYING VICTIMIZATION AS A RISK FACTOR FOR MENTAL HEALTH PROBLEMS AND SUICIDAL IDEATION IN ADOLESCENTS

RIENKE BANNINK, SUZANNE BROEREN, PETRA M. VAN DE LOOIJ-JANSEN, FROUWKJE G. DE WAART, AND HEIN RAAT

8.1 INTRODUCTION

Recent studies indicate that approximately 20–35% of adolescents report involvement in traditional, offline bullying either as a bully, a victim or both [1]. Bullying can be defined as an aggressive act that is carried out by a group or an individual repeatedly and over time against a victim who cannot easily defend himself or herself [2]. Traditionally, four main types of bullying are distinguished: physical (e.g., assault), verbal (e.g., threats), relational (e.g., social exclusion) and indirect (e.g., spreading rumors) [3]. With the increased use of Internet and mobile phones, a new form of bullying has emerged, often labeled "cyber bullying" [3]–[5]. In cyber bullying, aggression occurs via electronic forms of contact [6].

Increased exposure to the online environment has contributed to a heightened appreciation of the potential negative impact of cyber bullying [7]. Recent cross-sectional studies have shown an association between cyber bullying victimization and mental health problems, and even between cyber bullying victimization and suicide [4], [6], [8], [9]. Despite evidence from these cross-sectional studies, little is known with regard to the longitudinal impact of cyber bullying. To the best of our knowledge, only Schultze-Krumbholz et al. studied the longitudinal association between cyber bullying victimization and mental health problems in a relatively small sample (N = 233). They only showed a significant association between cyber bullying victimization and mental health problems in girls, not in boys [10].

The few available longitudinal studies examining the relationship between traditional bullying and mental health problems or suicide (ideation) show that being a victim of traditional bullying increases the risk of developing mental health problems and committing suicide later in life [6], [11]–[16]. However, longitudinal studies examining the associations between traditional bullying victimization and mental health problems or suicide (ideation) within large samples are still rare and further research is recommended [6].

Therefore, it is of interest to examine the longitudinal associations between traditional bullying and mental health and suicide (ideation), as well as the longitudinal associations between cyber bullying and mental health and suicide (ideation) in a large sample. The impact of traditional bullying victimization on mental health and suicide may be different than the impact of cyber bullying victimization on mental health. It is possible that for example blocking online bullying messages, an option not available for face-to-face bullying, lessens the impact of cyber bullying on mental health while, in contrast, the possible breadth of audience on for instance websites may heighten the impact [3].

Furthermore, the impact of bullying victimization on boys may differ from the impact on girls. Few longitudinal studies have examined gender differences in victimization and mental health. These longitudinal studies indicate that both genders may have different risk profiles [6], [17]–[21], with girls who are victimized at baseline developing symptoms of depression or suicidal ideation at follow-up [10], [17], [20], [21] and boys not [10], [18]–[23].

The purpose of the current study was to examine whether traditional and cyber bullying victimization were associated with mental health problems and suicidal ideation at two-year follow-up (when controlling for mental health problems or suicidal ideation at baseline) in a large sample of adolescents. In line with previous findings [6], [17]–[23], we hypothesize that being a victim of traditional bullying is associated with mental health problems and suicidal ideation at two-year follow-up. In line with cross-sectional studies on cyber bullying victimization [4], [6], [8], [9], we hypothesize that cyber bullying victimization is associated with mental health problems and suicidal ideation at two year follow-up. Additionally, we explored whether bullying affects boys and girls in a different way, as previously suggested [6], [17]–[21].

8.2 METHODS

8.2.1 DESIGN AND PARTICIPANTS

A prospective study with two-year follow-up was conducted as part of the Rotterdam Youth Monitor (RYM), a longitudinal youth health surveillance system. The RYM monitors the general health, well-being, behavior and related factors of youth aged 0 to 19 years living in Rotterdam and the surrounding region in the Netherlands. The RYM is incorporated in the care (regular health examinations) of the preventive youth healthcare system; the RYM is used to detect (potential) individual health risks and problems in order to take the necessary preventive measures (including referrals for treatment).

The current study used RYM data from students at secondary schools. At baseline, the students were in their first year of secondary education (M_{age} = 12.50 years, SD = 0.62), and at follow-up in their third year (M_{age} = 14.31 years, SD = 0.58). Data were collected throughout the school year, except for July and August (Dutch summer holidays). The students completed a baseline questionnaire between September 2008 and July 2009 and a follow-up questionnaire between September 2010 and July 2011. Administration of the questionnaire took place at schools and was conducted by specially trained researchers and school nurses from the Municipal Public Health Service and/or by a teacher. In 2008–2009, 8,272 adolescents participated (95% participation rate), of whom 3,181 participated again in 2010–2011 (38%). The main reason for non-response (62%) at follow-up was schools being unwilling to participate again, which led to 49% of adolescents not being invited to participate at follow-up. Other reasons were: students were absent at the time of administering the follow-up questionnaire (about 5%), students had transferred to a school that did not participate at follow-up or students had repeated a school year (about 8%).

8.2.2 ETHICS STATEMENT

The data became available in the context of the government approved routine health examinations of the preventive youth health care. Separate informed consent was therefore not requested. Only anonymous data were used and the questionnaires were completed on a voluntary basis. Adolescents received verbal information about these questionnaires each time they were applied, whereas their parents received written information at every assessment point. Adolescents and their parents were free to refuse participation. Observational research with data does not fall within the ambit of the Dutch Act on research involving human subjects and does not require the approval of an ethics review board. As the data was provided anonymously tothe researchers, the study is not covered by the WMA Declaration of Helsinki.

8.2.3 MEASURES

8.2.3.1 BULLYING VICTIMIZATION.

At baseline, two questions assessed whether the adolescent had been bullied in the past four week: 1) at school, and/or 2) via the Internet or via their telephone via Short Message Service (SMS). The response categories were: Never, Once or twice, Once a week, Several times a week, and Daily. For analysis purposes, being a victim of bullying at school (traditional victim), and being a victim on the Internet or via SMS (cyber victim) were dichotomized into the following categories: Never being victimized and Being victimized at least once or twice.

8.2.3.2 MENTAL HEALTH PROBLEMS.

At baseline and follow-up, mental health was assessed by the Dutch self-report version of the Strengths and Difficulties Questionnaire (SDQ) [24], [25]. The SDQ consists of 25 items describing positive and negative attributes of adolescents that can be divided into five subscales (five items each), i.e. emotional problems, conduct problems, hyperactivity-inattention, peer problems, and prosocial behavior. Each item is scored on a 3-point scale, with 0 = "not true", 1 = "somewhat true", and 2 = "certainly true". A total difficulties score is calculated by summing the scores on the emotional problems, conduct problems, hyperactivity-inattention and peer problems subscales (range 0–40; current study $\alpha = 0.74$).

In line with other authors who divided their sample into subgroups (normal versus borderline/abnormal) based on questionnaire scores [13], [17], [19]–[23], we created two "mental health" groups: normal (cut-off point SDQ total score at follow-up ≤80th percentile; score ≤13) and borderline/abnormal mental health problems (cut-off point SDQ total score at follow-up >80th percentile; score ≥14) [26]. These cut-off points were based on a large national survey in the Netherlands among 14–15 year-old adolescents [27].

8.2.3.3 SUICIDAL IDEATION.

Suicidal ideation during the past 12 months was examined with one question at baseline and follow-up: "In the past 12 months, have you ever seriously considered ending your life?". This item was scored on a 5-point scale: Never, Once in a while, Sometimes, Often and Very often. For analysis purposes, suicidal ideation was dichotomized in: Never had suicidal ideation over the last year; versus Had suicidal ideation at least once in a while over the last year.

8.2.3.4 CONFOUNDERS.

Age, gender, ethnicity, and level of education of the adolescent were measured at baseline and were incorporated as potential confounders in this study. Age was dichotomized into Below 13 years versus 13 years or older. Education was dichotomized into Basic or theoretical pre-vocational education versus, General secondary/pre-university education [28]. Ethnicity was classified as Dutch or non-Dutch in accordance with the definition of Statistics Netherlands [29]; i.e., adolescents with at least one parent born outside the Netherlands were classified as non-Dutch.

8.2.4 STATISTICAL ANALYSES

All analyses were conducted using the total sample. Descriptive statistics were used to describe general characteristics of the study population. Differences in age, ethnicity, educational level, bullying victimization, mental health problems, and suicidal ideation between boys and girls were evaluated using chi-square tests. A chi-square test was also conducted to assess the association between traditional and cyber bullying victimization.

Furthermore, binary logistic regression analyses were used to assess the association between bullying victimization and mental health status or suicidal ideation at follow-up. Model 1 tested the association between traditional or cyber bullying victimization and mental health status or suicidal ideation at follow-up, adjusting for confounders (i.e., gender, age, ethnicity, and education) and the other type of bullying victimization. Model 2 also adjusted for baseline mental health status or suicidal ideation. Model 2 corresponds with the purpose of the study to examine the two-year longitudinal association between bullying victimization and mental health status or suicidal ideation, while controlling for mental health problems or suicidal ideation at baseline. In addition, we tested whether there were gender differences on mental health and suicidal ideation for the two types of bullying by respectively adding a Gender × Traditional bullying victimization (Model 3a) or a Gender × Cyber bullying victimization (Model 3b) interaction term to Model 2. If there was a significant Gender × Bullying victimization interaction, the results were described separately for boys and girls. Finally, we explored whether there were significant interactions between traditional and cyber bullying victimization on mental health and suicidal ideation. Odds ratios (OR) and their corresponding 95% confidence intervals (95% CI) were calculated.

Analyses were conducted using SPSS version 20. Results were considered significant at $p<0.05$, with the exception of interactions which were considered significant at $p<0.10$, in line with recommendations of Twisk [30].

8.3 RESULTS

8.3.1 NON-RESPONSE ANALYSIS

Differences between the boys/girls included in this study (N = 3181) and the boys/girls who did not participate in the follow-up assessment (N = 5091) were examined using chi-square tests (Table 1). Chi-square tests did not yield significant age differences between adolescents who participated at follow-up and who were lost-to-follow-up. However, group differences were found for education, ethnicity, mental health problems, suicidal ideation, and bullying victimization, with the lost–to-follow-up group having a lower education level, more often being of Dutch ethnicity, having more mental health problems, more suicidal ideation, and more often being a traditional and cyber bullying victim (only for girls) than the adolescents who participated at follow-up.

8.3.2 DESCRIPTIVES

Mean age of adolescents in the current sample was 12.47 years (SD = 0.62); 51.0% of the sample consisted of boys and 48.4% was of Dutch ethnicity (Table 2). In total, 21.4% of the adolescents was a victim of traditional bullying and 5.1% was a victim of cyber bullying. No significant gender differences were found on bullying victimization (p = 0.10). Compared with boys, girls had significantly more mental health problems at follow-up (χ^2 = 10.04; p<0.002) and suicidal ideation at baseline (χ^2 = 52.42; p<0.001) and at follow-up (χ^2 = 58.69; p<0.001). Furthermore, cyber bullying victims were more likely to also be traditional bullying victims compared to non-cyber bullying victims (boys: χ^2 = 60.38; p<0.001; girls: χ^2 = 29.21; p<0.001).

TABLE 1: Differences between boys/girls who did and did not participate at follow-up (N = 8271).

	Boys			Girls		
	Participated n = 1623 %	Lost-to-follow-up n = 2645 %	p value (χ^2)	Participated n = 1558 %	Lost-to-follow-up n = 2445 %	p value (χ^2)
Age (mean = 12.50, SD = 0.62)						
<13 years	53.9	51.2	0.09	58.6	56.0	0.09
Ethnicity						
Dutch	50.4	56.9	<0.001	46.3	55.4	<0.001
Level of education						
Basic or theoretical pre-vocational education	49.3	63.6	<0.001	51.0	64.2	<0.001
Victim of bullying						
Traditional alone	22.4	25.8	0.01	20.3	24.4	0.002
Cyber alone	4.7	5.3	0.45	5.5	9.0	<0.001
Mental health problems	20.5	24.9	0.001	20.5	25.5	<0.001
Suicidal ideation	13.8	17.5	0.002	23.9	26.8	0.04

8.3.3 BULLYING VICTIMIZATION AND MENTAL HEALTH PROBLEMS

There was a significant interaction between gender and traditional bullying victimization (p = 0.08) (Model 3a) in the total sample (Table 3). Among boys, traditional bullying victimization was not significantly related to mental health problems in the fully-adjusted model (OR 1.03; 95% CI 0.72–1.47). Among girls, traditional bullying victimization was significantly related to mental health problems in the fully-adjusted model (OR 1.41; 95% CI 1.02–1.96).

TABLE 2: General characteristics of the total study population, and by gender (N = 3181).

	Total	Boys	Girls	p value
	N = 3181	n = 1623	n = 1558	(χ^2)
	%	%	%	
Age (mean = 12.47, SD = 0.62)				
<13 years	56.2	53.9	58.6	0.01
Ethnicity				
Dutch	48.4	50.4	46.3	0.02
Level of education				
Basic or theoretical pre-vocational education	50.1	49.3	51.0	0.33
Victim of bullying				0.10
Traditional alone	18.8	19.6	17.9	
Cyber alone	2.6	2.0	3.2	
Traditional and cyber	2.6	2.8	2.4	
Mental health problems				
At baseline	20.5	20.5	20.5	0.98
At follow-up	15.0	13.0	17.0	0.002
Suicidal ideation				
At baseline	18.8	13.8	23.9	<0.001
At follow-up	11.8	7.5	16.3	<0.001

There was a significant interaction between gender and cyber bullying victimization (p = 0.04) (Model 3b). Being a victim of cyber bullying was not related to mental health problems among boys (OR 1.18; 95% CI 0.64–2.17), whereas among girls, cyber bullying victimization was significantly related to mental health problems after controlling for baseline mental health (OR 2.38; 95% CI 1.45–3.91).

No significant interaction was found between traditional and cyber bullying victimization on mental health.

TABLE 3: Associations of bullying victimization and mental health problems (N = 3181).

	Model 1		Model 2		Model 3a		Model 3b	
	OR (95% CI)	p value	OR (95% CI)	p value	OR (95% CI)	p value	OR (95% CI)	p value
Sociodemographic characteristics								
Gender, boy	0.73 (0.60–0.89)	0.002	0.71 (0.58–0.88)	0.001	0.80 (0.63–1.02)	0.07	0.76 (0.61–0.95)	0.01
Age, <13 years[a]	1.13 (0.92–1.39)	0.25	1.10 (0.89–1.38)	0.34	1.11 (0.90–1.38)	0.34	1.11 (0.90–1.39)	0.33
Ethnicity, Dutch	0.95 (0.77–1.17)	0.62	0.89 (0.72–1.10)	0.29	0.89 (0.72–1.11)	0.30	0.88 (0.71–1.09)	0.24
Education, basic or theoretical prevocational education	1.58 (1.27–1.96)	<0.001	1.23 (0.98–1.54)	0.08	1.23 (0.98–1.54)	0.08	1.23 (0.98–1.54)	0.08
Bullying victimization								
Traditional victim	1.64 (1.31–2.05)	<0.001	1.20 (0.95–1.53)	0.13	1.45 (1.06–2.00)	0.02	1.22 (0.96–1.54)	0.11
Cyber victim	2.35 (1.64–3.36)	<0.001	1.79 (1.23–2.61)	0.003	1.81 (1.24–2.65)	0.002	2.53 (1.55–4.12)	<0.001
Mental health problems at baseline			4.59 (3.68–5.73)	<0.001	4.59 (3.68–5.73)	<0.001		
Gender × Traditional bullying victimization					0.66 (0.42–1.54)	0.08		
Gender × Cyber bullying victimization							0.44 (0.20–0.95)	0.04

Note: OR = odds ratio; CI = confidence interval. [a]Similar results were obtained when age was included as a continuous variable in the analysis. Model 1 is adjusted for sociodemographic characteristics and bulling victimization. Mental health problems is the dependent variable. Model 2 is the same as Model 1, but all also adjusted for mental health problems at baseline. Model 3a is the same as Model 2, but also includes a Gender × Traditional bullying victimization interaction term. Model 3b is the same as Model 2, but also includes a Gender × Cyber bullying victimization interaction term.

TABLE 4: Associations of bullying victimization and suicidal ideation (N = 3181).

	Model 1		Model 2		Model 3a		Model 3b	
	OR (95% CI)	p value	OR (95% CI)	p value	OR (95% CI)	p value	OR (95% CI)	p value
Sociodemographic characteristics								
Gender, boy	0.40 (0.32–0.51)	<0.001	0.48 (0.37–0.60)	<0.001	0.53 (0.40–0.70)	<0.001	0.49 (0.38–0.63)	<0.001
Age, <13 years[a]	0.89 (0.71–1.12)	0.31	0.90 (0.71–1.15)	0.39	0.90 (0.71–1.15)	0.39	0.90 (0.71–1.14)	0.39
Ethnicity, Dutch	1.06 (0.84–1.34)	0.63	1.10 (0.87–1.41)	0.42	1.11 (0.87–1.41)	0.41	1.10 (0.86–1.40)	0.44
Education, basic or theoretical prevocational education	1.32 (1.04–1.68)	0.02	1.17 (0.91–1.50)	0.22	1.17 (0.91–1.50)	0.22	1.17 (0.91–1.50)	0.22
Bullying victimization								
Traditional victim	1.95 (1.53–2.48)	<0.001	1.56 (1.21–2.02)	<0.001	1.77 (1.29–2.44)	<0.001	1.57 (1.21–2.03)	0.001
Cyber victim	1.74 (1.17–2.61)	0.007	1.22 (0.80–1.87)	0.36	1.23 (0.80–1.89)	0.34	1.36 (0.81–2.28)	0.24
Suicidal ideation at baseline			4.82 (3.79–6.12)	<0.001	4.84 (3.81–6.15)	<0.001	4.81 (3.79–6.10)	<0.001
Gender × Traditional bullying victimization					0.71 (0.43–1.20)	0.20		
Gender × Cyber bullying victimization							0.72 (0.29–1.79)	0.48

Note: OR = odds ratio; CI = confidence interval. [a]Similar results were obtained when age was included as a continuous variable in the analysis. Model 1 is adjusted for sociodemographic characteristics and bulling victimization. Suicidal ideation is the dependent variable. Model 2 is the same as Model 1, but all also adjusted for suicidal ideation at baseline. Model 3a is the same as Model 2, but also includes a Gender × Traditional bullying victimization interaction term. Model 3b is the same as Model 2, but also includes a Gender × Cyber bullying victimization interaction term.

8.3.4 BULLYING VICTIMIZATION AND SUICIDAL IDEATION

No significant interaction was found between gender and traditional bullying victimization (p = 0.20) (Model 3a) and between gender and cyber bullying victimization (p = 0.48) (Model 3b) (Table 4). In the total sample, traditional bullying victimization was significantly related to suicidal ideation in the fully-adjusted model (Model 2: OR 1.56; 95% CI 1.21–2.02). Cyber bullying victimization was not associated with suicidal ideation after controlling for baseline suicidal ideation (Model 2: OR 1.22; 95% CI 0.80–1.87).

A significant interaction was found between traditional and cyber bullying victimization on suicidal ideation (p = 0.01). Follow-up logistic regression analysis revealed that there was no further increased risk of developing suicidal ideation for adolescents being a victim of both types of bullying compared to adolescents being solely a victim of cyber (OR 1.35; 95% CI 0.86–2.12) or traditional bullying (OR 1.13; 95% CI 0.91–1.41).

8.4 DISCUSSION

This study shows that both traditional and cyber bullying victimization were associated with mental health problems in girls but not in boys, after controlling for baseline problems. Only traditional bullying victimization was associated with suicidal ideation after controlling for baseline suicidal ideation.

As hypothesized, but only among girls, traditional bullying victimization was associated with mental health problems after controlling for baseline mental health. This difference between boys and girls in the long-term effects of traditional bullying victimization on mental health is supported by various previous studies [6], [17]–[21]. The current study extends these findings to cyber bullying victimization, as we too found that the association between cyber bullying victimization and mental health problems was particularly driven by girls.

The gender differences in the impact of bullying on mental health found in our study may be partly explained by differences in the types of bullying (e.g. physical, relational) to which girls and boys are exposed.

Regarding to traditional bullying, previous studies have found that girls more often experience relational victimization and that relational victimization has a greater impact on mental health problems than overt victimization, which is more often experienced by boys [31]–[33]. However, as the present study did not distinguish between different types of traditional or cyber bullying, it remains unclear whether the gender differences found in our study can be explained by the type of bullying. Therefore, future research should focus on different types of traditional bullying, as well as cyber bullying (e.g., via photos or video clips, emails), as different types of cyber bullying may also have different associations with mental health problems and suicidal ideation, and girls and boys may be exposed to different types of cyber bullying as well.

Furthermore, this study confirms the results of earlier studies indicating an association between traditional bullying victimization and suicidal ideation [6], [12], [15]. In contrast with our hypothesis, being a cyber bullying victim was not related to suicidal ideation after controlling for baseline suicidal ideation. A possible explanation for this discrepancy is the small size of the group of adolescents who were either a cyber bullying victim and had suicidal ideation. This may have resulted in limited power to detect a significant relationship between cyber bullying and suicidal ideation. Another possible explanation could be the difference in duration of exposure to the two types of bullying. Adolescents in our sample may have been exposed to cyber bullying for a shorter period of time compared to the time that they have been exposed to traditional bullying. This is in line with previous research showing that traditional bullying victimization remains relatively stable over time (between the ages of 8 and 16 years) [34], whereas cyber bullying victimization may occur at a later age, around the age of 14 years [4], when children spend more time on their mobile phones and are more likely to participate on social network sites (e.g. Facebook, MySpace) which are likely places for cyber bullying to occur [35]. It is possible that on the long-term, suicidal ideation only develops as a result of more pronounced and further developed mental health problems [36] and/or after persistent long-term exposure to bullying, as may have been the case with traditional bullying, but perhaps not yet with cyber bullying in our sample. Future research is required to gain more insight into these associations.

The purpose of the current study was to examine if bullying victimization was associated with mental health problems and suicidal ideation at follow-up. Nevertheless, analyzing the cross-sectional associations and the change in the percentage of adolescents with problems between baseline and follow-up among the different bullying victimization subgroups could provide additional information. Exploratory analyses on the baseline data (cross-sectional analyses) showed similar results as the longitudinal analyses described in the results section of this manuscript. As often the case, our cross-sectional analyses yielded somewhat stronger associations between both types of bullying victimization and mental health and suicidal ideation than our longitudinal analyses. No significant interactions were found between gender and bullying victimization on mental health or suicidal ideation. This could indicate that the short term impact of bullying victimization on adolescents' mental health is similar for boys and girls, but that the long term impact of bullying on the mental health is different for boys and girls. Furthermore, additional analyses showed that the proportion of adolescents with mental health problems in the bullying victimization group significantly decreased more over the two year follow-up period compared to adolescents in the non-bullying victimization group (data not shown). However, it must be noted that percentage of mental health problems at two year follow-up was still higher in the bullying victimization group than in the non-bullying group. The same results were found for suicidal ideation. The only exception was that no significantly different change in the proportion of mental health problems in girls in the cyber bullying victimization group over the two-year follow-up period was found compared to girls who were not a cyber bullying victim at baseline.

The present study has both strengths and limitations that need to be addressed. A strength of the study is its longitudinal nature. The dataset provided the opportunity to explore relationships between the particular variables of interest within a large sample. Furthermore, many studies on cyber bullying are conducted online, and, therefore, may have a bias toward the experiences of adolescents who use the Internet more frequently. However, this study also has some limitations. First, not all adolescents in the study were available for analyses due to non-participation at follow-up. A non-response analysis showed that the adolescents who did not participate at follow-up had a lower educational level, were older, more often of Dutch ethnicity, more often a traditional or cyber bullying victim, and more often had mental health problems and suicidal ideation at baseline. Although we included these variables as confounders and adjusted for baseline problems in our analyses, it is possible that this selective drop out led to underestimation of the size of the association between bullying victimization and mental health problems or suicidal ideation, since a vulnerable group (i.e. a group with a high risk of mental health problems and suicidal ideation) dropped out. However, additional analyses showed that the relationship between both types of bullying victimization and mental health or suicidal ideation at baseline did not significantly differ between adolescents who dropped out and adolescents who did not drop out at follow-up. Nevertheless, the current findings should be generalized with caution, and we propose replication in large and varied populations. Second, traditional and cyber bullying victimization were assessed using single, self-reported items. Moreover, there is currently no consensus among researchers how to measure cyber bullying, and the changing nature of communication technology makes it difficult to establish a fixed definition. Third, mental health and suicidal ideation were also assessed using self-reported items, which may have resulted in less reliable outcomes. Nevertheless, research suggests that adolescents are better reporters of their own mental health status than parents and teachers [37].

In conclusion, our findings suggest that traditional bullying victimization is associated with an increased risk of suicidal ideation, and traditional and cyber bullying victimization are associated with an increased risk of mental health problems among girls. Future research should examine the mechanisms responsible for this differential response of girls and boys to the stress caused by bullying victimization. Furthermore, based on our results and results of other studies, studies on the current topic may want to consider differentiating between boys and girls. Our findings stress the importance of programs aimed at reducing bullying behavior in schools and online. These programs are particularly important because early-onset mental health problems may pose a risk for the development of psychiatric disorders in adulthood [38]–[40]. Moreover, although several intervention programs are available that reduce bullying behavior and victimization in schools [41], [42] such programs should not solely focus on school bullying. Prevention of cyber bullying should also be included in school anti-bullying policies [3], [4] since this is currently often lacking [43]. While some traditional methods for reducing bullying may be useful for cyber bullying too (e.g., peer support), more specific interventions will also be needed to reduce cyber bullying, such as how to contact mobile phone companies and internet service providers [3].

REFERENCES

1. Levy N, Cortesi S, Crowley E, Beaton M, Casey J, et al. (2012) Bullying in a Networked Era: A Literature Review. Harvard University: Berkman Center Research Publication.
2. Olweus D (1993) Bullying at school: What we know and what we can do. Cambridge, MA: Wiley-Blackwell.
3. Smith PK, Mahdavi J, Carvalho M, Fisher S, Russell S, et al. (2008) Cyberbullying: its nature and impact in secondary school pupils. J Child Psychol Psychiatry 49: 376–385. doi: 10.1111/j.1469-7610.2007.01846.x
4. Suzuki K, Asaga R, Sourander A, Hoven CW, Mandell D (2012) Cyberbullying and adolescent mental health. Int J Adolesc Med Health 24: 27–35. doi: 10.1515/ijamh.2012.005
5. Raskauskas J, Stoltz AD (2007) Involvement in traditional and electronic bullying among adolescents. Dev Psychol 43: 564–575. doi: 10.1037/0012-1649.43.3.564
6. Brunstein Klomek A, Sourander A, Gould M (2010) The association of suicide and bullying in childhood to young adulthood: a review of cross-sectional and longitudinal research findings. Can J Psychiatry 55: 282–288.
7. Ybarra ML, Mitchell KJ, Espelage DL (2012) Comparisons of bully and unwanted sexual experiences online and offline among a national sample of youth. In: Özdemir Ö, editor. Complementary pediatrics.Croatia: InTech.
8. Bonanno RA, Hymel S (2013) Cyber Bullying and Internalizing Difficulties: Above and Beyond the Impact of Traditional Forms of Bullying. J Youth Adolesc.
9. Schneider SK, O'Donnell L, Stueve A, Coulter RW (2012) Cyberbullying, school bullying, and psychological distress: a regional census of high school students. Am J Public Health 102: 171–177. doi: 10.2105/ajph.2011.300308
10. Schultze-Krumbholz A, Jäkel A, Schultze M, Scheithauer H (2012) Emotional and behavioural problems in the context of cyberbullying: a longitudinal study among German adolescents. Emotional and Behavioural Difficulties 17: 329–345. doi: 10.1080/13632752.2012.704317
11. Reijntjes A, Kamphuis JH, Prinzie P, Telch MJ (2010) Peer victimization and internalizing problems in children: a meta-analysis of longitudinal studies. Child Abuse Negl 34: 244–252. doi: 10.1016/j.chiabu.2009.07.009
12. Fisher HL, Moffitt TE, Houts RM, Belsky DW, Arseneault L, et al. (2012) Bullying victimisation and risk of self harm in early adolescence: longitudinal cohort study. BMJ 344: e2683. doi: 10.1136/bmj.e2683

13. Copeland WE, Wolke D, Angold A, Costello EJ (2013) Adult Psychiatric Outcomes of Bullying and Being Bullied by Peers in Childhood and Adolescence. JAMA Psychiatry: 1–8.

14. Schreier A, Wolke D, Thomas K, Horwood J, Hollis C, et al. (2009) Prospective study of peer victimization in childhood and psychotic symptoms in a nonclinical population at age 12 years. Arch Gen Psychiatry 66: 527–536. doi: 10.1001/archgenpsychiatry.2009.23

15. Heikkila HK, Vaananen J, Helminen M, Frojd S, Marttunen M, et al. (2013) Involvement in bullying and suicidal ideation in middle adolescence: a 2-year follow-up study. Eur Child Adolesc Psychiatry 22: 95–102. doi: 10.1007/s00787-012-0327-0

16. Lereya ST, Winsper C, Heron J, Lewis G, Gunnell D, et al. (2013) Being bullied during childhood and the prospective pathways to self-harm in late adolescence. J Am

17. Brunstein Klomek A, Marrocco F, Kleinman M, Schonfeld IS, Gould MS (2007) Bullying, depression, and suicidality in adolescents. J Am Acad Child Adolesc Psychiatry 46: 40–49. doi: 10.1097/01.chi.0000242237.84925.18

18. Klomek AB, Sourander A, Niemela S, Kumpulainen K, Piha J, et al. (2009) Childhood bullying behaviors as a risk for suicide attempts and completed suicides: a population-based birth cohort study. J Am Acad Child Adolesc Psychiatry 48: 254–261. doi: 10.1097/chi.0b013e318196b91f

19. Haavisto A, Sourander A, Multimaki P, Parkkola K, Santalahti P, et al. (2004) Factors associated with depressive symptoms among 18-year-old boys: a prospective 10-year follow-up study. J Affect Disord 83: 143–154. doi: 10.1016/j.jad.2004.06.008

20. Bond L, Carlin JB, Thomas L, Rubin K, Patton G (2001) Does bullying cause emotional problems? A prospective study of young teenagers. BMJ 323: 480–484. doi: 10.1136/bmj.323.7311.480

21. Sourander A, Ronning J, Brunstein-Klomek A, Gyllenberg D, Kumpulainen K, et al. (2009) Childhood bullying behavior and later psychiatric hospital and psychopharmacologic treatment: findings from the Finnish 1981 birth cohort study. Arch Gen Psychiatry 66: 1005–1012. doi: 10.1001/archgenpsychiatry.2009.122

22. Klomek AB, Sourander A, Kumpulainen K, Piha J, Tamminen T, et al. (2008) Childhood bullying as a risk for later depression and suicidal ideation among Finnish males. J Affect Disord 109: 47–55. doi: 10.1016/j.jad.2007.12.226

23. Sourander A, Jensen P, Ronning JA, Niemela S, Helenius H, et al. (2007) What is the early adulthood outcome of boys who bully or are bullied in childhood? The Finnish "From a Boy to a Man" study. Pediatrics 120: 397–404. doi: 10.1542/peds.2006-2704

24. Goodman R, Ford T, Simmons H, Gatward R, Meltzer H (2000) Using the Strengths and Difficulties Questionnaire (SDQ) to screen for child psychiatric disorders in a community sample. Br J Psychiatry 177: 534–539. doi: 10.1080/0954026021000046128

25. Muris P, Meesters C, van den Berg F (2003) The Strengths and Difficulties Questionnaire (SDQ)—further evidence for its reliability and validity in a community sample of Dutch children and adolescents. Eur Child Adolesc Psychiatry 12: 1–8. doi: 10.1007/s00787-003-0298-2

26. Scoring the SDQ. Instructions in English for scoring self-rated SDQs by hand. Available: http://www.sdqinfo.org/py/sdqinfo/c0.py. Accessed 2013 September 29.

27. van Dorsselaer S, de Looze M, Vermeulen-Smit E, de Roos S, Verdurmen J, et al. (2009) Gezondheid, welzijn en opvoeding van jongeren in Nederland. Utrecht: Trimbos-instituut, Universiteit Utrecht, Sociaal en cultureel planbureau.

28. van de Looij-Jansen PM, de Wilde EJ, Mieloo CL, Donker MC, Verhulst FC (2009) Seasonal variation in self-reported health and health-related behaviour in Dutch adolescents. Public Health 123: 686–688. doi: 10.1016/j.puhe.2009.07.015

29. Centraal Bureau voor de Statistiek. Allochtoon. Available at: http://www.cbs.nl/nl-NL/menu/methoden/begrippen/default.htm?ConceptID=37. Accessed 2013 June 18.

30. 30. Twisk JW (2006) Applied multilevel analysis: A Practical Guide (Practical Guides to Biostatistics and Epidemiology).Cambridge University Press.

31. Crick NR, Bigbee MA (1998) Relational and overt forms of peer victimization: a multiinformant approach. J Consult Clin Psychol 66: 337–347. doi: 10.1037//0022-006x.66.2.337

32. Cullerton-Sen C, Crick NR (2005) Understanding the effects of physical and relational victimization: the utility of multiple perspectives in prediction social-emotional adjustment. School Psych Rev 34: 147–160.

33. Baldry A (2004) The impact of direct and indirect bullying on the mental and physical health of Italian youngsters. Aggress Behav 30: 343–355. doi: 10.1002/ab.20043

34. Sourander A, Helstela L, Helenius H, Piha J (2000) Persistence of bullying from childhood to adolescence—a longitudinal 8-year follow-up study. Child Abuse Negl 24: 873–881. doi: 10.1016/s0145-2134(00)00146-0

35. Kowalski RM, Limber SP (2007) Electronic bullying among middle school students. J Adolesc Health 41: S22–30. doi: 10.1016/j.jadohealth.2007.08.017

36. Cash SJ, Bridge JA (2009) Epidemiology of youth suicide and suicidal behavior. Curr Opin Pediatr 21: 613–619. doi: 10.1097/mop.0b013e32833063e1

37. Rutter M (1986) The development of psychopathology of depression: Issues and perspectives. In: Rutter M, Izard CE, Read PB, editors. Depression in young people: Developmental and clinical perspectives. New York: Guilford Press.

38. Fergusson DM, Woodward LJ (2002) Mental health, educational, and social role outcomes of adolescents with depression. Arch Gen Psychiatry 59: 225–231. doi: 10.1001/archpsyc.59.3.225

39. Kim-Cohen J, Caspi A, Moffitt TE, Harrington H, Milne BJ, et al. (2003) Prior juvenile diagnoses in adults with mental disorder: developmental follow-back of a prospective-longitudinal cohort. Arch Gen Psychiatry 60: 709–717. doi: 10.1001/archpsyc.60.7.709

40. Hofstra MB, van der Ende J, Verhulst FC (2002) Child and adolescent problems predict DSM-IV disorders in adulthood: a 14-year follow-up of a Dutch epidemiological sample. J Am Acad Child Adolesc Psychiatry 41: 182–189. doi: 10.1097/00004583-200202000-00012

41. Smith PK, Ananiadou K, Cowie H (2003) Interventions to reduce school bullying. Can J Psychiatry 48: 591–599.

42. Ttofi MM, Farrington DP (2011) Effectiveness of school-based programs to reduce bullying: A systematic and meta-analytic review. J Exp Criminol.7: pp.

43. Bhat CS (2008) Cyber Bullying: Overview and Strategies for School Counsellors, Guidance Officers, and All School Personnel. Aust J Guid Counsell 18: 53–66. doi: 10.1375/ajgc.18.1.53

CHAPTER 9

ASSOCIATIONS BETWEEN PARENT-ADOLESCENT ATTACHMENT RELATIONSHIP QUALITY, NEGATIVE LIFE EVENTS, AND MENTAL HEALTH

RIENKE BANNINK, SUZANNE BROEREN, PETRA M. VAN DE LOOIJ-JANSEN, AND HEIN RAAT

9.1 INTRODUCTION

An estimated 15% of adolescents in the Netherlands have mental health problems [1]. Mental health problems often have their first manifestation during adolescence [2] and are associated with serious co-morbidity including underachievement in age-appropriate social skills, delinquency and an elevated risk of suicide [3], . Mental health problems in adolescence pose a risk for the development of psychiatric disorders in adulthood [5]–[8]. Understanding determinants of mental health problems, such as risk and protective factors, is important for the prevention of these problems.

One important risk factor for psychopathology that has been under investigation for many years is the impact of negative life events [9], [10].

Associations between Parent-Adolescent Attachment Relationship Quality, Negative Life Events and Mental Health. © *Bannink R, Broeren S, van de Looij-Jansen PM, and Raat H.* PLoS ONE **8,11** *(2013), doi:10.1371/journal.pone.0080812. Licensed under Creative Commons Attribution 3.0 Unported License, http://creativecommons.org/licenses/by/3.0/.*

Results from several studies indicate an association in adolescents between negative life events and mental health problems. Examples of such life events that have been posited as risk factors for developing mental health problems in previous studies are physical illness of a parent [11], parental psychiatric illness [12], [13], parental substance use [14], [15], family breakdown [16], parental conflicts [17], [18] and early parenthood [19].

Longitudinal studies have also identified factors positively influencing the mental health of adolescents [20]–[23]. One of these factors is parent-adolescent attachment relationship quality. Previous research has shown that a favourable parent-adolescent attachment relationship may serve as a protective factor for mental health problems [21], [22], [24], [25], with the quality of adolescents' attachment with parents having an impact on their current mental health status, as well as on their prospect of developing mental health problems, such as major depression, later in life [23].

Although there is a considerable amount of literature examining the simple association of life events and parent-adolescent attachment with mental health problems in isolation, most studies fail to examine the interaction between protective and risk factors such as parent-adolescent attachment and life events on mental health. Instead of concentrating on risks factors in isolation, increasing research attention is devoted to factors that promote health and their interaction with risk factors. This corresponds to research on resilience within the field of developmental psychology. Research on resilience focuses on adolescents who show positive developmental outcomes despite experiencing significant adversity [26], [27].

Social support, for example, is seen as one of these resilience factors and is theorized to protect adolescents from the impacts of stress. Support from parents is thought to operate by lessening the threat children experience when encountering stress, thereby leading to more adaptive coping efforts [28]. Finally, families who provide adequate support meet adolescent's needs for safety and security and may empower adolescents by bolstering their sense of self-esteem or control [29].

The parent-adolescent attachment relationship is another potential resilience factor that warrants further research attention. It is essential to understand the role that parent-adolescent attachment plays in the relationship between life events and mental health, because while life events often cannot be avoided, parent-adolescent attachment is amendable [30].

If a favourable parent-adolescent attachment could buffer the association between life events and mental health problems, this could help to distinguish vulnerable adolescents from those with good adaptation under extenuating circumstances, and could have implications for preventing and treating mental health problems in adolescents.

One initial study has examined the buffering role of multiple protective factors, including parental support, on mental health among adolescents with or without life events [31]. Wille et al. [31] compared the percentages of mental health problems in adolescents with different numbers of life events while taking into account the availability of protective factors. Protective factors were found to significantly buffer the association between adolescents exposed to one or two life events and mental health. Adolescents without a life event did not benefit from the availability of protective factors. The current study capitalizes on a large study and differs from Wille et al. by specifically quantifying the additional effect that the interaction between parent-child attachment and life events may have on mental health. In line with previous findings, we hypothesize that a favourable parent-adolescent attachment (i.e. the protective factor) will buffer the association between life events and mental health. The goals of this study were 1) to examine the association of negative life events and parent-adolescent attachment relationship quality with mental health problems and 2) to investigate if there is an interaction between the parent-adolescent attachment relationship and one or multiple negative life events on the mental health of adolescents.

9.2 METHODS

9.2.1 DESIGN AND PARTICIPANTS

A prospective study with a two-year follow-up was conducted as part of the Rotterdam Youth Monitor (RYM), a longitudinal youth health surveillance system. The RYM monitors the general health, well-being, behaviour and related factors of youth aged 0 to 19 years living in Rotterdam and the surrounding region in the Netherlands. The RYM is incorporated into the preventive care (regular health examinations) of the preventive youth healthcare system; the RYM is used to detect potential individual health risks and problems in order to take necessary preventive measures (including referrals for treatment).

The current study used RYM data from students at secondary schools. At baseline, the students were in the first year of secondary education (M_{age} = 12.5 years, SD = 0.62), and at follow-up (Year 2) in the third year (M_{age} = 14.3 years, SD = 0.58). Data were collected throughout the school year, except in the months of July and August (Dutch summer holidays). The students completed a baseline questionnaire between September 2008 and July 2009 and a follow-up questionnaire between September 2010 and July 2011. Administration of the questionnaire at schools was conducted by specially trained researchers and school nurses from the Municipal Public Health Service and/or by a teacher. In 2008–2009, 8,272 adolescents participated (95% participation rate), of whom 3,181 participated again in 2010–2011 (38%). The main reason for non-response at baseline was students' illness at the time of administering the questionnaire. The main reason for non-response at follow-up was that schools were not willing to participate at follow-up. Other reasons were: students had transferred to a school that did not participate at follow-up, students had repeated a school year or students were absent at the time of administering the follow-up questionnaire.

9.2.2 ETHICS STATEMENT

All data were gathered within and as part of the government approved routine health examinations of preventive youth health care; the RYM was completed on a voluntary basis; anonymous data were used in this study; separate informed consent was therefore not requested. Adolescents received verbal information on the RYM, each time it was applied; their parents received written information on the RYM, each time it was applied; both adolescents and their parents were free to object to participation.

9.2.3 MEASURES

Mental health problems. Mental health was assessed at follow-up by the Dutch self-report version of the Strengths and Difficulties Questionnaire

(SDQ) [32]–[36]. The SDQ consists of 25 items for describing positive and negative attributes of adolescents that can be allocated to five subscales of five items each. The subscales are: emotional problems, conduct problems, hyperactivity-inattention, peer problems, and prosocial behaviour. Each item has to be scored on a three-point scale, with 0 = 'not true', 1 = 'somewhat true', and 2 = 'certainly true'. A total difficulties score can be calculated by adding up the scores on the emotional problems, conduct problems, hyperactivity-inattention and peer problems subscales (range 0–40; current study $\alpha = 0.74$).

Two groups were created based on the total SDQ score: normal (cut-off point SDQ at follow-up ≤ 80th percentile; score ≤ 13) and borderline/abnormal mental health problems (cut-off point SDQ at follow-up > 80th percentile; score ≥ 14) [37]. Cut-off points were based on a previous large cross-national survey among 14–15 year old adolescents [1].

Life events. Adolescents were asked about 11 negative life events, which were measured using three different types of response categories. Each life event was assessed at baseline with one item. For six of the life events (i.e. chronic or severe illness of parent, chronic or severe illness of sibling, mental illness of parent, mental illness of sibling, addiction to alcohol, drugs and/or gambling of parent, addiction to alcohol, drugs and/or gambling of sibling), the possible responses were: not true, not currently true and true. For analysis, these items were dichotomized into: not (currently) true, and true. For two life events (i.e. regular conflicts between parents, parental divorce), possible responses were: not experienced, experienced > 2 years ago and experienced ≤ 2 years ago. For analysis, regular conflicts between parents was dichotomized into: not experienced or > 2 years ago, and experienced ≤ 2 years ago. Parental divorce, as well as three other life events (i.e. unwanted pregnancy, victim of sexual abuse and victim of violence), were categorized as: no and yes.

A total life event score was calculated by adding up the dichotomized item scores. Subsequently, three groups were created based on the total life event scores: no life event, one life event or multiple life events.

Parent-adolescent attachment relationship. Parent-adolescent attachment relationship quality was measured at baseline using the "Family attachment scale" of The Communities That Care Youth Survey [38], [39]. This scale consists of six items: three items about the adolescent's relationship with the mother and three items about the relationship with the father.

The items were scored on the four-point scale using: NO!, no, yes, YES!. A total score could be calculated by taking the average of the six items (range 0 – 3; current study α = 0.82). This scale was dichotomized based on the sample distribution in this study: unfavourable parent-adolescent attachment (cut-off point < 20th percentile; score < 2.00) and favourable parent-adolescent attachment (cut-off point ≥ 20th percentile; score ≥ 2.00).

Confounders. Age, gender, ethnicity, and education level of the adolescent were measured at baseline and are incorporated in this study as potential confounders. For analysis purposes, confounders were dichotomized. Age was dichotomized into the categories below 13 years and 13 years or older. Education was categorized into two groups: basic or theoretical pre-vocational education, and general secondary/pre-university education [40]. Ethnicity was classified as Dutch or non-Dutch. In accordance with the definitions of Statistics Netherlands [41], adolescents with at least one parent born outside the Netherlands were classified as non-Dutch.

9.2.4 STATISTICAL ANALYSIS

Descriptive statistics were calculated for general characteristics of the study population (Table 1). Differences in gender, age, ethnicity, education, life events and parent-adolescent attachment among adolescents with and without mental health problems were evaluated by chi-square test (Table 1). Binary logistic regression analyses were conducted to assess the association between life events, parent-adolescent attachment and mental health status at follow-up (Table 2).

Odds ratios (OR) and their corresponding 95% confidence intervals (95% CI) were calculated. First, bivariate analyses were used to assess the association between life events and mental health status at follow-up and to assess the association between parent-adolescent attachment and mental health status at follow-up, adjusting for confounders (i.e. age, gender ethnicity and education). Second, a multivariate analysis using an enter method was performed incorporating all life events, parent-adolescent attachment and all confounders. Life events were checked for multicollinearity (all Phi correlation coefficients ≤ 0.17). Because multicollinearity was not present among the life events, all life events were entered in the same model.

TABLE 1: General characteristics for the total study population at baseline and by mental health at follow-up (N = 3181).

| | Total | Mental health at follow-up | | P value (χ^2) |
| | | Normal | Borderline/ Abnormal | |
	(N = 3181)	(n = 2705)	(n = 476)	
Gender				
boys	51.0	52.2	44.3	0.002
Age (mean =12.5, SD = 0.62)				
<13 years	56.2	56.3	55.4	0.692
Ethnicity				
Dutch	48.4	49.0	44.6	0.076
Level of education				
Basic or theoretical pre-vocational education	50.1	48.3	60.7	<0.001
Life events				
Chronic or severe illness of parent	7.5	6.9	10.8	0.003
Chronic or severe illness of sibling	3.6	3.4	4.9	0.118
Mental illness of parent	2.4	1.7	5.9	<0.001
Mental illness of sibling	1.5	1.2	3.6	<0.001
Addiction to alcohol, drugs, and/or gambling of parent	2.9	2.1	7.6	<0.001
Addiction to alcohol, drugs, and/or gambling of sibling	1.6	1.4	2.5	0.082
Conflicts between parents	26.9	25.0	37.6	<0.001
Parental divorce	17.4	16.1	25.1	<0.001
Unwanted pregnancy	0.4	0.3	1.3	0.003
Victim of sexual abuse	1.3	0.9	3.2	<0.001
Victim of violence	4.9	3.6	12.0	<0.001
Number of life events				<0.001[a]
No life event	52.3	55.0	36.6	
One life event	32.0	32.2	31.2	
Multiple life events	15.7	12.9	32.1	
Parent-adolescent attachment				
Unfavorable	12.2	10.2	23.5	<0.001

[a]*The three groups with different number of life events differed significantly from each other, with the no life event group displaying the least mental health problems (10.4%) and the multiple life events group showing the highest rate of mental health problems (30.3%).*

TABLE 2: Bivariate and multivariate associations of life events and parent-adolescent attachment with mental health problems (N = 3181).

	Bivariate[1]		Multivariate[1]	
	OR	95% CI	OR	95% CI
Life events				
Chronic or severe illness of parent	**1.57**	**1.13–2.19****	1.34	0.94–1.90
Chronic or severe illness of sibling	1.43	0.89–2.29	1.23	0.75–2.04
Mental illness of parent	**3.37**	**2.08–5.47*****	**1.86**	**1.08–3.21***
Mental illness of sibling	**2.97**	**1.63–5.44*****	1.91	0.98–3.73
Addiction of parent	**3.64**	**2.36–5.63*****	**2.34**	**1.45–3.79****
Addiction of sibling	1.58	0.82–3.06	0.82	0.39–1.71
Conflicts between parents	**1.85**	**1.50–2.27*****	**1.51**	**1.21–1.88*****
Parental divorce	**1.64**	**1.30–2.08*****	1.25	0.97–1.62
Unwanted pregnancy	**4.22**	**1.44–12.33****	2.17	0.63–7.45
Victim of sexual abuse	**3.02**	**1.56–5.83****	1.11	0.50–2.50
Victim of violence	**3.66**	**2.59–5.19*****	**2.51**	**1.69–3.70*****
Unfavorable parent-adolescent attachment	**2.65**	**2.07–3.40*****	**2.03**	**1.55–2.65*****
Nagelkerke R²			0.10	

[1]*Bivariate and multivariate analyses included confounders: age, sex, ethnicity, and education level. *p<0.05, **p<0.01, ***p<0.001. Note: bold numbers indicated significant P-values.*

To study if and to what extent parent-adolescent attachment modified the effect of one life event or multiple life events on mental health status, interaction effects were analysed on the additive scale (Table 3). Interaction on an additive scale means that the combined effect of two risk factors is different from (larger or smaller than) the sum of the individual effects of the factors [42]. Because we included a protective factor in our study, i.e. parent-adolescent attachment, this factor was recoded to a risk factor before calculating the interaction effect [42]. As a measure of interaction on the additive scale we present the Relative Excess Risk due to Interaction (RERI) and their 95% confidence intervals, using the delta method in Excel [43], [44]. RERI considers absolute risk and is positive (> 0) when the joint effect of risk factors is greater than the product of the effects of the individual factors. RERIs were calculated with mental health status as outcome measure at follow-up. RERIs are calculated using the following formula [42]:

TABLE 3: Interaction effect of parent-adolescent attachment and life events on mental health (N = 3181).

Life events	Parent-adolescent attachment	Mental health		OR	95% CI	RERI	95% CI
		Total	Borderline/Abnormal				
		n	n				
One life event	Not present[1]	Favorable	1532	157	1.00		1.56	0.15–2.96
	Not present[1]	Unfavorable	101	13	1.29	0.70–2.36		
	Present	Favorable	850	105	1.23	0.95–1.60		
	Present	Unfavorable	143	38	3.07	2.04–4.63		
Multiple life events	Not present[1]	Favorable	1532	157	1.00		3.32	0.80–5.84
	Not present[1]	Unfavorable	101	13	1.29	0.70–2.37		
	Present	Favorable	360	92	2.86	2.14–3.84		
	Present	Unfavorable	131	57	6.47	4.39–9.55		

Analyses included confounders: age, sex, ethnicity, and education level. [1]The reference group is no life event.

$$RERI = OR_{A+B+} - OR_{A+B-} - OR_{A-B+} + 1$$

RERI = 0 means no interaction or exact additivity; RERI > 0 means positive interaction or more than additivity; RERI < 0 means negative interaction or less than additivity; RERI can range from − infinity to + infinity.

As part of this analysis we also calculated the proportion attributable to interaction (proportion of the combined effect that is due to interaction) using the following formula [42]:

$$AP = RERI/OR_{A+B+}$$

$AP = 0$ means no interaction or exact additivity; $AP > 0$ means positive interaction or more than additivity; $AP < 0$ means negative interaction or less than additivity; AP can range from -1 to +1.

Analyses were conducted using SPPS version 20 and Excel. Results were considered significant at $p<0.05$.

Non-response analysis. A comparison of adolescents included in this study (N = 3181) with adolescents who were excluded due to non-partic-ipation at follow-up (N = 5091) did not indicate significant differences in terms of gender ($\chi^2 = 0.70$; p = 0.40) and parent-adolescent attachment ($\chi^2 = 1.20$; p = 0.27). However, differences were found with regards to educa-tion, age, ethnicity and life events, with the excluded group being lower educated ($\chi^2 = 151.53$; p<0.001), older ($\chi^2 = 5.94$; p<0.05), more often of Dutch ethnicity ($\chi^2 = 47.68$; p<0.001), and with more life events ($\chi^2 = 55.22$; p<0.001) than the adolescents who were included.

9.3 RESULTS

9.3.1 DESCRIPTIVE INFORMATION

As can be seen in Table 1, the average age of adolescents in the current sample was 12.5 years (SD = 0.62); 51.0% of the sample consisted of boys and 48.4% was of Dutch ethnicity. Regular conflicts between parents during the past two years was the most frequently reported life event that adolescents had experi-enced (26.9%). At baseline, 32.0% of the adolescents reported one life event and 15.7% reported multiple life events. Girls and lower educated adolescents had significantly more mental health problems at follow-up than boys ($\chi^2 = 10.04$; p = 0.002) and higher educated adolescents ($\chi^2 = 25.03$; p<0.001).

9.3.2 LIFE EVENTS AND MENTAL HEALTH STATUS

Table 1 shows the distribution of specific life events and the number of life events for the total sample, and for adolescents with normal and borderline/abnormal mental health at follow-up. The three groups with different numbers of life events differed significantly from each other ($\chi^2 = 118.82$; $p<0.001$), with the no life event group displaying the least mental health problems (10.4%) and the multiple life events group showing the highest rate of mental health problems (30.3%).

The presence of each specific life event, with the exception of Chronic or severe illness of sibling and Addiction of sibling, was related to a significantly increased risk of mental health problems in bivariate analyses (Table 2). After adjusting for other life events and parent-adolescent attachment, all ORs decreased and only Addiction of a parent, Mental illness of a parent, Conflicts between parents and Victim of violence were still significantly associated with mental health problems.

9.3.3 PARENT-ADOLESCENT ATTACHMENT RELATIONSHIP AND MENTAL HEALTH STATUS

An unfavourable parent-adolescent attachment at baseline was related to an increased risk of mental health problems at follow-up (see Table 2). After adjusting for the life events, the OR remained significant (OR 2.03; 95% CI 1.55 – 2.65).

9.3.4 INTERACTION EFFECT OF PARENT-ADOLESCENT ATTACHMENT RELATIONSHIP AND LIFE EVENTS ON MENTAL HEALTH

As shown in Table 3, parent-adolescent attachment interacts with life events on mental health outcome. The combined effect of an unfavourable parent-adolescent attachment and life events on mental health was larger than the sum of the two individual effects. An unfavourable parent-adolescent attachment was associated with a higher risk of mental health problems among adolescents with one life event (RERI 1.56; 95% CI 0.15 – 2.96) and multiple life events (RERI 3.32; 95% CI 0.80 – 5.84) compared to those without a life event. Figure 1 displays the parent-adolescent attachment—multiple life events interaction effect on mental health outcome. The proportion of the combined effect that is due to interaction (AP) was 0.51 in the group with an unfavourable parent-adolescent attachment and one life event, and 0.51 in the group with an unfavourable parent-adolescent attachment and multiple life events. This indicates that 51% of the combined effect can be attributed to the interaction between parent-adolescent attachment and life events. Interaction analyses were repeated for the subgroups of age, gender, ethnicity and education; these analyses yielded similar results (data not shown, results available upon request).

9.4 DISCUSSION

This study shows that negative life events and parent-adolescent attachment relationship quality were associated with mental health problems in adolescents. More importantly, an interaction between the parent-adolescent attachment relationship and one and multiple life events on adolescents' mental health was found.

This study confirms the results of earlier studies indicating a clear relationship between life events and mental health problems among adolescents [11]–[19]. A particularly high impact on mental health was observed among victims of violence. Consistent with other studies, some life events were found to no longer be significantly linked to mental health after controlling for the other life events [31], thus reflecting that some life events often co-occur. Higher rates of mental health problems were shown when multiple life events occurred together. This is also in line with previous studies, suggesting a higher probability of mental health problems when several life events accumulate [31], [45]. Furthermore, the results fit with indications by other studies that a favourable parent-adolescent attachment may be a protective factor for mental health problems in adolescents [20]–[25].

We were particularly interested in the interaction effects of parent-adolescent attachment and life events on mental health because most studies fail to examine this effect. An interaction effect of parent-adolescent attachment and life events on mental health was observed in this study. The combined effect of an unfavourable parent-adolescent attachment and life events on mental health was larger than the sum of the two individual effects, with more than half of the combined effect being due to the interaction. Thus, it seems important to not only look at direct associations, but also to assess the presence of an interaction between these factors in future research. In line with our hypothesis, these results seems to suggest that a favourable parent-adolescent attachment may serve as a buffer on the association between one or multiple life events and the mental health of adolescents. A potential explanation of the interaction found in this study could be that a favourable parent-adolescent attachment enhances adolescent's coping abilities. Coping theory suggests that when individuals encounter potentially stressful situations one of the things they do is to evaluate their resources (e.g. parent-adolescent relationship) to handle the situation [46]. In this appraisal process, if individuals decide their internal or external resources are adequate to handle the situation, then they are not likely to feel threatened and thereby leading to more adaptive coping efforts. So, when adolescents are experiencing life events they possible could better cope with these life events if they have a favourable parent-adolescents attachment instead of an unfavourable parent-adolescent attachment.

Among adolescents who reported no life events, there was no association between the quality of the parent-adolescent attachment and their mental health status. This is in line with the findings from Wille et al. [31]. An explanation could be that individuals only benefit from protective factors, such as a favourable parent-adolescent attachment, in the presence of a risk factor [26].

There are strengths and limitations to this study that have to be mentioned. One strength of this study is that it was embedded in a longitudinal study. Also, the data set provided a unique opportunity to explore relations between particular variables of interest within a large sample. An innovative aspect of this study is that it looked not only at direct associations among the variables of interest but also at interaction effects.

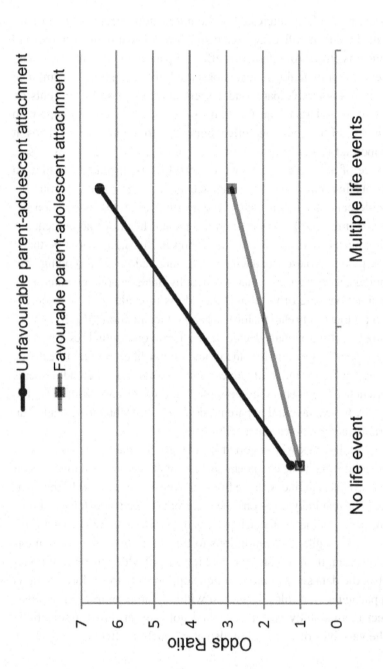

FIGURE 1: Interaction effect of parent-adolescent attachment and multiple life events on mental health.

However, this study also has some limitations. First, adolescents were excluded due to non-participation at follow-up. In a non-response analysis we showed that the excluded group was lower educated, older and more often of Dutch ethnicity. Although we included these variables as confounders in our analyses, the current findings should be generalized with caution, and we propose replication in large and varied populations. Second, as with any self-report survey, adolescents' self-report could be biased. Although it would have been preferably to use multiple informants, research suggests that adolescents are better reporters of their own mental health status than parents and teacher. For example, adolescents' self-reported mental health status corresponded better with independent psychiatric assessment than parent or teacher [47]. Nevertheless, results of this study have to be interpreted with caution and we recommend future studies to use multiple informants. Third, a total life event score was calculated, which makes it not possible to distinguish, for example, the interaction between parent-adolescent attachment and life events that are (at least partly) related to the adolescents' own behaviour (behaviour-dependent events), such as conflicts with parents or peers, and those that are independent of their behaviour (behaviour-independent), such as natural disasters. Therefore we cannot distinguish if a favourable parent-adolescent attachment may be particularly beneficial for adolescents exposed to particular life events, and/or not beneficial for adolescents exposed to other life events.

Furthermore, as our main aim was to predict the occurrence of mental health problems at follow-up. Therefore, we choose not to adjust for baseline mental health in the analyses because this would have only allow us to draw conclusions about the influences of an unfavourable parent-adolescent attachment and life events on changes in mental health between follow-up and baseline. In that case, we would not have taken into account the impact that an unfavourable parent-adolescent attachment and life events already had on the mental health of adolescents at baseline. The unfavourable parent-adolescent attachment and life events could have been present earlier than at baseline. So, due to the nature of our research question (i.e. about the occurrence of mental health), and not changes in mental health (i.e. incidence), we did not adjust for baseline mental health in this study. Thereby, we studied whether there is a long term relationship and interaction effect between parent-adolescent attachment, life events and mental health. However, it must be noted that causality cannot be inferred from these analyses, because it is unknown for example whether mental health problems were already present when life events occurred or wether life events, parent-adolescent attachment and mental health problems have mutually influenced each other.

To disentangle the questions posed above, future research with a prospective design that enables researchers to examine the temporal ordering of the variables is needed. However, this is difficult, because life events and mental health issues are often already present at very young age. Long-term longitudinal cohort studies that follow children from fetal life onwards are therefore desirable. Furthermore, better understanding of why the parent-adolescent attachment could serve as a buffer on the relation between life events and mental health problems is necessary. As we mentioned before, it is possible, for example, that a favourable parent-adolescent attachment enhance adolescent's coping abilities, which mediates the relation between life events and mental health problems. Therefore, future studies should integrate moderator and mediator research by testing for specific mediators (e.g. threat or coping abilities) in relation to parent-adolescent attachment as a moderator, so that we can further test our hypotheses and better understand the complex way in which life events affect the mental health of adolescents. Further, experimental studies in which the parental-adolescent attachment will be enhanced by an intervention can give more information about the causal influence the parent-adolescent attachment relationship may have on mental health problems.

In conclusion, results from the current study support earlier studies indicating an association of negative life events and parent-adolescent attachment with mental health problems. Results also support an interaction effect between parent-adolescent attachment and negative life events on mental health. This seems to support the hypothesis that a favourable parent-adolescent attachment relationship may serve as a buffer for adolescents with one or multiple life events. However, conclusions about causality cannot be drawn from this study and examining the effects of life events and an unfavourable parent-adolescent attachment on adolescents' mental health simplifies the complex processes in the development of mental health problems in which a large number of factors play a role. Nonetheless, it enables the identification of adolescents with a high probability of displaying disturbed development. Adolescents with one or multiple life events and an unfavourable parent-adolescent attachment seems to be a vulnerable group for mental health problems. Future research needs to continue to probe the reasons why some adolescents with life events are functioning better than others. This knowledge would be helpful in designing effective prevention and intervention programs for adolescents exposed to life events.

REFERENCES

1. van Dorsselaer S, de Looze M, Vermeulen-Smit E, de Roos S, Verdurmen J, et al.. (2009) Gezondheid, welzijn en opvoeding van jongeren in Nederland. Utrecht: Trimbos-instituut, Universiteit Utrecht, Sociaal en cultureel planbureau.
2. Costello EJ, Pine DS, Hammen C, March JS, Plotsky PM, et al. (2002) Development and natural history of mood disorders. Biol Psychiatry 52: 529–542. doi: 10.1016/s0006-3223(02)01372-0
3. Jaycox LH, Stein BD, Paddock S, Miles JN, Chandra A, et al. (2009) Impact of teen depression on academic, social, and physical functioning. Pediatrics 124: e596–605. doi: 10.1542/peds.2008-3348
4. Suicide and suicide attempts in adolescents. Committee on Adolescents. American Academy of Pediatrics. Pediatrics 105: 871–874. doi: 10.1542/peds.105.4.871
5. Fergusson DM, Woodward LJ (2002) Mental health, educational, and social role outcomes of adolescents with depression. Arch Gen Psychiatry 59: 225–231. doi: 10.1001/archpsyc.59.3.225
6. Pine DS, Cohen P, Gurley D, Brook J, Ma Y (1998) The risk for early-adulthood anxiety and depressive disorders in adolescents with anxiety and depressive disorders. Arch Gen Psychiatry 55: 56–64. doi: 10.1001/archpsyc.55.1.56
7. Kim-Cohen J, Caspi A, Moffitt TE, Harrington H, Milne BJ, et al. (2003) Prior juvenile diagnoses in adults with mental disorder: developmental follow-back of a prospective-longitudinal cohort. Arch Gen Psychiatry 60: 709–717. doi: 10.1001/archpsyc.60.7.709
8. Hofstra MB, van der Ende J, Verhulst FC (2002) Child and adolescent problems predict DSM-IV disorders in adulthood: a 14-year follow-up of a Dutch epidemiological sample. J Am Acad Child Adolesc Psychiatry 41: 182–189. doi: 10.1097/00004583-200202000-00012
9. Compas BE (1987) Coping with stress during childhood and adolescence. Psychol Bull 101: 393–403. doi: 10.1037//0033-2909.101.3.393
10. Grant KE, Compas BE, Thurm AE, McMahon SD, Gipson PY, et al. (2006) Stressors and child and adolescent psychopathology: evidence of moderating and mediating effects. Clin Psychol Rev 26: 257–283. doi: 10.1016/j.cpr.2005.06.011
11. Barkmann C, Romer G, Watson M, Schulte-Markwort M (2007) Parental physical illness as a risk for psychosocial maladjustment in children and adolescents:

epidemiological findings from a National Survey in Germany. Psychosomatics 48: 226–236. doi: 10.1176/appi.psy.48.6.476

12. Hammen C, Burge D, Burney E, Adrian C (1990) Longitudinal study of diagnoses in children of women with unipolar and bipolar affective disorder. Arch Gen Psychiatry 47: 1112–1117. doi: 10.1001/archpsyc.1990.01810240032006

13. Rutter M, Quinton D (1984) Parental psychiatric disorder: effects on children. Psychol Med 14: 853–880. doi: 10.1017/s0033291700019838

14. Diaz R, Gual A, García M, Arnau J, Pascual F, et al. (2008) Children of alcoholics in Spain: from risk to pathology: results from the ALFIL program. Soc Psychiatry Psychiatr Epidemiol 43: 1–10. doi: 10.1007/s00127-007-0264-2

15. Hanson RF, Self-Brown S, Fricker-Elhai A, Kilpatrick DG, Saunders BE, et al. (2006) Relations among parental substance use, violence exposure and mental health: the national survey of adolescents. Addict Behav 31: 1988–2001. doi: 10.1016/j.addbeh.2006.01.012

16. Amato PR (2001) Children of divorce in the 1990s: an update of the Amato and Keith (1991) meta-analysis. J Fam Psychol 15: 355–370. doi: 10.1037/0893-3200.15.3.355

17. Jenkins JM, Smith MA (1991) Marital disharmony and children's behaviour problems: aspects of a poor marriage that affect children adversely. J Child Psychol Psychiatry 32: 793–810. doi: 10.1111/j.1469-7610.1991.tb01903.x

18. Herrenkohl TI, Kosterman R, Hawkins JD, Mason WA (2009) Effects of growth in family conflict in adolescence on adult depressive symptoms: mediating and moderating effects of stress and school bonding. J Adolesc Health 44: 146–152. doi: 10.1016/j.jadohealth.2008.07.005

19. Hofferth SL, Reid L (2002) Early childbearing and children's achievement and behavior over time. Perspect Sex Reprod Health 34: 41–49. doi: 10.2307/3030231

20. Werner EE (1997) Vulnerable but invincible: high-risk children from birth to adulthood. Acta Paediatr Suppl 422: 103–105.

21. Herrenkohl TI, Lee JO, Kosterman R, Hawkins JD (2012) Family influences related to adult substance use and mental health problems: a developmental analysis of child and adolescent predictors. J Adolesc Health 51: 129–135. doi: 10.1016/j.jadohealth.2011.11.003

22. Lewinsohn PM, Rohde P, Seeley JR, Klein DN, Gotlib IH (2000) Natural course of adolescent major depressive disorder in a community sample: predictors of recurrence in young adults. Am J Psychiatry 157: 1584–1591. doi: 10.1176/appi.ajp.157.10.1584

23. Reinherz HZ, Giaconia RM, Pakiz B, Silverman AB, Frost AK, et al. (1993) Psychosocial risks for major depression in late adolescence: a longitudinal community study. J Am Acad Child Adolesc Psychiatry 32: 1155–1163. doi: 10.1097/00004583-199311000-00007

24. Prinstein MJ, Boergers J, Spirito A, Little TD, Grapentine WL (2000) Peer functioning, family dysfunction, and psychological symptoms in a risk factor model for adolescent inpatients' suicidal ideation severity. J Clin Child Psychol 29: 392–405. doi: 10.1207/s15374424jccp2903_10

25. Walsh SD, Harel-Fish Y, Fogel-Grinvald H (2010) Parents, teachers and peer relations as predictors of risk behaviors and mental well-being among immigrant and

Israeli born adolescents. Social Science & Medicine 70: 976–984. doi: 10.1016/j. socscimed.2009.12.010

26. Masten AS, Reed M-GJ (2002) Resilience in development. In: Snyder CR, Lopez SJ, editors. The handbook of positive psychology. Oxford: University Press. pp. 74–88.

27. Rutter M (1979) Protective factors in children's responoses to stress and disadvantage. In: Kent MW, Rolf JE, editors. Primary prevention in psychopathology: social competence in children. Hanover: University Press of New England. pp. 49–74.

28. Kliewer W, Sandler IN, Wolchik SA (1994) Family socialization of threat appraisal and coping: coaching, modeling, and family context. In: Nestmann F, Hurrelmann K, editors. Social networks and social support in childhood and adolescence. Berlin: Walter de Gruyter. pp. 271–291.

29. Sandler IN, Miller P, Short J, Wolchik SA (1989) Social support as a protective factor for children in stress. In: Belle D, editor. Children's social networks and social supports. New York: Wiley. pp. 277–301.

30. Toumbourou JW, Gregg ME (2002) Impact of an empowerment-based parent education program on the reduction of youth suicide risk factors. J Adolesc Health 31: 277–285. doi: 10.1016/s1054-139x(02)00384-1

31. Wille N, Bettge S, Ravens-Sieberer U (2008) group Bs (2008) Risk and protective factors for children's and adolescents' mental health: results of the BELLA study. Eur Child Adolesc Psychiatry 17 Suppl 1 133–147. doi: 10.1007/s00787-008-1015-y

32. Goodman R, Ford T, Simmons H, Gatward R, Meltzer H (2000) Using the Strengths and Difficulties Questionnaire (SDQ) to screen for child psychiatric disorders in a community sample. Br J Psychiatry 177: 534–539. doi: 10.1080/0954026021000046128

33. Goodman R, Meltzer H, Bailey V (1998) The Strengths and Difficulties Questionnaire: a pilot study on the validity of the self-report version. Eur Child Adolesc Psychiatry 7: 125–130. doi: 10.1007/s007870050057

34. Muris P, Meesters C, van den Berg F (2003) The Strengths and Difficulties Questionnaire (SDQ)--further evidence for its reliability and validity in a community sample of Dutch children and adolescents. Eur Child Adolesc Psychiatry 12: 1–8. doi: 10.1007/s00787-003-0298-2

35. van Widenfelt BM, Goedhart AW, Treffers PD, Goodman R (2003) Dutch version of the Strengths and Difficulties Questionnaire (SDQ). Eur Child Adolesc Psychiatry 12: 281–289. doi: 10.1007/s00787-003-0341-3

36. Janssens A, Deboutte D (2009) Screening for psychopathology in child welfare: the Strengths and Difficulties Questionnaire (SDQ) compared with the Achenbach System of Empirically Based Assessment (ASEBA). Eur Child Adolesc Psychiatry 18: 691–700. doi: 10.1007/s00787-009-0030-y

37. Scoring the SDQ. Instructions in English for scoring self-rated SDQs by hand. Available: http://www.sdqinfo.org/py/sdqinfo/c0.py. Accessed 19 March 2013.

38. Arthur MW, Hawkins JD, Pollard JA, Catalano RF, Baglioni AJj (2002) Measuring risk and protective factors for substance use, delinquency, and other adolescent problem behaviors. The Communities That Care Youth Survey. Evaluation review 26: 575–601. doi: 10.1177/019384102237850

39. Jonkman H, Boers R, van Dijk B, Rietveld M (2006) Wijken gewogen. Gedrag van jongeren in kaart gebracht. Amsterdam: SWP.

40. van de Looij-Jansen PM, de Wilde EJ, Mieloo CL, Donker MC, Verhulst FC (2009) Seasonal variation in self-reported health and health-related behaviour in Dutch adolescents. Public Health 123: 686–688. doi: 10.1016/j.puhe.2009.07.015

41. Centraal Bureau voor de Statistiek. Allochtoon. Available: http://www.cbs.nl/nl-NL/menu/methoden/begrippen/default.htm?ConceptID=37. Accessed 19 March 2013.

42. Knol MJ, VanderWeele TJ, Groenwold RH, Klungel OH, Rovers MM, et al. (2011) Estimating measures of interaction on an additive scale for preventive exposures. Eur J Epidemiol 26: 433–438. doi: 10.1007/s10654-011-9554-9

43. Andersson T, Alfredsson L, Kallberg H, Zdravkovic S, Ahlbom A (2005) Calculating measures of biological interaction. Eur J Epidemiol 20: 575–579. doi: 10.1007/s10654-005-7835-x

44. Hosmer DW, Lemeshow S (1992) Confidence interval estimation of interaction. Epidemiology 3: 452–456. doi: 10.1097/00001648-199209000-00012

45. Forehand R, Wierson M, Thomas AM, Armistead L, Kempton T, et al. (1991) The role of family stressors and parent relationships on adolescent functioning. J Am Acad Child Adolesc Psychiatry 30: 316–322. doi: 10.1097/00004583-199103000-00023

46. Lazarus RS, Folkman S (1984) Stress, appraisal, and coping. New York: Springer.

47. Rutter M (1986) The development of psychopathology of depression: issues and perspectives. In: Rutter M, Izard CE, Read PB, editors. Depression in young people: developmental and clinical perspectives. New York: Guilford Press.

CHAPTER 10

SUICIDAL BEHAVIORS IN DEPRESSED ADOLESCENTS: ROLE OF PERCEIVED RELATIONSHIPS IN THE FAMILY

ANGÈLE CONSOLI, HUGO PEYRE, MARIO SPERANZA, CHRISTINE HASSLER, BRUNO FALISSARD5, EVELYNE TOUCHETTE, DAVID COHEN, MARIE-ROSE MORO, AND ANNE RÉVAH-LÉVY

10.1 BACKGROUND

Suicide is the third leading cause of death in adolescents and young adults in the United States and the second leading cause in European countries [1]. Suicidal behaviors are also the most common reason for adolescent psychiatric hospitalizations in many countries [2]. Reducing suicide and suicide attempts is therefore a key public health target. In the United States, the death rate by suicide is 6.9/100 000 in adolescents aged 15 to 19 [3]. In France, recent epidemiological data showed that the suicide rate in adolescents aged 15 to 19 is 4.1/100 000 inhabitants [4]. Considerable variability exists among the European countries that published their statistics regarding death rates by suicide in 2008 [5]. Prevalence of suicidal

Suicidal Behaviors in Depressed Adolescents: Role of Perceived Relationships in the Family. Consoli A, Peyre H, Speranza M, Hassler C, Falissard B, Touchette E, Cohen D, Moro M-R, and Révah-Lévy A. Child and Adolescent Psychiatry and Mental Health, 7,8 (2013), doi:10.1186/1753-2000-7-8. Licensed under Creative Commons Attribution 2.0 Generic License, http://creativecommons.org/licenses/by/2.0/.

ideations ranges from 15 to 25% in the general population, whereas the lifetime estimates of suicide attempts among adolescents range from 1.3 to 3.8% in males and from 1.5 to 10.1% in females, with higher rates in females than in males in the older age range [6].

Current models of suicide phenomena in adolescents emphasize: (i) the importance of distinguishing suicidal ideation, non-suicidal self-harm, suicide attempt and completed suicide [7,8] (ii) the key role of depression in the transition from suicidal ideations to suicide attempts, in which depression is a strong proximal factor [9]; (iii) the fact that the numerous risk factors identified do not capture the whole risk leading to the idea that protective factors should be taken into account for suicide risk prediction [10]. Risk factors for completed and attempted suicide have been widely studied. First, psychiatric disorders are present in about 90% of suicidal adolescents [6]. Depressive disorders are consistently the most prevalent psychiatric disorder among adolescents who commit suicide with a prevalence ranging from 49% to 64% and among adolescents who attempt suicide [6,11,12]. Secondly, adolescents who attempted suicide in the past are up to 60 times more likely to commit suicide than those who have not [6]. Also, self-harm is an important predictor of future completed suicide [13]. Thirdly, substance abuse plays a significant role in adolescent suicide and in suicide attempts, especially in older adolescent males when it is comorbid with mood disorders or disruptive disorders [14,15]. Fourthly, social factors such as socio-economic status, school exclusion and social isolation have been also implicated [16,17]. Finally, several studies pointed a significant association with family factors, including family psychopathology, abuse, loss of a parent (death, divorce), intrafamilial relationships, familial cohesion, support and suicidality [16,18-20].

Indeed, the family factors, and especially the perceived quality of family relationships, have been pinpointed as an important risk or protective factor in clinical and community samples of adolescents [1,2,6,21-26]. However, only few population-based studies have examined family factors [19]. They showed several predictive or associated factors, like: poor family environment (low satisfaction with support, communication, leisure time, low parental monitoring) [27], low family support [28], low family cohesion [29], poor family functioning, poor parent–child attachment and problems of parental adjustment [1,19]. On the contrary, higher family cohesion has been reported as a protective factor against future suicide attempt [26] as well as having positive relationships with a parent [30,31]. Improved family connectedness was related to less severe depressive symptoms and suicidal ideation [32]. Nevertheless, equivocal findings exist with regard to the relationship between adolescents' suicidal behaviours and family variables. This is mainly due to methodological limitations, such as considering only parental marital status (e.g. [22]) or parents together (e.g. [33]), and ignoring other common risk factors from multivariate analysis (e.g. [16,19,34]). Moreover, data suggest a different effect of family factors on suicidal behaviours according to gender (e.g. [34]), clinical severity (e.g. [34]), parental marital status (e.g. [22]), dissatisfaction with relationship with parents (e.g. [33]), and different relationship with mother vs. father (e.g. [34]).

Notwithstanding these interesting results, the complex association between family factors, depression and suicidal behaviors among adolescents remains to be explored in samples large enough to allow multivariate analysis, so as to understand specific contributions (e.g. mother vs. father; conflict vs. no conflict; separation vs. no separation) taking into account other risk factors and severity of depression and suicidal behaviors. The aim of the present study was to assess the link between family factors and suicidal behaviors, adjusting for several potential confounding factors, in a large community-based sample of adolescents aged 17 years. Given that the prevalence of suicide differs substantially between boys and girls, we hypothesized that the impact of familial risk factors would differ according to gender. Similarly, given the role of current depression, we hypothesized that family risk would be related to depression severity, defined as depression associated with suicidal ideation in the last year and/ or life-time suicide attempt.

10.2 METHODS

10.2.1 PARTICIPANTS

Participants were recruited in a representative sample of young people from metropolitan France (i.e. all European parts of France, excluding overseas territories) between March 15th and March 31st 2008 during the National Defense Preparation Day *"Journée d'Appel de Préparation à la Défense"* (JAPD) [35]. The JAPD is a civic and military information session that is required of all adolescents aged 17, and required to sit public examinations (e.g., driving license, university exams). All 764,000 French adolescents aged 17 and living in metropolitan France in 2008 are called to participate in these national days in one of the 250 Centers [36]. Two days were randomly selected during which all adolescents (n=44, 733, 5.9%) were invited to participate anonymously in the Survey on Health and Behaviour: "Enquête sur la Santé et les Consommations lors de l'Appel de Préparation A la Défense" (ESCAPAD) [35,37], a cross-sectional survey conducted by the French Monitoring Center for Drugs and Drug Addictions or *"Observatoire Français des Drogues et des Toxicomanies"* (OFDT), and administered during JAPD days in collaboration with the Army National Service Office. The participation rate for this survey was 88.4%. Thus, the total sample included 36,757 French subjects living in metropolitan France (n=18,590 girls and 18,163 boys). This represents 4.8% of adolescents aged 17 living in metropolitan France. Among the total sample, we excluded adolescents without current depression but presenting suicidal ideations or a history of suicide attempts (n=5,328). We excluded these subjects because we were interested in studying the role of current depression as a proximal variable of suicidality and its association with familial risk factors. Our sample finally included n=31,429 adolescents (see flowchart in Figure 1). The same analyses conducted in this study were additionally performed on the excluded sample, and showed similar results for family risk factor (see Additional file 1: Figure S1). The survey obtained the public statistics general interest and statistical quality seal from "Comité National de l'Information Statistique" (CNIS) as well as the approval of ethics committee.

10.2.2 ASSESSMENT

The ESCAPAD survey is a self-administered questionnaire which takes 35 minutes to complete. The response rates for socio-demographic characteristics, familial variables, suicidal behaviors and potential confounding factors were higher than 90%.

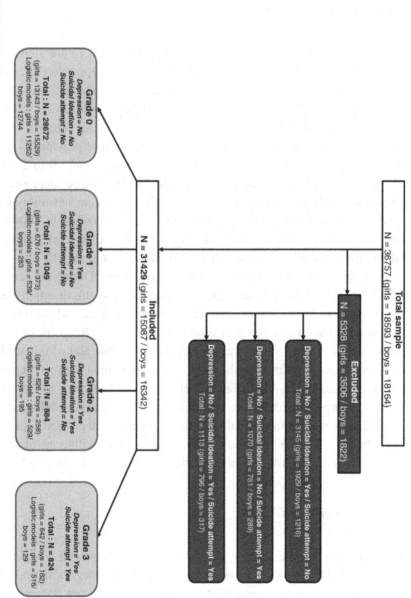

FIGURE 1: Flowchart.

10.2.3 DEPRESSION, SUICIDAL IDEATION, AND SUICIDE ATTEMPTS

Current depression was assessed using the "Adolescent Depression Rating Scale" (ADRS), specifically developed to assess depression intensity among adolescents. This scale has been previously validated on young people aged 12 to 20 and published with an official cut-off [38]. It is a 10-item self-administered questionnaire with yes/no responses concerning the two weeks preceding completion. The sum of item scores provides a score that divides the population into three distinct groups: score 0 to 2 "not depressed", 3 to 5 "sub-threshold depression", and 6 or more "depressed". The cut-off of 6 was chosen because it provides maximum sensitivity and specificity in screening for major depressive states according to DSM-IV with clinically relevant intensity corresponding to a CGI score (Clinical Global Impression) of 5 or more (i.e. markedly ill or more) [38].

Suicidal ideations were measured by one question: "During the past 12 months, have you had suicidal thoughts?" Responses to this question were never, once, and several times. Suicide attempts (SA) were also explored by one question: "Have you ever tried to kill yourself?" Responses to this question were: never, once, and several times. For the aim of our study, three groups were defined on the basis of the association between depression (i.e. score > 6 on ADRS) and levels of suicidal severity, as follows: grade 1: depressed without suicidal ideation and without suicidal attempt, grade 2: depressed with suicidal ideations and grade 3: depressed with suicide attempts. The control group included adolescents with none of these problems (i.e. < 6 ADRS, no suicidal ideations nor suicide attempts).

10.2.4 FAMILY FACTORS

Parental status was measured by the question: "Do your parents live together?" answered by yes or no. Parental harmony had four categorical levels: 1) Living together and good agreement, 2) Separated and discord, 3) Separated and good agreement, and 4) Living together and discord, and was measured by the combination of two questions: 1) "Do your parents live together?" answered by yes or no and 2) "How your parents get along?" with responses scored on a 4-point Likert scale which were dichotomized to increase the clinical relevance of results (i.e."very well, well, and fairly well" and "badly, and very badly"). The quality of the perceived relationship with the mother and with the father was assessed by the questions: "How do you get along with your mother?" and "How do you get along with your father?" on the same Likert scales and with the same dichotomization as the previous variable. Cohabitation status was measured by a yes or no answer to the question: "Do you live with your parents most of the time?"

10.2.5 POTENTIAL CONFOUNDING VARIABLES

The following covariates were included because of their potential association with depression, suicidal ideations and suicidal behaviors in adolescence. First, the adolescent's educational level was assessed in three categories: 1) normal high school attainment, 2) vocational school or apprenticeship and 3) out of school. Secondly, repeat school years were explored via a specific question (it can be noted that it is a more frequent practice in France than in the US and other European countries). Thirdly, socio-economic status (SES) was based on the higher occupational category of the two parents reported by the adolescent, based on the typology of the National institute for statistics and economic studies [39] and grouped into 4 categories: 1) managerial, or intellectual professions, 2) small to medium business owners or farmers, 3) manual, office or sales workers, and 4) unemployed. Finally, alcohol consumption was measured with a cut-off of 10 times or more per month, regular smoking was assessed with a cut-off of 11 cigarettes per day, and cannabis use was measured with a cut-off of 10 times or more per year [40]. These cut-off have been determined by the French Monitoring Center for Drugs and Drug Addictions or "*Observatoire Français des Drogues et des Toxicomanies*" (OFDT).

10.2.6 STATISTICAL ANALYSES

The prevalence rates for depression, suicidal ideations, suicide attempts and suicide risk severity were calculated by frequencies. Statistical analyses were performed separately for boys and girls on SAS V9.2. Chi-square tests were used to compare adolescent characteristics between suicide risk severity subgroups and family factors variables. Multivariate regressions were performed to assess the association between suicide risk severity and familial context variables adjusted on educational level, repeat school years, SES status, alcohol, tobacco, and cannabis use. A significant difference was considered to exist at $p < 0.05$. Odds Ratios were calculated with their 95% Confidence Interval.

10.3 RESULTS

10.3.1 SOCIO-DEMOGRAPHIC CHARACTERISTICS, FAMILY FACTORS AND CLINICAL DATA

The sample (n=31,429) included 49.7% girls and 50.3% boys. The mean age was 17.4 years ±0.3. A large majority of the sample (98%) had followed classic or vocational school educational career at age 17. Around 44% had repeated a school year at least once. 7.2% of the parents were unemployed. Regarding family factors, 87.8% of the adolescents were living in their parents' home and 12.2% of adolescents reported not living with their parents at age 17. In the entire sample, nearly 5% reported a negative relationship with their mother and 11.8% with their father. There were 24.4% of adolescents who had separated parents. When the parents were living together, 12.1% of the adolescents reported negative parental harmony.

Regarding substance use, we found that 7.8% of the adolescents were tobacco users, 8.9% were alcohol users and 13.5% were marijuana users. For depression, 7.5% of the adolescents had ADRS scores compatible with current depression (10.4% of the girls versus 4.5% of the boys, Chi-2=466, df =1, p<.001). Sixteen percent reported suicidal ideations (of whom 9.4% reported having suicidal ideations once and 6.8% reported having suicidal ideations several times) in the past 12 months. Eight percent reported lifetime suicide attempts (of whom 5.6% reported one suicide attempt and 2.7% several). The results are presented in Table 1.

10.3.2 SUICIDE RISK SEVERITY GRADE COMBINING DEPRESSION AND SUICIDALITY

Three severity subgroups were defined: grade 1 (n=1049, 3.4%) were depressed without suicidal ideations or attempts, grade 2 (n=884, 2.8%) were depressed and reported suicidal ideations but no suicide attempts, and grade 3 (n=824, 2.6%) were depressed and reported suicide attempts. The control group, grade 0, included 28,672 adolescents (91.2%) who were not depressed and had not reported suicide ideation in the past year or lifetime SA. The results are presented in Table 2.

10.3.3 ASSOCIATIONS BETWEEN FAMILY VARIABLES AND SEVERITY GRADE OF SUICIDE RISK ADJUSTING FOR EDUCATIONAL LEVEL, REPEAT SCHOOL YEARS, SOCIO-ECONOMIC STATUS AND SUBSTANCE USE

Associations between family variables, educational data, substance use and suicide risk severity grade combining depression and suicidality were assessed using multivariate analysis. Three severity subgroups were defined: grade 1 (depressed without suicidal ideations or attempts), grade 2 (depressed with suicidal ideations) and grade 3 (depressed with suicide attempts). The control group, grade 0, included adolescents not depressed and without suicidal ideations or attempts. We ran a series of multivariate logistic regression analyses to assess the association between suicide risk severity and family factors adjusted on educational level, repeated school years, SES status and substance use. In the model 1, the dependant variable was grade 1 versus grade 0, in the model 2: grade 2 versus grade 0 and in the model 3: grade 3 versus grade 0. Models were performed separately for boys and girls. Backward selection was used until all remaining variables had a p value <0.1. A significant difference was considered to exist at $p < 0.05$. Odds Ratios were calculated with their 95% Confidence Interval. The results are presented in Figures 2.

TABLE 1: Socio-demographic characteristics, family factors and clinical data

		Total (N=31429)		Girls (N=15087)		Boys (N=16342)	
		N	%	N	%	N	%
Socio-demographic characteristics							
Education	Typical or vocational school	37817	97.9	18988	98.5	18829	97.37
	Out of school	799	2.1	290	1.5	509	2.63
Grade repetition	No	21894	55.6	11903	60.8	9991	50.5
	Yes	17467	44.4	7677	39.2	9790	49.5
Parental occupation status	Working	34767	92.8	17416	92.4	17351	93.2
	Unmployed	2702	7.2	1439	7.6	1263	6.8
Family factors							
Not living at parent's home	Yes	4785	12.2	2306	11.9	2479	12.6
	No	34293	87.8	17136	88.1	17157	87.4
Negative relationship with the mother	Yes	1860	4.8	1039	5.3	821	4.2
	No	37232	95.2	18428	94.7	18804	95.8
Negative relationship with the father	Yes	4584	11.8	2656	13.8	1928	9.9
	No	34112	88.2	16598	86.2	17514	90.1
Parental status and harmony	Parents living together/ positive relationship	22731	63.5	11074	61.8	11657	65.1
	Separated parents/ negative relationship	6030	16.8	3149	17.6	2881	16.1
	Separated parents/ positive relationship	2713	7.6	1228	6.9	1485	8.3
	Parents living together/ negative relationship	4346	12.1	2457	13.7	1889	10.6
Drug use							
Alcohol use	No	35663	91.1	18729	96.0	16934	86.3
	Yes	3473	8.9	784	4.0	2689	13.7
Tabacco use	No	35856	92.2	18193	93.7	17663	90.8
	Yes	3023	7.8	1227	6.3	1796	9.2

TABLE 1: *Cont.*

		Total (N=31429)		Girls (N=15087)		Boys (N=16342)	
		N	%	N	%	N	%
Marijuana use	No	33917	86.5	17813	91.2	16104	81.9
	Yes	5290	13.5	1725	8.8	3565	18.1
Depression and suicidal risk							
Depression	No	34637	92.5	16903	89.6	17734	95.5
	Yes	2816	7.5	1970	10.4	846	4.5
Suicidal ideations	No	31847	83.8	15115	78.8	16732	89.0
	Yes	6151	16.2	4074	21.2	2077	11.0
Suicidal attempts	No	35090	91.8	16971	88.0	18119	95.6
	Yes	3146	8.2	2317	12.0	829	4.4
Suicidal risk	Grade 0	28672	91.2	13143	87.1	15529	95.0
	Grade 1	1049	3.3	676	4.5	373	2.3
	Grade 2	884	2.8	626	4.1	258	1.6
	Grade 3	824	2.7	642	4.3		

Regarding girls (Figure 2), all substance use appeared to be associated with the severity grade combining depression and suicidality (grade 1=depressed without suicidal ideation and without suicidal attempts, grade 2=depressed with suicidal ideations and grade 3=depressed with suicide attempts). Tobacco use reported by girls was associated with greater likelihood of belonging to risk severity grades 2 and 3 compared to controls (OR=2.09 [1.55 – 2.81], p<0.05 for both). Marijuana use was more likely to be associated with severity grade 3 compared to controls (OR=2.09 [1.60 – 2.73], p<0.05). Regarding educational data, repeat school years was associated with greater likelihood of risk severity grades 1 and 3 compared to the control group (grade 1: OR=1.54 [1.28 – 1.83], p<0.05 and grade 3: OR=2.57 [2.13 – 3.11], p<0.05). Regarding family variables, girls reporting a negative maternal relationship were more at risk for all severity grades compared to controls (grade 1: OR=2.6 [1.84 – 3.73], p<0.05, grade 2: OR=4.4 [3.32 – 5.97], p<0.05 and grade 3: OR=4.9 [3.69 – 6.57], p<0.05). Girls reporting a negative paternal relationship were also more at risk for all severity grades compared to controls (grade 1: OR=1.7 [1.32 – 2.30], p<0.05, grade 2: OR=2.4 [1.91 – 3.14], p<0.05 and grade 3: OR=3 [2.38 – 4.85], p<0.05). We also found that girls reporting that their parents were living together but in parental discord were more at risk for all severity grades compared to controls (grade 1: OR=1.81 [1.42 – 2.29], p<0.05, grade 2: OR=2.02 [1.59 – 2.57], p<0.05 and grade 3: OR=2.26 [1.76 – 2.89], p<0.05). The odds ratios for most family variables increased with severity (Figure 3). No significant statistical difference was found for girls reporting that their parents were divorced but did not have a negative relationship compared to controls.

Results for boys (Figure 4) were very similar to those for girls. However, for boys two associations were slightly different regarding family factors. First, boys not living with their parents were significantly more likely to belong to grade 3 risk compared to controls (OR=1.9 [1.26 – 2.95], p<0.05). Second, having parents not living together and with a negative relationship was more associated with grade 2 risk compared to controls (OR=1.6 [1.10 – 2.38], p<0.05).

10.4 DISCUSSION

This study assessed the associations between depression, family factors and suicidality in a large representative community-based sample of adolescents aged 17 (n=39,542), adjusting for confounding variables. Given data in the literature regarding depression as a proximal risk factor in suicidality [9] and the relevance of classifying suicidality (ideations and suicide attempt) [7], we divided the sample into 3 grades of suicide risk severity combining depression and suicidality (grade 1=depressed without suicidal ideation and without suicide attempts, grade 2=depressed with suicidal ideations and grade 3=depressed with suicide attempts). The results confirmed previous risk factors for depression/suicidality in adolescents. Previously, school exclusion and academic difficulties have been implicated in suicidality in young people [17,41]. In France, given the high frequency of repeated years in school, this educational data also needs to be taken into account in assessment of suicidality among adolescents. All substance use including tobacco and marijuana use was associated with increased suicide risk in depressed adolescents. It has been shown that, unless comorbid, substance abuse disorders were not proximally associated with suicidality [9]. Adjusting on confounding variables (educational data, socio economic status, substance use), the results here showed that negative relationships with either or both parents, and parents' living together with a negative relationship were significantly associated with depression and/or suicide risk in both genders (all risk severity grades) and that odds ratios increased according to risk severity grade. This means that what affects depression and suicidality is not parental separation per se, but rather parental harmony on the one hand, and perceived quality of the adolescents' relationships with mother and father, on the other. Although we hypothesized different familial risk factors between girls and boys because of differential epidemiology, we found similar family risk factors in the two genders.

We found depression rates similar to those reported in the literature (e.g. the Center for Disease Control, for the year 2005–2006, found a depression prevalence between 4% and 6.4% in adolescents aged 12 to 17, without testing for gender differences) [42]. We also had a higher prevalence in girls than boys, as found in many epidemiological studies [43-45]. Therefore, the higher prevalence of depression in girls than boys may not be a consequence of differential perceptions of family relationships. It should rather be interpreted as a consequence of other factors that were not assessed in the current study: e.g. genetic vulnerability, hormonal changes, gender specific social constraints, differential comorbid psychopathology [45-49].

The importance of family factors is strengthened by the fact that we found increases in odds ratios for most factors according to severity grade. Recent data suggested that defining and classifying suicidality could provide a better understanding of risk factors (proximal and distal) and interactions among them [7]. The recommended classification distinguishes depression, suicidal ideation and suicidal behavior in a hierarchical model [7,50]. Previous studies have underlined the role of family factors in suicidality in young people. First, adolescents who commit suicide are more likely to come from a family with a history of suicide and/or family psychopathology [17,19,20,51]. Second, childhood abuse, a history of separation and loss (by death or divorce) and exposure to physical and/

or sexual violence are also associated with suicidality [16,52-55]. Third, adolescents with suicidal behaviors are more likely to be living in non-intact families [17,22,33,56-59] and their environment is characterized by problematic communication, poor attachment and high levels of conflict [14,16,17,28,29,34,51,57,60-62]. In depressed adolescents, poor family function is predictor of suicide attempts [1], and suicidal ideations and family conflict were independently associated with a suicidal event over a one-year follow-up [26]. Another recent study showed that the most common proximal risk factor for completed suicide for subjects younger than 30 years was conflict with family members, partners or friends [63]. Here, we focused on perceived intrafamilial relationships and found that negative relationship with either or both parents, and parents living together but with discord were significantly associated with suicide risk and/or depression in the two genders.

The current results have important clinical implications. Practitioners working with young people presenting depression and suicidal behaviors (ideation and/or attempts) should take the family factors into account, in particular aspects such as the adolescent's relationships with either or both parents and relationships between parents whether or not they are living together. Assessing suicide risk in adolescents should include the assessment of family relationships and this could enable appropriate care to be provided for the adolescent and his family. A recent study assessed treatment of adolescent suicide attempters [64]. Depressed adolescents with prior suicide attempts were treated with a combination of medication and psychotherapy. After treatment, rates of improvement and remission of depression appeared comparable to those in non-suicidal depressed adolescents. The treatment included antidepressant medication and CBT (specifically developed to address suicide risk) including both individual and parent-adolescent sessions. Parent-adolescent sessions had probably contributed to this improvement. Of course, other psychotherapies have empirical evidences for its effectiveness such as family therapy.

The current study has several limitations. First, we could only focus on and assess a limited number of risk factors. Regarding adolescent psychopathology, 70 to 91% of young people who attempt or commit suicide present a psychiatric disorder [60,65]. Depression is the most common diagnosis in adolescents who commit suicide and it is highly prevalent in those with suicidal ideations and suicide attempts [15,65]. However, other conditions can interfere, but were not assessed in the current study (e.g. generalized anxiety disorder; disruptive behaviors; borderline personality disorder) [9,15,49,66,67]. Similarly, many non-clinical risk factors were not assessed (e.g. life stressors, problems with authorities, relationship problems with peers, sexual and physical abuse, low socio-economic status) [7]. Second, as our study was cross sectional, meaning that the assessment of suicidal behaviors and changes in family structure was retrospective and that the mechanisms underpinning the associations could not be investigated. Only longitudinal studies are able to explore the different effects of the potential moderators of associations. Third, we had no data available on ethnicity because in France it is not allowed by ethics committees. It can however be noted that the present data only concerned French people from metropolitan France (i.e. excluding overseas territories). The sample nevertheless included 5% of the French metropolitan population aged 17 and was representative of it. Fourth, we had a differential temporal focus for our clinical variables. Current depression was measured for the previous 2 weeks, suicide ideations concerned the past 12 months and suicide attempts concerned lifetime. However, (1) given that subjects were 17 years old, suicide attempts mostly concerned the previous 5 years; (2) prior suicide attempt is an important risk factor for suicidality in young people. In addition, we did not differentiate single suicide attempt and lifetime history of several attempts because of the small numbers of subjects in each subgroup. Thus, grade 3 risk severity included adolescents with a history of one or several suicide attempts. Finally, our aim to investigate current depression as a proximal risk factor led us to exclude many adolescents who had experienced suicidal ideations in the past 12 months and/or lifetime suicide attempt(s) but were not depressed at the time of assessment (see Figure 1). The same analyses (multivariate analysis) as those conducted in this study were performed on the excluded sample and showed similar results for family risk factor (see Additional file 1: Figure S1). Therefore the exclusion of these subjects did not radically modify our results. Finally, self-report of family functioning was also a limitation because depression may lead to a negative perception bias regarding relationships with parents.

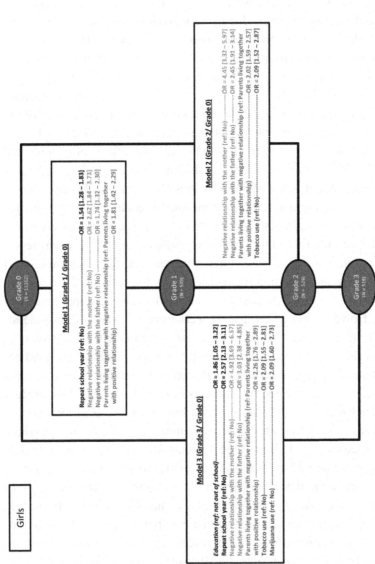

Girls

Grade 0
(N = 1126)

Grade 1
(N = 928)

Grade 2
(N = 524)

Grade 3
(N = 516)

Model 1 (Grade 1 / Grade 0)

Repeat school year (ref: No) ———————— OR = 1.54 [1.28 – 1.83]
Negative relationship with the mother (ref: No) ———— OR = 2.62 [1.84 – 3.73]
Negative relationship with the father (ref: No) ———— OR = 1.74 [1.32 – 2.30]
Parents living together with negative relationship (ref: Parents living together
with positive relationship) ————————— OR = 1.81 [1.42 – 2.29]

Model 2 (Grade 2 / Grade 0)

Negative relationship with the mother (ref: No) ———— OR = 4.45 [3.32 – 5.97]
Negative relationship with the father (ref: No) ———— OR = 2.45 [1.91 – 3.14]
Parents living together with negative relationship (ref: Parents living together
with positive relationship) ————————— OR = 2.02 [1.59 – 2.57]
Tobacco use (ref: No) ——————————— OR = 2.09 [1.52 – 2.87]

Model 3 (Grade 3 / Grade 0)

Education (ref: not out of school) ——————— OR = 1.86 [1.05 – 3.22]
Repeat school year (ref: No) ————————— OR = 2.57 [2.13 – 3.11]
Negative relationship with the mother (ref: No) ———— OR = 4.92 [3.69 – 6.57]
Negative relationship with the father (ref: No) ———— OR = 3.03 [2.38 – 4.85]
Parents living together with negative relationship (ref: Parents living together
with positive relationship) ————————— OR = 2.26 [1.76 – 2.89]
Tobacco use (ref: No) ——————————— OR = 2.09 [1.55 – 2.81]
Marijuana use (ref: No) ——————————— OR = 2.09 [1.60 – 2.73]

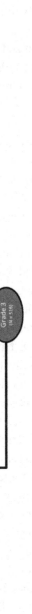

FIGURE 2: Associations between family variables and severity grade in girls adjusting for educational level, repeat school years, socio-economic status and substance use.

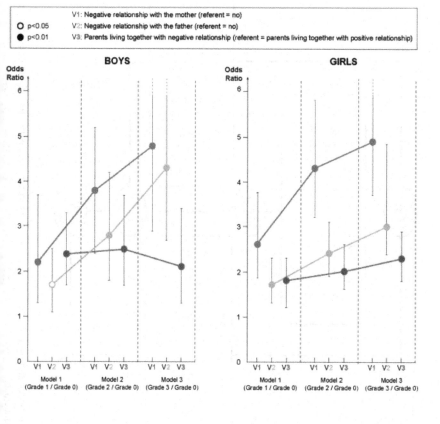

FIGURE 3: Associations between family variables and severity grade in girls and boys adjusting for confounding variables (graph).

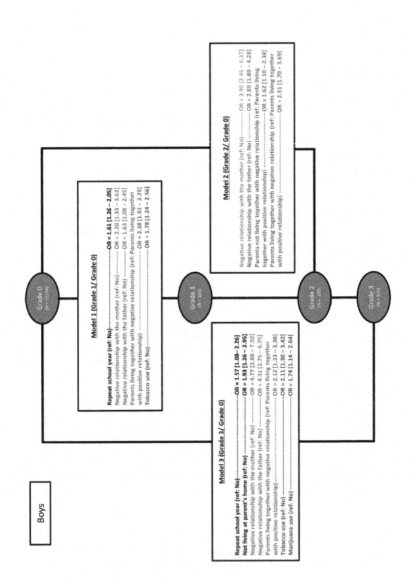

FIGURE 4: Associations between family variables and severity grade in boys adjusting for educational level, repeat school years, socio-economic status and substance use.

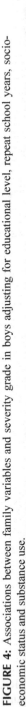

TABLE 2: Risk severity grade combining depression and suicidality in girls and boys

Girls		Grade 0 (N=13143)		Grade 1 (N=676)		Grade 2 (N=626)		Grade 3 (N=642)	
		N	%	N	%	N	%	N	%
Socio-demographic characteristics									
Education	Out of school	137	1.1	.4	0.6	14	2.3	24	3.8
Grade repetition	Yes	4542	34.7	307	46.0	264	42.3	386	60.2
Parental occupation status	Unmployed	866	6.8	54	8.4	58	9.7	70	11.6
Family factors									
Not living at parent's home	Yes	1327	10.2	77	11.6	82	13.3	98	15.5
Negative relationship with the mother	Yes	405	3.1	51	4.5	96	15.5	117	18.4
Negative relationship with the father	Yes	1325	10.3	125	19.0	151	24.4	196	31.2
Parental status and harmony	Parents living together with positive relationship	8074	66.7	334	54.6	277	47.8	236	41.5
	Separated parents with negative relationship	1838	15.2	114	18.6	127	21.9	147	25.8
	Separated parents with positive relationship	809	6.7	41	6.7	43	7.4	33	5.8
	Parents living together with negative relationship	1378	11.4	123	20.1	133	22.9	153	26.9
Drug use									
Alcohol use	Yes	395	3.0	28	4.2	34	5.5	112	9.0
Tabacco use	Yes	542	4.2	40	6.0	65	10.5	93	17.5
Marijuana use	Yes	878	6.7	67	10.0	77	12.4	134	20.9
Boys		Grade 0 (N=15529)		Grade 1 (N=373)		Grade 2 (N=258)		Grade 3 (N=182)	
		N	%	N	%	N	%	N	%
Socio-demographic characteristics									
Education	Out of school	315	2.1	11	3.0	.9	3.6	.8	4.5
Grade repetition	Yes	7211	46.6	228	61.6	114	44.5	113	62.4
Parental occupation status	Unmployed	928	6.3	34	10.0	20	8.4	.10	6.1
Family factors									
Not living at parent's home	Yes	1814	11.8	41	11.1	43	16.8	47	26.5

TABLE 2: *Cont.*

Boys		Grade 0 (N=15529)		Grade 1 (N=373)		Grade 2 (N=258)		Grade 3 (N=182)	
		N	%	N	%	N	%	N	%
Negative relationship with the mother	Yes	464	3.0	34	9.2	38	14.9	40	22.6
Negative relationship with the father	Yes	1228	8.1	57	15.8	59	23.3	56	31.8
Parental status and harmony	Parents living together with positive relationship	9574	67.7	172	54.3	106	47.1	77	50.0
	Separated parents with negative relationship	2104	14.9	63	19.9	52	23.1	40	25.6
	Separated parents with positive relationship	1173	8.3	22	6.9	15	6.7	.6	3.9
	Parents living together with negative relationship	1280	9.1	60	18.9	52	23.1	31	20.1
Drug use									
Alcohol use	Yes	1949	12.7	55	14.9	41	16.0	50	27.9
Tabacco use	Yes	1135	7.4	49	13.5	31	12.3	53	29.8
Marijuana use	Yes	2522	16.3	74	20.0	55	21.5	74	41.3

The study also has some strength. First, the study included a large representative population-based sample of French adolescents aged 17 which allowed an exhaustive investigation of suicide risk severity in depressed adolescents. In addition, the setting in which the study was implemented (JAPD) was a good guarantee of methodological thoroughness for sampling and conditions of administration. Compared to studies conducted in adult populations, we were able to restrict recall bias because subjects were all 17 years old. Second, depression assessment was performed on a scale specific to adolescents [38]. In previous studies, depression has often been lifetime depression so that it was difficult to know if depression reported by a subject was present before, during or after suicide attempts. Third, results regarding family factors were adjusted on several confounding variables (educational level, repeat school years, socio-economic status, and substance use). Fourth, because of the good statistical power, we were able to (1) run multivariate analyses on each gender; (2) distinguish family separation, family discord and perceived parental relationship.

10.5 CONCLUSION

This study has provided keys regarding the epidemiology of suicidal behaviours in a large community-based sample of French adolescents aged 17. Substance use, repeat school years and family factors were associated with an increased suicide risk in depressed adolescents, with no difference according to gender. Specifically, perceived negative relationships with either or both parents, and a negative relationship between parents, whether living together or not, were associated with suicidality. So it appears essential to take into account real and perceived intrafamilial relationships among depressed adolescents to assess and prevent suicidal behaviours.

REFERENCES

1. Wilkinson P, Kelvin R, Roberts C, Dubicka B, Goodyer I: Clinical and psychosocial predictors of suicide attempts and nonsuicidal self-injury in the Adolescent Depression Antidepressants and Psychotherapy Trial (ADAPT). Am J Psychiatry 2011, 168(5):495-501.
2. Zalsman G, Levy T, Shoval G: Interaction of child and family psychopathology leading to suicidal behavior. Psychiatr Clin North Am 2008, 31(2):237-246.
3. Centers for Disease Control and Prevention, National Center for Injury Prevention and Control. Web-based Injury Statistics Query and Reporting System (WISQARS). 2007. http://www.cdc.gov/ncipc/wisqars
4. de Tournemire R: [Teenagers' suicides and suicide attempts: finding one's way in epidemiologic data]. Arch Pediatr 2010, 17(8):1202-1209.
5. Eurostat. http://epp.eurostat.ec.europa.eu
6. Bridge JA, Goldstein TR, Brent DA: Adolescent suicide and suicidal behavior. J Child Psychol Psychiatry 2006, 47(3–4):372-394.
7. Posner K, Melvin GA, Stanley B, Oquendo MA, Gould M: Factors in the assessment of suicidality in youth. CNS Spectr 2007, 12(2):156-162.
8. Posner K, Oquendo MA, Gould M, Stanley B, Davies M: Columbia Classification Algorithm of Suicide Assessment (C-CASA): classification of suicidal events in the FDA's pediatric suicidal risk analysis of antidepressants. Am J Psychiatry 2007, 164(7):1035-1043.

9.   Foley DL, Goldston DB, Costello EJ, Angold A: Proximal psychiatric risk factors for suicidality in youth: the Great Smoky Mountains Study. Arch Gen Psychiatry 2006, 63(9):1017-1024.

10. Breton JJ, Boyer R, Bilodeau H, Raymond S, Joubert N, Nantel MA: Is evaluative research on youth suicide programs theory-driven? The Canadian experience. Suicide Life Threat Behav 2002, 32(2):176-190.

11. Gould MS, Greenberg T, Velting DM, Shaffer D: Youth suicide risk and preventive interventions: a review of the past 10 years. J Am Acad Child Adolesc Psychiatry 2003, 42(4):386-405.

12. Brent DA, Mann JJ: Familial pathways to suicidal behavior–understanding and preventing suicide among adolescents. N Engl J Med 2006, 355(26):2719-2721.

13. Cavanagh JT, Carson AJ, Sharpe M, Lawrie SM: Psychological autopsy studies of suicide: a systematic review. Psychol Med 2003, 33(3):395-405.

14. Brent DA, Baugher M, Bridge J, Chen T, Chiappetta L: Age- and sex-related risk factors for adolescent suicide. J Am Acad Child Adolesc Psychiatry 1999, 38(12):1497-1505.

15. Shaffer D, Gould MS, Fisher P, Trautman P, Moreau D, Kleinman M, Flory M: Psychiatric diagnosis in child and adolescent suicide. Arch Gen Psychiatry 1996, 53(4):339-348.

16. Fergusson DM, Woodward LJ, Horwood LJ: Risk factors and life processes associated with the onset of suicidal behaviour during adolescence and early adulthood. Psychol Med 2000, 30(1):23-39.

17. Gould MS, Fisher P, Parides M, Flory M, Shaffer D: Psychosocial risk factors of child and adolescent completed suicide. Arch Gen Psychiatry 1996, 53(12):1155-1162.

18. O'Donnell L, Stueve A, Wardlaw D, O'Donnell C: Adolescent suicidality and adult support: the reach for health study of urban youth. Am J Health Behav 2003, 27(6):633-644.

19. King CA, Merchant CR: Social and interpersonal factors relating to adolescent suicidality: a review of the literature. Arch Suicide Res 2008, 12(3):181-196.

20. Hawton K, James A: Suicide and deliberate self harm in young people. BMJ 2005, 330(7496):891-894.

21. Prinstein MJ, Boergers J, Spirito A, Little TD, Grapentine WL: Peer functioning, family dysfunction, and psychological symptoms in a risk factor model for adolescent inpatients' suicidal ideation severity. J Clin Child Psychol 2000, 29(3):392-405.

22. Ponnet K, Vermeiren R, Jespers I, Mussche B, Ruchkin V, Schwab-Stone M, Deboutte D: Suicidal behaviour in adolescents: associations with parental marital status and perceived parent-adolescent relationship. J Affect Disord 2005, 89(1–3):107-113.

23. Fotti SA, Katz LY, Afifi TO, Cox BJ: The associations between peer and parental relationships and suicidal behaviours in early adolescents. Can J Psychiatry 2006, 51(11):698-703.

24. Ackard DM, Neumark-Sztainer D, Story M, Perry C: Parent–child connectedness and behavioral and emotional health among adolescents. Am J Prev Med 2006, 30(1):59-66.

25. Brent DA, Emslie GJ, Clarke GN, Asarnow J, Spirito A, Ritz L, Vitiello B, Iyengar S, Birmaher B, Ryan ND, et al.: Predictors of spontaneous and systematically assessed suicidal adverse events in the treatment of SSRI-resistant depression in adolescents (TORDIA) study. Am J Psychiatry 2009, 166(4):418-426.

26. Brent DA, Greenhill LL, Compton S, Emslie G, Wells K, Walkup JT, Vitiello B, Bukstein O, Stanley B, Posner K, et al.: The Treatment of Adolescent Suicide Attempters study (TASA): predictors of suicidal events in an open treatment trial. J Am Acad Child Adolesc Psychiatry 2009, 48(10):987-996.

27. King RA, Schwab-Stone M, Flisher AJ, Greenwald S, Kramer RA, Goodman SH, Lahey BB, Shaffer D, Gould MS: Psychosocial and risk behavior correlates of youth suicide attempts and suicidal ideation. J Am Acad Child Adolesc Psychiatry 2001, 40(7):837-846.

28. Lewinsohn PM, Rohde P, Seeley JR: Psychosocial risk factors for future adolescent suicide attempts. J Consult Clin Psychol 1994, 62(2):297-305.

29. McKeown RE, Garrison CZ, Cuffe SP, Waller JL, Jackson KL, Addy CL: Incidence and predictors of suicidal behaviors in a longitudinal sample of young adolescents. J Am Acad Child Adolesc Psychiatry 1998, 37(6):612-619.

30. Lynskey MT, Fergusson DM: Factors protecting against the development of adjustment difficulties in young adults exposed to childhood sexual abuse. Child Abuse Negl 1997, 21(12):1177-1190.

31. Borowsky IW, Ireland M, Resnick MD: Adolescent suicide attempts: risks and protectors. Pediatrics 2001, 107(3):485-493.

32. Czyz EK, Liu Z, King CA: Social connectedness and one-year trajectories among suicidal adolescents following psychiatric hospitalization. J Clin Child Adolesc Psychol 2012, 41(2):214-226.

33. Kokkevi A, Rotsika V, Arapaki A, Richardson C: Changes in associations between psychosocial factors and suicide attempts by adolescents in Greece from1984 to 2007. Eur J Public Health 2011, 21(6):694-698.

34. Samm A, Tooding LM, Sisask M, Kolves K, Aasvee K, Varnik A: Suicidal thoughts and depressive feelings amongst Estonian schoolchildren: effect of family relationship and family structure. Eur Child Adolesc Psychiatry 2010, 19(5):457-468.

35. Beck F, Legleye S, Peretti-Watel P: Les usages des substances psychoactives à la fin de l'adolescence: mise en place d'une enquête annuelle (The use of psychoactive substances among adolescents in their late teens: setting up an annual survey). Tendances 2000, 10:.

36. Bulletin statistique. INSEE; 2011. http://www.indices.insee.fr

37. Beck F, Costes J-M, Legleye S, Spilka S: L'enquête ESCAPAD sur les consommations de drogues des jeunes français: un dispositif original de recueil de l'information sur un sujet sensible. In Méthodes d'enquêtes et sondages - Pratiques européennne et nord-américaine. Edited by Lavallée P, Rivest L. Dunod, Québec; 2006:56-60. collection Sciences Sup

38. Revah-Levy A, Birmaher B, Gasquet I, Falissard B: The Adolescent Depression Rating Scale (ADRS): a validation study. BMC Psychiatry 2007, 7:2.

39. INSEE: Nomenclature des Professions et Catégories socioprofessionnelles (PCS). Nationale Institute of Statistics and Economic studies, France; 2012. http://www.insee.fr

40. Observatoire français des drogues et des toxicomanies. http://www.ofdt.fr
41. Brent DA, Perper JA, Moritz G, Allman C, Friend A, Roth C, Schweers J, Balach L, Baugher M: Psychiatric risk factors for adolescent suicide: a case–control study. J Am Acad Child Adolesc Psychiatry 1993, 32(3):521-529.
42. Centers for Disease Control and Prevention, National Center for Injury Prevention and Control. Web-based Injury Statistics Query and Reporting System (WISQARS). 2006. http://www.cdc.gov/ncipc/wisqars
43. Compas BE, Oppedisano G, Connor JK, Gerhardt CA, Hinden BR, Achenbach TM, Hammen C: Gender differences in depressive symptoms in adolescence: comparison of national samples of clinically referred and nonreferred youths. J Consult Clin Psychol 1997, 65(4):617-626.
44. Essau CA, Lewinsohn PM, Seeley JR, Sasagawa S: Gender differences in the developmental course of depression. J Affect Disord 2010, 127(1–3):185-190.
45. Garber J: Depression in children and adolescents: linking risk research and prevention. Am J Prev Med 2006, 31(6 Suppl 1):S104-S125.
46. Uddin M, Koenen KC, de Los SR, Bakshis E, Aiello AE, Galea S: Gender differences in the genetic and environmental determinants of adolescent depression. Depress Anxiety 2010, 27(7):658-666.
47. Hankin BL, Abramson LY: Development of gender differences in depression: description and possible explanations. Ann Med 1999, 31(6):372-379.
48. Angold A, Costello EJ, Erkanli A, Worthman CM: Pubertal changes in hormone levels and depression in girls. Psychol Med 1999, 29(5):1043-1053.
49. Brent DA, Johnson B, Bartle S, Bridge J, Rather C, Matta J, Connolly J, Constantine D: Personality disorder, tendency to impulsive violence, and suicidal behavior in adolescents. J Am Acad Child Adolesc Psychiatry 1993, 32(1):69-75.
50. Perez VW: The relationship between seriously considering, planning, and attempting suicide in the youth risk behavior survey. Suicide Life Threat Behav 2005, 35(1):35-49.
51. Beautrais AL, Joyce PR, Mulder RT: Risk factors for serious suicide attempts among youths aged 13 through 24 years. J Am Acad Child Adolesc Psychiatry 1996, 35(9):1174-1182.
52. Johnson JG, Cohen P, Gould MS, Kasen S, Brown J, Brook JS: Childhood adversities, interpersonal difficulties, and risk for suicide attempts during late adolescence and early adulthood. Arch Gen Psychiatry 2002, 59(8):741-749.
53. Seguin M, Renaud J, Lesage A, Robert M, Turecki G: Youth and young adult suicide: a study of life trajectory. J Psychiatr Res 2011, 45(7):863-870.
54. Beautrais AL, Gibb SJ, Faulkner A, Fergusson DM, Mulder RT: Postcard intervention for repeat self-harm: randomised controlled trial. Br J Psychiatry 2010, 197(1):55-60.
55. Nock MK, Kessler RC: Prevalence of and risk factors for suicide attempts versus suicide gestures: analysis of the National Comorbidity Survey. J Abnorm Psychol 2006, 115(3):616-623.
56. Beautrais AL: Suicides and serious suicide attempts: two populations or one? Psychol Med 2001, 31(5):837-845.

57. Brent DA, Perper JA, Moritz G, Liotus L, Schweers J, Balach L, Roth C: Familial risk factors for adolescent suicide: a case–control study. Acta Psychiatr Scand 1994, 89(1):52-58.

58. Groholt B, Ekeberg O, Wichstrom L, Haldorsen T: Suicide among children and younger and older adolescents in Norway: a comparative study. J Am Acad Child Adolesc Psychiatry 1998, 37(5):473-481.

59. Sauvola A, Rasanen PK, Joukamaa MI, Jokelainen J, Jarvelin MR, Isohanni MK: Mortality of young adults in relation to single-parent family background. A prospective study of the northern Finland 1966 birth cohort. Eur J Public Health 2001, 11(3):284-286.

60. Fergusson DM, Lynskey MT: Suicide attempts and suicidal ideation in a birth cohort of 16-year-old New Zealanders. J Am Acad Child Adolesc Psychiatry 1995, 34(10):1308-1317.

61. Lewinsohn PM, Rohde P, Seeley JR: Psychosocial characteristics of adolescents with a history of suicide attempt. J Am Acad Child Adolesc Psychiatry 1993, 32(1):60-68.

62. Tousignant M, Bastien MF, Hamel S: Suicidal attempts and ideations among adolescents and young adults: the contribution of the father's and mother's care and of parental separation. Soc Psychiatry Psychiatr Epidemiol 1993, 28(5):256-261.

63. Im JS, Choi SH, Hong D, Seo HJ, Park S, Hong JP: Proximal risk factors and suicide methods among suicide completers from national suicide mortality data 2004–2006 in Korea. Compr Psychiatry 2011, 52(3):231-237.

64. Vitiello B, Brent DA, Greenhill LL, Emslie G, Wells K, Walkup JT, Stanley B, Bukstein O, Kennard BD, Compton S, et al.: Depressive symptoms and clinical status during the Treatment of Adolescent Suicide Attempters (TASA) Study. J Am Acad Child Adolesc Psychiatry 2009, 48(10):997-1004.

65. Gould MS, King R, Greenwald S, Fisher P, Schwab-Stone M, Kramer R, Flisher AJ, Goodman S, Canino G, Shaffer D: Psychopathology associated with suicidal ideation and attempts among children and adolescents. J Am Acad Child Adolesc Psychiatry 1998, 37(9):915-923.

66. Jacobson CM, Muehlenkamp JJ, Miller AL, Turner JB: Psychiatric impairment among adolescents engaging in different types of deliberate self-harm. J Clin Child Adolesc Psychol 2008, 37(2):363-375.

67. Muehlenkamp JJ, Ertelt TW, Miller AL, Claes L: Borderline personality symptoms differentiate non-suicidal and suicidal self-injury in ethnically diverse adolescent outpatients. J Child Psychol Psychiatry 2011, 52(2):148-155.

There is a supplemental file that is not available in this version of the article. To view this additional information, please use the citation on the first page of this chapter.

PART IV

COMMUNITY-BASED INTERVENTIONS

CHAPTER 11

A SYSTEMATIC REVIEW OF THE EFFECTIVENESS OF MENTAL HEALTH PROMOTION INTERVENTIONS FOR YOUNG PEOPLE IN LOW AND MIDDLE INCOME COUNTRIES

MARGARET M. BARRY, ALEISHA M. CLARKE, RACHEL JENKINS, AND VIKRAM PATEL

11.1 BACKGROUND

Mental health is fundamental to good health and wellbeing and influences social and economic outcomes across the lifespan [1-3]. Childhood and adolescence are crucial periods for laying the foundations for healthy development and good mental health. It is estimated that 10-20% of young people worldwide experience mental health problems [4]. Poor mental health in childhood is associated with health and social problems such as school failure, delinquency and substance misuse, and increases the risk of poverty and other adverse outcomes in adulthood [3]. Interventions that promote positive mental health equip young people with the necessary

A Systematic Review of the Effectiveness of Mental Health Promotion Interventions for Young People in Low and Middle Income Countries. Barry MM, Clarke AM, Jenkins R, and Patel V. EBMC Public Health, *13,835 (2013), doi:10.1186/1471-2458-13-835. Licensed under Creative Commons Attribution 2.0 Generic License, http://creativecommons.org/licenses/by/2.0/.*

life skills, supports and resources to fulfill their potential and overcome adversity. Systematic reviews of the international evidence, which come predominantly from high income countries (HICs), show that comprehensive mental health promotion interventions carried out in collaboration with families, schools and communities, lead to improvements not only in mental health but also improved social functioning, academic and work performance, and general health behaviours [5-13].

Despite the recognition of the importance of mental health promotion for children and adolescents, mental health remains a neglected public health issue, especially in low and middle-income countries (LMICs). Mental health is inequitably distributed as people living in poverty and other forms of social disadvantage bear a disproportionate burden of mental disorders and their adverse consequences [14-17]. There is increasing recognition of the relevance of mental health to global development strategies, and in particular to the achievement of the Millennium Development Goals (MDGs), including improving child and maternal health, universal education, combating HIV/AIDS and other diseases, and eradicating poverty [18,19]. As 90% of the world's children and adolescents live in LMICs, where they constitute up to 50% of the population [20], there is an urgent need to address the mental health of young people as part of the wider health promotion and development agenda.

Schools are one of the most important community settings for promoting the mental health of young people [21]. The school setting provides a forum for promoting emotional and social competence as well as academic learning and offers a means of reaching the significant number of young people who experience mental health problems [22-25]. Educational opportunities throughout life are associated with improved mental health outcomes. The promotion of emotional health and wellbeing is a core feature of the WHO's Health Promoting Schools initiative [26]. There is good evidence that mental health promotion programmes in schools, especially those adopting a whole school approach, lead to positive mental health, social and educational outcomes [13,27-29]. Programmes incorporating life skills, social and emotional learning and early interventions to address emotional and behavioural problems, produce long-term benefits for young people, including improved emotional and social functioning, positive health behaviours, and improved academic performance [5,13,25,27-

31]. To date there has been comparatively little research on school and community-based mental health promotion interventions for young people in LMIC settings and no systematic attempt to synthesize the evidence from such settings. This is the goal of this paper. The work described here was undertaken in 2011–2012 as part of the World Health Organization Task Force on Mainstreaming Health Promotion. Established on foot of the WHO 7th Global Conference on Health Promotion [32], the Task Force sought to develop a package of evidence-based health promotion actions addressing priority public health conditions in LMICs.

The objectives of the review were:

- To synthesize evidence on the effectiveness of mental health promotion interventions for young people that have been implemented in LMICs.
- To identify gaps in the existing evidence and highlight areas where further research is needed.

11.2 METHODS

11.2.1 STUDY SELECTION

This systematic review conforms to the guidelines outlined by the PRIS-MA 2009 checklist. A research protocol for the original review was agreed with the Members of the WHO Task Force and the Cochrane Public Health Group (CPHG). Studies were eligible for inclusion if the intervention was designed to promote positive mental health for young people in LMIC settings. For the purpose of this review, mental health promotion interventions were defined as any planned action, programme or policy, which was undertaken with the aim of improving mental health or modifying its determinants. Evidence in relation to the studies for young people aged 6–18 years across all school and community settings was included, with no exclusions based on gender or ethnicity. Academic and grey literature published from 2000 onwards in printed or electronic format was deemed eligible for inclusion. In order to include studies of comparable quality, we considered study designs including randomized controlled trials, cluster randomized controlled trials, and quasi-experimental study designs. The primary outcomes of interest were mental health and wellbeing benefits including; indicators of positive mental health such as self-esteem, self-efficacy, coping skills, resilience, emotional wellbeing; negative mental health such as depression, anxiety, psychological distress, suicidal behaviour; and wellbeing indicators such as social participation, empowerment, communication and social support. Secondary health related outcomes were also noted. Studies with the following characteristics were excluded from the review; (i) selective and indicated prevention interventions, as defined by Mrazek and Haggerty [33], (ii) studies with no control/comparison group, and (iii) qualitative only studies.

TABLE 1: Original search strategy for electronic databases (+ denotes terms used for updated search in Sept 2012)

Mental health terms	Origin	Population	Setting	Intervention terms	Related outcomes
Mental health +	Middle income country+	Infant	Home	Promotion+	Gender
Psychosocial+	Low income country+	Child+	Pre-school+	Prevention+	Child health
Wellbeing+	Developing world+	Adolescent+	School+	Intervention+	Stigma+
Lifeskills+	Developing country+	Young people+	Classroom+	Program+	Discrimination
Empowerment+		outh+	Community+	Policy+	Primary care
Mental capital+		Adult	Out-of-school+	Implementa-tion +	Maternal health
Resilience+		Worker	Health service	Evaluation+	Violence+
Social emotional+		Employee	Workplace	Home visiting	Sexual health+
Mental health literacy+		Family		Early years	HIV prevention+
		Indigenous community		Parenting	Social capital
		Population group		Organiza-tional	Social networks
					Social functioning
					Microfinance+
					Micro-credit+

Searches included: (* denotes multiple word endings including singular and plural). Mental health terms AND Origin AND Population AND Intervention Terms. e.g. mental *health OR psychosocial OR wellbeing OR lifeskills OR empowerment OR mental capital OR resilience OR social emotional OR mental health literacy AND middle income countr* OR low income countr* OR developing world OR developing countr* AND child* OR adolescent* OR young people OR youth AND Promotion OR prevention OR intervention OR program* OR policy OR implementation OR evaluat*. Mental health terms AND Origin AND Population AND Setting. Mental health terms AND Origin AND Population AND Related Outcomes. Mental health terms AND Origin AND Setting AND Related Outcomes. Mental health terms AND Origin AND Related outcomes AND Intervention Terms. Mental health terms AND Origin AND Related outcomes AND Setting. Mental health terms AND Origin AND Related outcomes AND Population.*

11.2.2 SEARCH STRATEGY

Academic databases including PubMed, PsychInfo, Scopus, ISI Web of Knowledge, Cochrane database of systematic reviews were searched. Health Promotion and Public Health Review databases were also searched including Evidence for Policy and Practice information and Coordinating (EPPI) Centre; University of York National Health Service Centre for reviews and dissemination; National Institute of Clinical Excellence (NICE); Effective Public Health Practice, Health Evidence Canada; WHO programmes and projects. Additional sources included Google Scholar and reference list of relevant articles, book chapters and reviews. Key individuals and organizations identified through the search process were contacted to identify further details on publications. The electronic search strategy used across all databases is provided in Table 1. The last search for the original systematic review of mental health promotion interventions was completed on 11th March 2011 and included articles published between January 2000 – December 2010. A repeated search was conducted on 7th September 2012 to update results and included articles published between January 2011 – June 2012.

11.2.3 STUDY SELECTION AND DATA COLLECTION

Using the search strategy described above, all titles and abstracts retrieved were scanned for relevance. Duplicates, articles not relevant, and articles that did not meet the inclusion criteria were removed. Full text papers were obtained for studies that were selected for inclusion. Studies were subsequently selected relating to young people and were classified according to (i) school-based programmes (ii) community-based programmes for adolescents. Two reviewers assessed the studies in order to ensure that they met the inclusion criteria set out for this review.

11.2.4 DATA ANALYSIS

As the interventions and outcomes evaluated in the included studies were too diverse to allow a quantitative synthesis of the study findings, a narrative synthesis was undertaken. Following the guidelines of the Cochrane Public Health Group, the methodological quality of the intervention evaluations was assessed using the Quality Assessment Tool for Quantitative Studies developed by the Effective Public Health Practice Project [34]. Studies were assessed for selection bias, study design, confounders, blinding, data collection and withdrawals and drop-outs. Each study was rated independently by two reviewers (MB and AC). The quality assessments were compared and disagreements were resolved through discussion. Based on the ratings of each of the six components, each study received an overall global rating of strong, moderate or weak. Following the quality assessment stage, the inclusion of studies and extraction of key findings was finalized. Extracted data were entered into a table of study characteristics (Table 2) including the quality assessment ratings for each study.

11.3 RESULTS

The results of the search and study selection are shown in Figure 1. The original search process carried out in 2011 produced 10,471 articles, 188 articles of which were selected for full review and exported to Endnote. Of these, 146 were either contextual articles related to mental health promotion in LMICs or studies that did not meet one of our inclusion criteria. Seven articles were systematic/summary reviews of the evidence base in LMICs, five of which were reviews of interventions for young people. A total of 35 primary studies were selected for review. Of these, 14 studies evaluated school or community-based interventions for young people in LMICs. During the repeated search performed in September 2012, a further eight studies evaluating school-based interventions were identified. The combined searches resulted in a total of 22 studies (14 school and eight community-based studies) undergoing quality assessment. No studies in non-English language specific to school and community based-interventions were identified in the review process.

The five systematic review articles from LMICs that were identified examined the effectiveness of HIV related lifeskills interventions [69,70] and psychosocial interventions for children and adolescents affected by armed conflict in LMICs [71-73]. All relevant interventions across the reviews were identified and cross-referenced with the primary articles retrieved through the electronic search. Given the specific focus of this systematic review on mental health promotion and primary prevention, several studies from these systematic reviews did not meet the inclusion criteria for this review.

Regarding the number and percentage of evaluation studies carried out across LMICs, 18.2% (N = 4) of the interventions were carried out in low income countries, 36.4% (N = 8) were carried out in lower middle income countries and 45.4% (N = 10) were carried out in upper middle income countries. Just under one third of the interventions (N = 7) were carried out in South Africa alone.

11.3.1 SCHOOL-BASED PROGRAMMES

Fourteen studies describing thirteen interventions implemented in school settings in eight LMIC countries were identified. Four studies were carried out in Gaza/Palestine [48,50,55,56], three were carried out in South Africa [37,38,41,44], two in Uganda [45,49] and one intervention was carried out in India [35], Chile [36], Mauritius [42], Nepal [47], and the Lebanon [54]. The majority of studies (>60%) were published between 2010–2012. The quality of evidence from the majority of studies was strong. A total of eight studies received a strong quality rating [42,45,47,48,50,54-56], five studies received a moderate quality assessment rating as a result of selection bias [36,44] and not reporting the percentage of withdrawals/dropouts [35,38,49]. One study received a weak quality assessment rating due to selection bias, not reporting confounders and not reporting level of withdrawals [41].

The programmes were mental health promotion and universal pre-vention interventions designed for all children and adolescents of school going age. Interventions varied slightly in their focus from the develop-ment of social, emotional, problem solving and coping skills [35,41] to a combined mental health promotion with physical fitness programme [36], combined mental health promotion and sexuality education [37,38] and a universal depression prevention intervention [42]. Two interventions were designed specifically to support AIDS orphaned children, one was an art intervention [44], another was a peer support intervention led by teachers [45]. Seven interventions (eight studies) were school-based psychosocial interventions implemented in countries affected by armed conflict [47-50,54-56]. These interventions were designed to reduce distress, enhance resilience and coping skills. Four of these interventions incorporated cog-nitive behavioural techniques (CBT) and trauma related psychoeducation modules [47-50,54]. One intervention consisted of short writing sessions [55], another provided structured recreational activities [56].

Seven of the school-based interventions were designed for post-primary school students (>12 years of age). Four interventions were implemented with a broad age range from 6 – 18 years [44,48,54,56]. Three interven-tions were implemented with children in the senior end of primary school (>10 years of age) [45,49,50]. Eight interventions were implemented by the class teacher [35-38,42,44,49,54,55], with the remaining interventions implemented by mental health professionals [41,48,50], locally trained paraprofessionals [47] and local youth workers [44,56]. The majority of session ranged in length from 11 – 16 sessions implemented weekly. One intervention provided six booster sessions at 12 months following comple-tion of the programme [37,38]. Eight school interventions were developed in the implementing country. Five interventions were adapted versions of evidence-based interventions from high income countries [37,38,42,47-49].

Regarding intervention outcomes, in terms of the seven universal pro-grammes implemented with children affected by armed conflict, the find-ings are generally positive but with some studies reporting mixed effects. Loughry et al. [56] reported that the after-school recreational activities implemented over one year had a significant positive impact on children and adolescents' externalising and internalising problem scores and also improved parental support as a result of parental involvement in the structured activities. Khamis et al. [48] reported that the Classroom-Based Intervention (CBI) had a significant positive effect on children (age 6–11) and adolescents (age 13–16) in terms of improved social and emotional wellbeing, communication skills and reduced conduct and peer problems and hyperactivity levels. Ager et al. [49] reported similar findings for the school-based Psychosocial Structures Activities intervention (PSSA) which is based on principles of the CBI, with the intervention having a significant positive effect on primary school children's (mean age 10 years) wellbeing. Interestingly, the CBI study carried out in Nepal reported specific gender effects, with significant reductions in psychological difficulties and aggression among males only and improved prosocial behaviour among females only [47]. Two studies reported less positive findings. Karam et al. [54] found that the cognitive behavioural therapy intervention (CBT) implemented over 12 consecutive days had no significant effect on participant rates of depression, separation anxiety and post-traumatic stress disorder (PTSD). Lange-Nielsen et al. [55] reported that the three day short-term writing intervention had no effect on participants' PTSD symptoms and anxiety scores. This study also reported that the writing intervention lead initially to significantly increased depression symptoms for participants between pre and post-intervention but that symptoms significantly declined at five months follow up. Contrasting findings in terms of gender effects were reported across three studies; two studies reported that the interventions have a more positive effect on girls [48,49] while another intervention reported no programme effect for girls with PTSD scores improving only in male participants [50].

Regarding the universal lifeskills and resilience school-based interventions, all six studies reported significant positive effects on students' mental health and wellbeing in terms of improved self-esteem [35,36,42], motivation [38] and self-efficacy [44]. The peer-group support intervention implemented with AIDS orphan children resulted in significant improvements in participants' depression, anger and anxiety scores but not for self-concept [45]. The combined fitness lifeskills education intervention reported improvements in anxiety symptoms, however, there was no change in participants' depression scores [36]. The depression prevention intervention on the other hand reported a significant reduction in depressive symptoms (medium effect size) and hopelessness (medium effect size) and a significant increase in coping skills (medium effect size) amongst participants in the intervention group [42]. Long-term findings from this depression prevention intervention included improved self-esteem and coping skills (medium effect size) at six months follow up. In addition, the resilience intervention in South Africa also reported long-term findings with improved self-appraisal scores maintained at three months follow up [41]. Additional outcomes from these studies include improved behaviour [35], school adjustment [35], fitness [36], attitudes about reproductive and sexual health [37] and a reduction in the level of substance misuse [37]. The art intervention for AIDS orphan children reported the least positive findings with a significant improvement reported in the intervention groups' self-efficacy score but no change in participants' depression, self-esteem and emotional and behavioural scores [44]. While the results from the resiliency intervention indicated significant improvements in participants' emotional reactivity, self appraisal and interpersonal strength, the weak quality of this study must be considered when interpreting these findings.

11.3.2 COMMUNITY-BASED INTERVENTIONS

This review identified eight studies evaluating seven out-of-school community interventions for adolescents in five countries. Four studies were carried out in South Africa [60,61,63,64], one study was carried out in India [57], Honduras [58], Egypt [59] and Uganda [65-68]. All eight studies were published between 2006 and 2010. The quality of evidence from these studies was moderate to strong. Four studies received a strong quality assessment rating [57,60,61,65] and four studies received a moderate quality assessment rating due to small sample size [58] and failure to report validity and reliability of measures used in three studies [59,63,64].

Interventions included a multi-component school and community-based intervention for youth aged 16–24 years [57]; a family-based strengthening programme (Familias Fuertas) for parents and their adolescent children [58]; a multidimensional programme (Ishraq) aimed at improving the life skills, literacy, recreational activities and health knowledge of 13–15 year old girls in Egypt [59] and combined HIV prevention and lifeskills interventions (Stepping Stones and CHAMPSA) for adolescents in South Africa [60,61]. Two studies evaluated the Intervention with Microfinance for AIDS and Gender Equity (IMAGE), a poverty-focused microfinance initiative for women that is combined with a 12–15 month gender and HIV education curriculum [63,64]. One study examined the effects of small individual loans and mentorship on health and mental health functioning of primary school children [65-68]. Five of the seven interventions were designed for young people aged 13+. The Familias Fuertas intervention was designed for children age 10–14 and one of the evaluations of the IMAGE microfinance intervention was implemented with females aged 18 and over. Two interventions provided parent training [58,61] and two interventions were designed specifically for females [59,63,64]. Five of the interventions were implemented by local trained community caregivers [59-61,63-68]. The Familias Fuertas intervention was implemented by a local nurse [58] and the multi-component school and community intervention in India was implemented by a team of social workers, psychologists and peer educators [57]. Five of the interventions were developed in the implementing country. Two interventions were adapted versions of evidence-based interventions that were developed in the United States [58,61].

Collectively, the results from these studies indicate the significant positive effect of community-based mental health promotion interventions on young people's mental health and social wellbeing. Five interventions provided strong evidence of their positive impact on mental health. Balaji et al. [57] reported that the community-based youth health intervention in India resulted in significant improvements in participants' depression scores, reported levels of suicidal behaviour, and knowledge and attitudes about mental health. South Africa's IMAGE intervention resulted in significant improvements in empowerment, social participation and levels of openness among women in the combined IMAGE-microfinance intervention, with no change evident the microfinance only intervention [64]. In addition, Pronijk et al. [64] reported that participants in the IMAGE intervention were significantly more likely to participate in training, and had greater participation in social and community groups. Ssewamala et al. [65,66] reported that the SUUBI economic empowerment intervention for AIDS orphaned children had a significant positive impact on participants' self-esteem and levels of depression. Results from the parent-youth interventions indicate the significant effect of the programmes on positive parenting communication and behaviours, parental self-esteem and family relations [58,61].

Other reported outcomes also included significantly improved: peer relations [59]; academic performance [59,68]; student-teacher relations [57]; communication [64]; improved gender roles [64] and significantly reduced sexual risk behaviour [60,63] one year follow up; physical and sexual partner violence [57,60,63,64]; and substance abuse [57,60]. Bell et al., [61] reported medium effect sizes for improved caregiver communication comfort. Long-term findings from the Stepping Stones intervention include reduced physical and sexual partner violence at two years follow-up, and reduced substance abuse at one year follow up [60].

11.4 DISCUSSION

This review sought to determine the effectiveness of mental health promotion interventions designed for young people (aged 6–18 years) in LMICs. A total of 22 studies evaluating 20 interventions were identified. The majority of interventions were implemented in upper and lower middle income countries, thus highlighting the paucity of evidence from low income countries. Four interventions were carried out in low income countries, three of which were conducted in Uganda. It is encouraging to note, however, the significant increase in publications from LMICs in the last four years, with the majority of interventions identified in this review published since 2008.

With regard to the school-based interventions, the quality of evidence from the 14 studies is moderate to strong. Findings from these studies indicate that there is reasonably robust evidence that school-based programmes implemented across diverse LMICs can have significant positive effects on students' emotional and behavioural wellbeing, including reduced depression and anxiety and improved coping skills. Promising interventions include the Resourceful Adolescent Program (RAP-A), which was implemented by teachers in Mauritius [42]. This study is an example of an evidence-based intervention adapted from a HIC for implementation in a LMIC and points to the potential of such interventions when adapted to meet the cultural needs of young people in LMICs. Another promising intervention is the teacher led peer-group support intervention for AIDs orphaned children which was implemented in a low-income country [45]. The findings from this study suggest the potential of peer support mental health promotion interventions in optimizing adjustment and decreasing the psychological distress associated with AIDS orphanhood in the adolescent age group. Such interventions may have great potential in addressing the increased risk of depression, peer relationship problems, post-traumatic stress and conduct problems among AIDS orphans [74-76]. There is also some encouraging evidence that interventions which combine lifeskills with reproductive and sexual health education [37,38] and physical health and fitness [36] can have a significant positive effect on pupils' risk-taking and prosocial behaviour. These findings are consistent with the substantive evidence from multiple reviews of school-based interventions in HICs which report the greater effectiveness of multi-component interventions (i.e. interventions that adopt a social competence approach and develop supportive environments), when compared with interventions that focus on specific problem behaviours [8,28,77-79]. The integration of multicomponent programmes within a whole school approach [13] based on generic social and emotional skills training addressing common risk and protective factors, delivered within a supportive school environment in partnership with parents and the local community, has the potential to reach larger population groups with fewer resources.

The evidence for universal interventions implemented with young people affected by war attests to the important role of the school as an accessible setting for such interventions. Similar to previous reviews [72,73], the heterogeneity across the studies in terms of programme content, delivery, duration, and study sample makes it difficult to draw general conclusions about the effectiveness of these interventions as a whole. However, there is evidence that the more structured interventions of longer duration can have a significant positive effect on mental health and wellbeing. The results from the Classroom-Based Intervention (CBI) and the school-based Psychosocial Structured Activities intervention (PSSA), which is based on CBI principles, highlight the positive effect of these interventions on young people's social, emotional and behavioural wellbeing. The differential effects according to gender reported across these interventions, however, calls for further investigation into possible gender specific components. The optimum age for programme implementation also needs further examination. There is evidence from Khamis et al. [48] that CBI did not yield the same significant positive changes with older males (12–16 years) as with the younger group (aged 6–11). This finding is in line with substantive evidence from HICs regarding the need to reach children when they are young in order to sustain their existing resilience and strengthen their coping capabilities [4,12,80-82].

Non-significant findings were also found for a writing intervention implemented with young people aged 12–17 [55] and a CBT intervention implemented with children and adolescents aged 5–16 [54]. It is important to note the initial negative impact of the writing intervention on participants' depression symptoms, which then subsequently declined at follow-up. Common characteristics of these interventions were their short duration and the broad age range of the intervention participants. This is in contrast to the year long after-school intervention implemented with children and adolescents and their parents living in Gaza and the West Bank, which resulted in significant improvement in participants' social and emotional wellbeing and parenting behaviours [56]. The results from these studies underscore the importance of understanding optimum programme components in terms of content, duration, and target age range in order to ensure the development of effective school-based interventions in conflict areas. This is in line with recommendations from previous reviews of school-based interventions implemented in war exposed countries [71,72] including those from secondary prevention interventions, not covered in this review, which also point to the need for more rigorous research on the differential intervention effects related to age, gender and war-related experiences [73,83]. The studies in this review support previous findings concerning the role of universal school programmes for children living in conflict areas as an effective, accessible and efficient means of enhancing and protecting good mental health alongside more targeted approaches for students at higher risk [84]. The exploration of a whole school approach to interventions in this area carries potential for reaching the wider community through the school setting.

The majority of the school-based interventions included in this review were implemented with young people age 12–16 years. In view of the

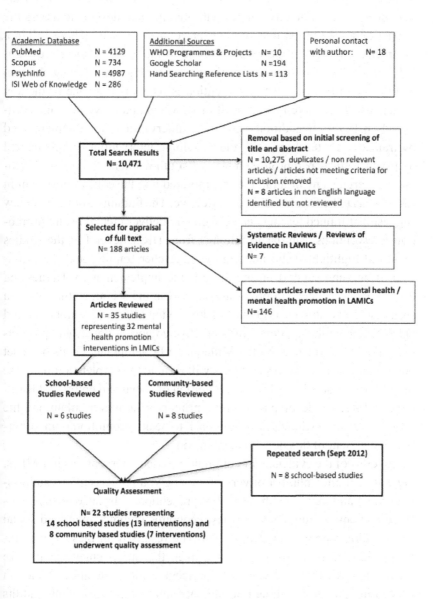

FIGURE 1: Search results from original search of mental health promotion interventions in LMICs.

paucity of evidence of mental health promotion interventions for young children in primary schools in LMICs (age 5–10 years), there is an urgent need for high quality studies with longitudinal designs to assess the impact of school-based intervention for younger primary school children in order to strengthen the evidence base in this area. Schools are arguably one of the most important settings for reaching out to young children and their families and early intervention is recognised as one of the key principles of effective mental health promotion and prevention interventions [4,8,12,80]. In addition, eight of the interventions were implemented by trained class teachers, with the remaining interventions implemented by psychologists, paraprofessionals and youth workers. As Srikala & Kumar [35] argue, any programme incorporated into the education system in LMICs has to be feasible and cost-effective. The findings from this review suggest that trained teachers can effectively deliver mental health promotion interventions. Similar to findings from HICs, several of the studies reviewed highlighted the importance of teacher training and the provision of ongoing support during programme implementation. Harnessing the skills of teachers and providing support in the school setting offers a sustainable and low cost method of improving children's emotional and behavioural wellbeing, developing positive coping strategies and promoting school performance. As the Millennium Development Goals have set out as a target that all boys and girls will be able to complete a full course of primary schools by 2015, the integration of social and emotional learning and lifeskills development in the primary school curriculum and the development of a whole school approach to health promotion is an important component of this development agenda.

In terms of the evidence for community-based interventions in LMICs, there are a limited number of very promising youth interventions addressing sexual and emotional health, HIV prevention, substance misuse, violence prevention, functional literacy, economic empowerment and social participation among excluded groups. The results from these multicomponent interventions are impressive given the improvements that were shown across a broad range of adolescent health outcomes. Although limited in number, the three microfinance interventions for young adults and primary school children included in this review, provide encouraging evidence that combined microfinance and training interventions promoting essential lifeskills, asset building and reourcefulness, can result in significant mental health and wellbeing benefits. Further evaluations of such multicomponent community-based interventions are needed to determine the long-term impact on more specific mental health outcomes.

11.4.1 STUDY LIMITATIONS

This systematic review has a number of important limitations, which impact on its validity. Firstly, there are limitations relating to the scope of the systematic search, which impact on the validity of the findings. Due to the timescale and resources available, a systematic search for studies published in the grey literature was not included, and neither was effort made to find well-designed studies that had not been reported at all due to nonsignificant findings. Furthermore, a search in languages other than English was not undertaken and, therefore, key studies in the other former colonial languages of French, Spanish, Portuguese and Dutch were not included.

Secondly, there are limitations relating to the selection criteria, which also impact on the validity of the findings. Studies not employing traditional experimental or quasi-experimental designs were excluded from the search and therefore, qualitative and other such study designs were discarded in the search process. Of the studies that were included, justification of sample size and validation of the outcome measures employed were not reported in a small number of the papers. It could be argued that such studies should also have been excluded from the review, but in our methodology they were included but received lower quality assessment ratings due to the absence of information on these issues. Finally, as a narrative synthesis the review is not designed to generate summary statistics derived from meta-analyses. Despite these limitations, the studies included in this review clearly demonstrate that high quality and effective mental health promotion interventions, and their evaluation through well-designed research studies, are feasible in LMIC settings.

11.5 CONCLUSIONS

The review findings indicate that mental health promotion interventions for young people can be implemented effectively in LMIC settings. There is good quality evidence regarding the impact of school-based programmes and promising evidence from multicomponent community-based studies that such interventions offer a viable means of promoting the mental health and wellbeing of young people. Notably, the studies reviewed demonstrate the feasibility and effectiveness of integrating mental health promotion interventions into education and community programmes such as community empowerment, poverty reduction, HIV/AIDS prevention, reproductive and sexual health. While the mental health promotion interventions identified in this review have achieved success across a diverse range of countries, relatively few have been systematically scaled up to serve the needs of young people at a regional or national level. Thus, evidence for their sustainability and effectiveness when scaled up through the educational system and community settings in LMICs needs to be strengthened, especially in low-income countries. In addition, the short-term follow-up periods of many of the studies point to the need for future research to evaluate long-term outcomes. Research is also needed to strengthen the evidence-base on the interrelationship between mental health and other health, educational and social wellbeing outcomes. Such research would strengthen the case for mainstreaming the integration of mental health into key health, education and development priorities for young people in LMICs.

The studies reviewed demonstrate the feasibility and potential sustainability of implementing mental health promotion interventions in LMICs through employing existing infrastructures and resources, working with local teachers, community workers, young people and their families. Further research is needed on the contextual factors influencing the adoption and adaptation in LMICs of well-validated interventions that have been developed in low resource settings in HIC countries. In particular, implementation research is needed to ensure the successful adaptation and transfer of school-based interventions for younger primary school children across educational, cultural and socio-economic settings. The development of culturally valid measures of mental health, that will support the evaluation of culturally appropriate interventions in LMICs, is also identified as an area for methodological development. Existing standardized mental health measures from HICs need to be locally validated and the development of culturally sensitive indicators of positive mental health and wellbeing will be particularly important in determining the benefits of mental health promotion interventions delivered in diverse cultural contexts. Developing capacity in LMICs for the implementation and evaluation of mental health promotion policies and practices is fundamental to promoting and sustaining action for positive youth mental health development.

REFERENCES

1. Herrman H, Jané-Llopis E: The status of mental health promotion. Publ Health Rev 2012, 34(2):1-21.
2. Barry MM, Friedli L: The influence of social, demographic and physical factors on positive mental health in children, adults and older people. In Foresight Mental Capital and Wellbeing Project. State-of-Science Review: SR-B3. London: Government Office of Science and Innovation; 2008.
3. Jenkins R, Baingana F, Ahmad R, McDaid D, Atun R: Social, economic, human rights and political challenges to global mental health. Mental Health Fam Med 2011, 8:87-96.
4. Kieling C, Baker-Henningham H, Belfer M, Conti G, Ertem I, Omigbodun O, Rohde LA, Srinath S: Child and adolescent mental health worldwide: evidence for action. Lancet 2011, 378:1515-1525.
5. Durlak JA, Wells AM: Primary prevention mental health programs for children and adolescents: a meta-analytic review. Am J Community Psychol 1997, 25(2):115-152.
6. Hosman C, Jané-Llopis E: Political challenge 2: mental health. Paris: International Union for Health Promotion and Education; 1999. [The Evidence of Health Promotion Effectiveness: Shaping Public Health in a new Europe, A Report for the European Commission]
7. Jané-Llopis E, Barry MM, Hosman C, Patel V: Mental health promotion works: a review. In The Evidence of Mental Health Promotion Effectiveness Strategies for Action Edited by Jane-Llopis E, Barry MM, Hosman C, Patel V. 2005, 2:9-25. [Promotion and Education Supplement]
8. Herrman H, Saxena S, Moodie R: Promoting Mental Health: Concepts, Emerging Evidence, Practice. Geneva: World Health Organization: A report of the World Health Organization, Department of Mental Health and Substance Abuse in collaboration with the Victorian Health Promotion Foundation and Univeristy of Melbourne; 2005.

9.   Barry MM, Jenkins R: Implementing Mental Health Promotion. Oxford: Churchill Livingstone Elsevier; 2007.

10. Nores M, Barnett WS: Benefits of early childhood interventions across the world: (Under) Investing in the very young. Econ Educ Rev 2010, 29(2):271-282.

11. Baker-Henningham H, Lopez Boo F: Early Childhood Stimulation Interventions in Developing Countries: A comprehensive literature review. Washington, DC: Inter-American Development Bank; 2010.

12. Stewart-Brown SL, Schrader-McMillan A: Parenting for mental health: What does the evidence say we need to do? Report of Workpackage 2 of the DataPrev project. Health Promot Int 2011, 26(SUPPL. 1):i10-i28.

13. Weare K, Nind M: Mental health promotion and problem prevention in schools: what does the evidence say? Health Promot Int 2011, 26(SUPPL. 1):i29-i69.

14. Melzer D, Fryers T, Jenkins R: Social Inequalities and the Distribution of Common Mental Disorders. Hove: Psychology Press; 2004. [Maudsley Monographs]

15. Jenkins R, Bhugra D, Bebbington P, Brugha T, Farrell M, Coid J, Fryers T, Weich S, Singleton N, Meltzer H: Debt, income and mental disorder in the general population. Psychol Med 2008, 38(10):1485-1493.

16. Lund C, Breen A, Flisher AJ, Kakuma R, Corrigall J, Joska JA, Swartz L, Patel V: Poverty and common mental disorders in low and middle income countries: a systematic review. Soc Sci Med 2010, 71(3):517-528.

17. Patel V, Lund C, Hatherill S, Plagerson S, Corrigall J, Fundl M, Flisher AJ: Mental disorders: equity and social determinants. In Equity, Social Determinants and Public Health Programmes. Edited by Blas E, Sivasankara Kurup A. Geneva: World Health Organization; 2010:115-134.

18. Miranda JJ, Patel V: Achieving the millennium development goals: does mental health play a role? PLoS Med 2005, 2(10):0962-0965.

19. United Nations General Assembly, 65th Session: Global Health and Foreign Policy Resolution. A/65/L.27.New York, 9th December 2010. Accessible at: http://www.un.org/ga/search/view_doc.asp?symbol=A/65/95

20. Patel V, Flisher AJ, Nikapota A, Malhotra S: Promoting child and adolescent mental health in low and middle income countries. J Child Psychol Psychiatr 2008, 49(3):313-334.

21. World Health Organization: Mental Health: New Understanding, New Hope. Geneva: World Health Organization; 2001. [The World Health Report]

22. Weare K: Promoting mental, emotional and social health: A whole school approach. London: Routledge; 2000.

23. Rowling L: Mental health promotion. In Mental health promotion and young people: concepts and practice. Edited by Rowling L. Australia: McGraw-Hill; 2002:10-23.

24. Zins J, Weissberg R, Wang M, Walberg H: Building academic success on social and emotional learning: What does the research say?. Columbia University New York and London: Teachers College Press; 2004.

25. Payton J, Weissberg RP, Durlak JA, Dymnicki AB, Taylor RD, Schellinger KB, Pachan M: The positive impact of social and emotional learning for kindergarten to eight-grade students: Findings from three scientific reviews. Chicago, IL: Collaborative for Academic, Social, and Emotional Learning; 2008.

26. World Health Organization: WHO's Global School Health Initiative: Health Promoting Schools. Geneva: World Health Organization; 1998. PubMed Abstract

27. Lister-Sharp D, Chapman S, Stewart-Brown S, Sowden A: Health promoting schools and health promotion in schools: two systematic reviews. Health Technol Assess 1999, 3(22):1-207.

28. Wells J, Barlow J, Stewart-Brown S: A systematic review of universal approaches to mental health promotion in schools. Health Educ 2003, 103(4):197-220.

29. Tennant R, Goens C, Barlow J, Day C, Stewart-Brown S: A systematic review of reviews of interventions to promote mental health and prevent mental health problems in children and young people. J Publ Mental Health 2007, 6(1):25-32.

30. Harden A, Rees R, Shepherd J, Brunton G, Oliver S, Oakley A: Young people and mental health: a systematic review of research on barriers and facilitators. London: EPPI Centre; 2001.

31. Wells J, Barlow J, Stewart-Brown S: A systematic review of universal approaches to mental health promotion in schools. Oxford: Health Service Research Unit; 2001.

32. World Health Organization: Seventh Global Conference on Health Promotion: Promoting Health and Development: closing the Implementation Gap. Nairobi, Kenya; 26th-30th October 2009. Accessible at: http://www.who.int/healthpromotion/conferences/7gchp/en/index.html

33. Mrazek CJ, Haggerty RJ: Reducing risks for mental disorders: frontiers for prevention intervention research. Washington DC: National Academic Press; 1994.

34. Jackson N, Waters E, Anderson L, Bailie R, Hawe P, Naccarella L, Norris S, Oliver S, Petticrew M, Pienaar E, Popay J, Roberts H, Rogers W, Shepherd J, Sowden A, Thomas H: The challenges of systematically reviewing public health interventions. J Publ Health 2004, 26(3):303-307.

35. Srikala B, Kumar KV: Empowering adolescents with life skills education in schools-School mental health program: Does it work. Indian J Psychiatr 2010, 52(4):344-349.

36. Bonhauser M, Fernandez G, Püschel K, Yañez F, Montero J, Thompson B, Coronado G: Improving physical fitness and emotional well-being in adolescents of low socioeconomic status in Chile: results of a school-based controlled trial. Health Promot Int 2005, 20(2):113-122.

37. Smith EA, Palen LA, Caldwell LL, Flisher AJ, Graham JW, Mathews C, Wegner L, Vergnani T: Substance use and sexual risk prevention in Cape Town, South Africa: an evaluation of the HealthWise program. Prev Sci 2008, 9(4):311-321.

38. Caldwell LL, Patrick ME, Smith EA, Palen LA, Wegner L: Influencing Adolescent Leisure Motivation: Intervention Effects of HealthWise South Africa. J Leis Res 2010, 42(2):203-220.

39. Caldwell LL, Smith EA, Wegner L, Vernani T, Mpofu E, Flisher AJ, Matthews C: HealthWise South Africa: development of a life skills curriculum for young adults. World Leisure 2004, 3:4-17.

40. Botvin GJ, Schinke S, Orlandi MA: Drug abuse prevention with multiethnic youth. Thousand Oaks, CA: Sage; 1995.

41. De Villiers M, van den Berg H: The implementation and evaluation of a resiliency programme for children. South Afr J Psychol 2012, 42(1):93-102.

42. Rivet-Duval E, Heriot S, Hunt C: Preventing Adolescent Depression in Mauritius: A Universal School-Based Program. Child Adolesc Mental Health 2011, 16(2):86-91.
43. Shochet IM, Ham D: Universal school-based approaches to preventing adolescent depression: Past findings and future directions of the Resourceful Adolescent Program. Int J Ment Heal Promot 2004, 6:17-25.
44. Mueller J, Alie C, Jonas B, Brown E, Sherr L: A quasi-experimental evaluation of a community-based art therapy intervention exploring the psychosocial health of children affected by HIV in South Africa. Trop Med Int Health 2011, 16(1):57-66.
45. Kumakech E, Cantor-Graae E, Maling S, Bajunirwe F: Peer-group support intervention improves the psychosocial well-being of AIDS orphans: Cluster randomized trial. Soc Sci Med 2009, 68(6):1038-1043.
46. Hope A, Trimmel S: Training for transformation, a handbook for community workers. Vols. 1–3. Nairobi: Gweru Mambo Press; 1995.
47. Jordans MJD, Komproe IH, Tol WA, Kohrt BA, Luitel NP, Macy RD, De Jong JT: Evaluation of a classroom-based psychosocial intervention in conflict-affected Nepal: a cluster randomized controlled trial. J Child Psychol Psychiatr 2010, 51(7):818-826.
48. Khamis V, Macy R, Coignez V: The Impact of the Classroom/Community/Camp-Based Intervention (CBI) Program on Palestinian Children. USA: Save the Children; 2004.
49. Ager A, Akesson B, Stark L, Flouri E, Okot B, McCollister F, Boothby N: The impact of the school-based Psychosocial Structured Activities (PSSA) program on conflict-affected children in northern Uganda. J Child Psychol Psychiatr 2011, 52(11):1124-1133.
50. Qouta SR, Palosaari E, Diab M, Punamaki RL: Intervention effectiveness among war-affected children: a cluster randomized controlled trial on improving mental health. J Trauma Stress 2012 2012, 25(3):288-298.
51. Smith P, Dyregrov A, Yule W: Children and war: Teaching recovery techniques. Bergen, Norway: Foundation for Children and War; 2000.
52. Ehntholt KA, Smith PA, Yule W: School-based cognitive-behavioral therapy group intervention for refugee children who have experienced war related trauma. Clin Child Psychol Psychiatr 2005, 10:235-250.
53. Giannopoulo J, Dikaiakou A, Yule W: Cognitive-behavioural group intervention for PTSD symptoms in children following the Athens 1999 earthquake: a pilot study. Clin Child Psychol Psychiatr 2006, 11:543-553.
54. Karam EG, Fayyad J, Karam AN, Tabet CC, Melhem N, Mneimneh Z, Dimassi H: Effectiveness and specificity of a classroom-based group intervention in children and adolescents exposed to war in Lebanon. World Psychiatr 2008, 7(2):103-109.
55. Lange-Nielsen II, Kolltveit S, Thabet AAM, Dyregrov A, Pallesen S, Johnsen TB, Christian J: Short-Term Effects of a Writing Intervention Among Adolescents in Gaza. J Loss Trauma 2012, 17(5):403-422.
56. Loughry M, Ager A, Flouri E, Khamis V, Afana AH, Qouta S: The impact of structured activities among Palestinian children in a time of conflict. J Child Psychol Psychiatr 2006, 47(12):1211-1218.

57. Balaji M, Andrews T, Andrew G, Patel V: The acceptability, feasibility, and effectiveness of a population-based intervention to promote youth health: an exploratory study in Goa, India. J Adolesc Heal 2011, 48(5):453-460.

58. Vasquez M, Meza L, Almandarez O, Santos A, Matute RC, Canaca LD, Cruz A, Cacosta A, Bacilla MEG, Wilson L: Evaluation of a Strengthening Families (Familias Fuertes) Intervention for Parents and Adolescents in Hondurus. Nurs Res South Online J 2010., 10(3)

59. Brady M, Assaad R, Ibrahim B, Salem A, Salem R, Zibani N: Providing new opportunities to adolescent girls in socially conservative settings: the Ishraq program in rural upper Egypt. New York: Population Council; 2007.

60. Jewkes R, Nduna M, Levin J, Jama N, Dunkle K, Puren A, Duvvury N: Impact of stepping stones on incidence of HIV and HSV-2 and sexual behaviour in rural South Africa: cluster randomised controlled trial. BMJ 2008, 337:a507.

61. Bell CC, Bhana A, Petersen I, McKay MM, Gibbons R, Bannon W, Amatya A: Building protective factors to offset sexually risky behaviors among black youths: a randomized control trial. J Natl Med Assoc 2008, 100(8):936-944.

62. McKay MM, Chasse KT, Paikoff R, McKinney LD, Baptiste D, Coleman D, Madison S, Bell CC: Family-level impact of the CHAMP Family Program: a community collaborative effort to support urban families and reduce youth HIV risk exposure. Fam Process 2004, 43(1):79-93.

63. Kim J, Ferrari G, Abramsky T, Watts C, Hargreaves J, Morison L, Phetla G, Porter J, Pronyk P: Assessing the incremental effects of combining economic and health interventions: The IMAGE study in South Africa. Bull World Health Organ 2009, 87(11):824-832.

64. Pronyk PM, Hargreaves JR, Kim JC, Morison LA, Phetla G, Watts C, Busza J, Porter JD: Effect of a structural intervention for the prevention of intimate-partner violence and HIV in rural South Africa: a cluster randomised trial. Lancet 2006, 368(9551):1973-1983.

65. Ssewamala FM, Neilands TB, Waldfogel J, Ismayilova L: The impact of a comprehensive microfinance intervention on depression levels of AIDS-orphaned children in Uganda. J Adolesc Heal 2012, 50(4):346-352.

66. Ssewamala FM, Han CK, Neilands TB: Asset ownership and health and mental health functioning among AIDS-orphaned adolescents: Findings from a randomized clinical trial in rural Uganda. Soc Sci Med 2009, 69(2):191-198.

67. Ssewamala FM, Karimli L, Han CK, Ismayilova L: Social capital, savings, and educational performance of orphaned adolescents in Sub-Saharan Africa. Child Youth Serv Rev 2010, 32(12):1704-1710.

68. Ssewamala FM, Ismayilova L: Integrating children's savings accounts in the care and support of orphaned adolescents in rural Uganda. Soc Serv Rev 2009, 83(3):453-472.

69. Paul-Ebhohimhen VA, Poobalan A, Van Teijlingen ER: A systematic review of school-based sexual health interventions to prevent STI/HIV in sub-Saharan Africa. BMC Publ Health 2008, 8:4.

70. Harrison A, Newell ML, Imrie J, Hoddinott G: HIV prevention for South African youth: which interventions work? A systematic review of current evidence. BMC Publ Health 2010, 10:102.

71. Persson TJ, Rousseau C: School-based interventions for minors in war-exposed countries: a review of targeted and general programmes. Torture Q J Rehabil Torture Victims Prev Torture 2009, 19(2):88-101.

72. Jordans MJD, Tol WA, Komproe IH, De Jong JVTM: Systematic review of evidence and treatment approaches: psychosocial and mental health care for children in war. Child Adolesc Mental Health 2009, 14(1):2-14.

73. Tol WA, Barbui C, Galappatti A, Silove D, Betancourt TS, Souza R, Golaz A, Van Ommeren M: Mental health and psychosocial support in humanitarian settings: linking practice and research. Lancet 2011, 378(9802):1581-1591.

74. Cluver L, Gardner F, Operario D: Psychological distress amongst AIDS-orphaned children in urban South Africa. J Child Psychol Psychiatr 2007, 48(8):755-763.

75. Nyamukapa CA, Gregson S, Lopman B, Saito S, Watts HJ, Monasch R, Jukes MCH: HIV-associated orphanhood and children's psychosocial distress: theoretical framework tested with data from Zimbabwe. Am J Publ Health 2008, 98(1):133-141.

76. Atwine B, Cantor-Graae E, Bajunirwe F: Psychological distress among AIDS orphans in rural Uganda. Soc Sci Med 2005, 61(3):555-564.

77. Green J, Howes F, Waters E, Maher E, Oberklaid F: Promoting the social and emotional health of primary school-aged children: reviewing the evidence base for school-based interventions. Int J Ment Heal Promot 2005, 7(3):30-36.

78. Adi Y: Systematic review of the effectiveness of interventions to promote mental wellbeing in primary schools Report 1: Universal approaches which do not focus on violence or bullying. London: National Institute of Clinical Excellence; 2007.

79. Stewart-Brown S: What is the evidence on school health promotion in improving health or preventing disease and, specifically, what is the effectiveness of the health promoting schools approach. Copenhagen: WHO Regional Office for Europe; 2006.

80. Greenberg M, Domitrovich C, Bumbarger B: The prevention of mental disorders in school-aged children: current state of the field. Prev Treatment 2001, 4(1):1-52.

81. Browne G, Gafni A, Roberts J, Byrne C, Majumdar B: Effective/efficient mental health programs for school-age children: a synthesis of reviews. Soc Sci Med 2004, 58(7):1367-1384.

82. Shucksmith J, Summerbell C, Jones S, Whittaker V: Mental wellbeing of children in primary education (targeted/indicated activities). London: National Institute of Clinical Excellence; 2007.

83. Tol WA, Komproe IH, Jordans MJD, Vallipuram A, Sipsma H, Sivayokan S, Macy RD, deJong JT: Outcomes and moderators of a preventive school-based mental health intervention for children affected by war in Sri Lanka: a cluster randomized trial. World Psychiatr 2012, 11(2):114-122.

84. Layne CM, Saltzman WR, Poppleton L, Burlingame GM, Pasalic A, Durakovic E, Music M, Campara N, Dapo N, Arslanagic B, Steinberg AM, Pynoos RS: Effectiveness of a school-based group psychotherapy program for war-exposed adolescents: a randomized controlled trial. J Am Acad Child Adolesc Psychiatr 2008, 47(9):1048-1062.

CHAPTER 12

PUZZLING FINDINGS IN STUDYING THE OUTCOME OF "REAL WORLD" ADOLESCENT MENTAL HEALTH SERVICES: THE TRAILS STUDY

FREDERIKE JÖRG, JOHAN ORMEL, SIJMEN A. REIJNEVELD, DANIËLLE E.M.C. JANSEN, FRANK C. VERHULST, AND ALBERTINE J. OLDEHINKEL

12.1 INTRODUCTION

Adolescence is a period in which many boys and girls suffer from emotional and behavioural problems, without these problems always posing a long-term health threat [1]. When problems are severe or persistent, however, mental health care may be indicated. Help seeking behaviour is determined by, among other things, whether or not adolescents or their parents perceive the problems as significant and in need of professional help [2]. At preadolescence, the pathway to care relies on parents' recognition of problems [3]. As adolescents mature, the pathway becomes less certain.

Puzzling Findings in Studying the Outcome of "Real World" Adolescent Mental Health Services: The TRAILS Study. © Jörg F, Ormel J, Reijneveld SA, Jansen DEMC, Verhulst FC, and AJ Oldehinkel. PLoS ONE, 7,9 (2012), doi:10.1371/journal.pone.0044704. Licensed under Creative Commons Attribution License, http://creativecommons.org/licenses/by/3.0/.*

Adolescents are probably better informants of their problems [4], but seem less inclined to seek professional help [5].

The increased use and accompanying costs of specialist child and adolescents mental health services (MHS) have heightened the importance of assessing efficacy and cost-effectiveness of services [6]. RCTs in the field typically test one specific intervention in a small, homogeneous sample without complex or co-morbid problems, limiting external validity [7]. There is some evidence from studies comparing care as usual to evidence based treatments [8], [9] that points towards negligible effectiveness of care as usual. Similar results were found in a one-year follow-up study comparing referred to non-referred children [10].

However, studies on outcomes of services provided in a naturalistic setting often suffer from methodological flaws, such as the absence of randomisation, the inclusion of different services and the presence of possible confounding factors [10]. These methodological shortcomings may be dealt with by using sophisticated statistical methods such as propensity score matching, multiple measurement waves, and outcomes on various domains. Using these strategies, we studied the course of emotional and behavioural problems in a population-based cohort of 2230 (pre)adolescents who used or did not use MHS.

The study is carried out in the Netherlands, where mental health care is organised in echelons. For MHS services a referral from the general practitioner (GP) is needed. In the Dutch health care system, everybody is insured for both GP and MHS services; there is no fee for service. The term MHS services includes all inpatient, outpatient and community mental health and social care services for children and adolescents.

12.2 METHODS

12.2.1 ETHICS STATEMENT

The study was approved by the Dutch Central Committee on Research Involving Human Subjects. Written informed consent was obtained of all adolescents and their parents after the nature of the study had been fully explained.

12.2.2 PARTICIPANTS

This study is part of the TRacking Adolescents' Individual Lives Survey (TRAILS), a prospective cohort study of Dutch preadolescents with the aim to explain the development of mental health from preadolescence into adulthood [11]. The present study involves data from the first, second and third assessment wave of TRAILS, which ran from March 2001 to July 2002 (T1), September 2003 to December 2004 (T2), and September 2005 to August 2008 (T3), respectively. TRAILS participants were selected from five municipalities in the North of the Netherlands, including both urban and rural areas. Children born between 1 October 1989 and 30 September 1991 were eligible for inclusion (N = 3483), providing that their schools were willing to cooperate and that they met the inclusion criteria. Over 90% of the schools accommodating 2935 eligible children agreed to participate in the study. 76.0% of these children (N = 2230, mean age = 11.09 years, SD = 0.56, 50.8% girls) were enrolled in the study (i.e., both child and parent agreed to participate). Teacher reports were available for 40.7% of the non-responders, and revealed that they did not differ from responders with respect to the prevalence of problem behaviour, nor regarding associations between socio-demographic variables and mental health outcomes, but were more likely to be boys, have a low socioeconomic background, and perform poorly at school [12]. Of the 2230 T1 participants, 96.4% (N = 2149, 51.0% girls) participated in the first follow-up assessment (T2), which was held two years after T1. Mean age at T2 was 13.56 years (SD = 0.53). The response at T3 was 81.4% (N = 1816, 52.3% girls); mean age was 16.27 years (SD = 0.73).

12.2.3 MEASURES

Emotional and behavioural problem score was the primary outcome measure. Parent-reported emotional and behavioural problems were assessed by the Child Behaviour Checklist (CBCL) [13] which parents filled in at home. Self-reported emotional and behavioural problems were assessed with the Youth Self Report (YSR) [14], which was filled in at school under supervision of one or more TRAILS assistants. Both questionnaires contain a list of 112 emotional and behavioural problems which can be rated as 0 = not true, 1 = somewhat or sometimes true and 2 = often or very true in the past six months. Total problem scores were derived by averaging the scores on all items.

The main predictor variable was mental health service (MHS) use. Parents were asked to report whether they had ever (T1), during the past year (T1), or during the past two years (T2 and T3) visited any MHS for emotional or behavioural problems of their child, and if they had, whether they had also visited this service in the past six months. MHS included child and adolescent inpatient and outpatient services, psychiatrists or psychologists in private practice, community (social) services, psychiatric emergency care, and youth protection services. Scores were dichotomised into having visited at least one MHS or not. Separate scores were made for use prior to T1 and for use in the past six months. Data on MHS use were available for 1885 respondents at T2 and 1464 at T3.

Additional measures included: temperament, which was measured during T1 by the parent version of the Early Adolescent Temperament Questionnaire-Revised (EATQ-R) [15]. The EATQ-R is a 62-item questionnaire containing eight domains: Effortful control, Affiliation, Fearfulness, Frustration, Surgency, Shyness, Aggression and Depressed Mood. Temperament is considered a multi-dimensional concept in which low scores on effortful control and affiliation as well as high scores on frustration and fear are associated with emotional and behavioural problems, whereas high scores on effortful control and affiliation have been shown to protect against these problems [16]–[18].

Preschool behaviour was assessed retrospectively during T1 with a questionnaire developed for TRAILS, on preschool (age 4–5) child characteristics. The questionnaire contained 17 behavioural, emotional and motor items that parents rate on a five-point scale in relation to their child's peers. Examples are: "Was your child bossy, compared to other children?" and "Was your child anxious, compared to other children?". Factor analysis yielded five dimensions: Anxiety, Motor Behaviour, Aggression, Social Behaviour, and Concentration [19].

Parental psychopathology was measured during T1 with the Brief TRAILS Family History Interview, which was administered at home with one of the parents. The questionnaire covered several domains of psychopathology: depression, anxiety, substance abuse, antisocial behaviour and psychosis. The syndromes were introduced by a vignette describing the main DSM-IV characteristics of the disorder, followed by a series of questions assessing lifetime occurrence, professional treatment and medication use. Prevalence rates were comparable to CIDI DSM-IV rates found by direct interviewing in a large population survey [20]. The scores for substance abuse and antisocial behaviour were used to construct a familial vulnerability index for behavioural disorder. The scores for depression and anxiety were used to construct a vulnerability index for emotional disorder [17].

Socioeconomic position (SEP) was constructed based on the educational and occupational level of both parents and family income level during T1. Educational level of parents was classified in five categories; occupational level was based on the International Standard Classification for Occupations [21]. Parents reported on the family income. SEP was constructed as the average of the five items, standardised. The SEP scale captured 61.2% of the variance in the five items and had an internal consistency of 0.84.

Intelligence Quotient (IQ) was estimated during T1 using the Vocabulary and Block Design subtests from the Revised Wechsler Intelligence Scales for Children [22].

Stressful life events were assessed during T2, using a list of 25 life events of which respondents rated whether the event had happened since T1 and how unpleasant it had been. Events were summed to create an overall stress score for the period between T1 and T2, excluding those rated as 'not unpleasant at all'. At T3 the Event History Calendar (EHC, cf. Caspi et al [23]) was administered. The EHC is an interview on important life events, either stressful or pleasant, during the past five years. Both instruments included life events such as death of close relatives, parental divorce, romantic breakup, loss of important friendship and bullying. In addition, the EHC included events such truancy and conflicts between family members. Stressful life events that had occurred between the second and third wave were summed to create an overall stress score during this period.

Self-esteem was measured with the Self-Perception Profile for Children (SPPC) [24] during T1. The SPPC evaluates self-esteem in five domains: scholastic competence, social acceptance, athletic competence, physical appearance, and behavioural conduct, as well as global self-worth. Research in a large sample of Dutch adolescents has confirmed the factor structure of the five domains. The questionnaire showed good psychometric properties [25].

Social skills were assessed with the Social Skills Rating System (SSRS) during T1. The SSRS is a multi-rater social behaviour assessment package with separate rating forms for teachers and parents [26]. Both teacher and parent forms contain three subscales: Cooperation, Assertion and Self Control. The parent version contains an additional Responsibility subscale. Psychometric properties of the SSRS are satisfactory [26]; an earlier TRAILS study with the SSRS has confirmed its reliability in the current sample [27].

Peer Acceptance and Rejection was assessed with peer nominations during T1 [28]. Children were asked which classmates they liked and disliked, for which they could nominate an unlimited number of same-gender and cross-gender classmates. The nominations received for being liked and being disliked were divided by the total number of classmates, that is, the maximum number of possible nominations. This way, the scores were transformed into proportions meaning that differences in class-size are taken into account. Scores for peer acceptance (like) and peer rejection (dislike) thus ranged from 0 to 1 [29].

Perceived parenting was assessed during T1 with the the Egna Minnen Beträffande Uppfostran (My Memories of Upbringing) for Children (EMBU-C). We used the shortened version [30], of which the psychometric properties are satisfactory [30], [31]. The EMCU-C contains three subscales: emotional warmth, rejection and overprotection. The scale Emotional Warmth is characterised by giving special attention, praising for approved behaviour, unconditional love, and being supportive and affectionately demonstrative ("Do your parents make it obvious that they love you?"). Rejection is characterised by hostility, punishment, derogation and blaming of child ("Do your parents sometimes punish you even though you have done nothing wrong"). Overprotection is characterised by fearfulness and anxiety for the child's safety, guilt engendering, and intrusiveness ("Do you feel that your parents are extremely anxious that something will happen to you?"). The answers for both parents were highly correlated, so we combined them into a single score [32].

12.2.4 STATISTICAL ANALYSIS

In mental health care research, randomized controlled trials (RCTs) are considered the golden standard when studying the effectiveness of treatment. Randomization minimizes pretreatment differences between the experimental groups, so that any posttreatment differences can be assumed to be due to the treatment condition. However, randomization is not always possible or desirable [33], [34] and RCTs are often conducted in highly selective patient samples, which threatens the external validity of these studies [35]. Observational studies therefore offer valuable complementary information about treatment outcomes. Since observational studies run the risk of (unmeasured) pretreatment differences between the intervention and control group, a phenomenon often referred to as confounding by indication, specific statistical techniques need to be applied to be able to draw valid conclusions about treatment effectiveness [36]. Three of these techniques, which are described below, were used in the current study on differences in the naturalistic course of emotional and behavioural problems between adolescents who had received mental health treatment and those who had not.

12.2.4.1 ADJUSTING FOR POSSIBLE CONFOUNDERS.

We first performed a multivariate linear regression analysis with MHS use as primary predictor and emotional and behavioural problems at follow up as outcome variables, adjusting for a wide range of potential confounders. In order to be a confounder, a variable should be associated with both the predictor (receiving treatment) and the outcome (follow-up problem score). In our analyses, the most important confounder was pretreatment severity of emotional and behavioural problems. In addition, we selected various other vulnerability markers (i.e., variables assumed to increase both the likelihood of treatment and mental health problems) as putative confounders, as well as a number of resilience markers, which might protect against treatment and mental health problems. Vulnerability markers included an unfavourable temperament (low scores on effortful control and affiliation, high on fearfulness and aggression [16]), difficult preschool behaviour (high scores on aggression, low on social behaviour [19]), low IQ [22], low SEP [37], parental rejection or overprotection [32], mental health care use prior to T1, parental emotional or behavioural disorders [17], poor social skills [27], and peer rejection [29]. Selected resilience markers were a favourable temperament (high scores on effortful control and affiliation, low on fearfulness and aggression [16]), self-esteem, parental warmth [38], and peer acceptance [32]. A final putative confounder was exposure to stressful life events [39]. The effect of all putative confounders on mental health problems and mental health care use was tested univariately. When statistically significant ($p<0.05$) the variable was included in the multivariate linear regression analysis. In the multivariate linear regression analysis, we adopted a stepwise approach to predict mental health problem scores at follow up. First, we included only MHS use (the predictor of interest) and baseline severity of emotional and behavioural problems. In the second step, we additionally included all other vulnerability and resilience markers that had been shown to be related to mental health problems and mental health care use (see above). Third, we added stressful life events.

12.2.4.2 PROPENSITY SCORE MATCHING.

The second technique used to prevent confounding by indication is called propensity score matching [36], [40], [41]. This method has been used in various fields, among which medicine [42], [43], social sciences [44] and mental health care research [45]. In this approach, treated cases are matched to control cases based on a so-called propensity score, that is, the likelihood of being assigned treatment, given a set of pre-treatment observed characteristics [41]. Propensity score matching thus mimics a randomized control trial, although unobserved differences between cases and controls are not accounted for. The propensity score can be derived from a logistic regression analysis in which treatment is predicted by a set of preselected variables known to influence help-seeking and service use [2]. A person's propensity score is the predicted treatment probability, which can range from 0 (lowest probability) to 1(highest probability).

Please note that the propensity score reflects a probability (i.e., having characteristics generally associated with treatment), not actual service use: theoretically, a respondent could have a propensity score of .99 but not have received treatment. The variables that were selected to derive the propensity score in the present study are presented in Appendix 1. After having derived the propensity scores, treated adolescents were matched to non-treated adolescents with a comparable (the same or nearest by) propensity score. Hence, this approach implied a reduction of the dataset because we used only controls (i.e., untreated adolescents) that could be matched to a treated adolescent. In total, 188 adolescents used MHS, of whom 11% (N = 21) could not be matched to a control with a comparable propensity score. These cases were excluded, leaving 167 MHS users and 167 MHS non-users, assumed to be comparable with respect to the likelihood of receiving treatment for emotional and behavioural problems. All covariates were equally distributed across the two groups, indicating that they were comparable in all respects, except for treatment condition. These two groups were compared with regard to the course of their emotional and behavioural problems.

Adolescents were considered "controls" if they did not receive treatment between T1 and T2. Some of the controls, however, did receive treatment two-to-four years later, between T2 and T3. Likewise, some cases received treatment only between T1 and T2, others also between T2 and T3. To examine treatment effects throughout the three measurement waves, we divided the treated adolescents and their matched controls each into two subcategories, yielding four groups. The first group (N = 146) consisted of controls who did not receive treatment between T2 and T3 either, hence did not use MHS throughout the waves. The second group (N = 114) consisted of adolescents who received treatment between T1 and T2, but did not between T2 and T3. The third group (N = 21) consisted of controls who started using MHS after T2, and the fourth group (N = 53) of treated adolescents who continued to receive treatment between T2 and T3. These four groups were compared with regard to their course of emotional and behavioural problems throughout the waves.

12.2.4.3 SENSITIVITY ANALYSES.

The third approach to enhance the validity of the conclusions consisted of sensitivity analyses to examine the robustness of the findings. We conducted four robustness checks. First, we used both parent- and self-reported emotional and behavioural problems to reduce informant bias. Second, we performed the multivariate linear regression analysis (approach 1) with regard to not only MHS use between T1 and T2, but also MHS use between T2 and T3. Third, because mental health care use can concern various types of care, we repeated the linear multivariate regression analysis for clinical (24 hours) mental health care and outpatient mental health care separately. Fourth, to investigate possible bias because of selective dropout, we compared the results with those after multiple imputation of missing data. Missing data were estimated by linear regression analysis using all relevant observations. Five new datasets were created, which were used for the analyses described above. Estimates from all datasets were then pooled, using Rubin's rules [46]

12.3 RESULTS

12.3.1 DESCRIPTIVE STATISTICS

Adolescents who used MHS were, on average, more often male, had higher total problem scores on the CBCL and the YSR, had higher familial loadings on both internalizing and externalizing disorders, and had a lower IQ than those who did not. Of the T1 respondents who scored above the 85th percentile of the CBCL, which is considered a clinical cut-off, 38% visited MHS services, versus 3% of the respondents with the lowest (<P25) CBCL scores.

12.3.2 RESULTS APPROACH 1

Table 1 shows the regression coefficients of the putative predictors of parent-reported problems at T2, tested univariately. Results of the univariate regression analysis predicting mental health care use (available upon request) show statistically significant associations between all putative predictors and mental health care use, except for SEP which was marginally significant. The associations were in the same direction as the associations presented in Table 1, with baseline parent-reported emotional and behavioural problem scores and previous mental health care use being important predictors, and a favourable temperament, social skills and emotional warmth of parents protecting against both emotional and behavioural problems at follow up as well as against mental health care use.

Table 2 shows the result of the multivariate linear regression model with MHS use as predictor of problems at follow up, adjusted for T1 severity, markers of adolescent vulnerability and resilience, and life events between the assessment waves.

MHS use predicted increased total problems as reported by parents at T2, adjusted for severity of symptoms at T1. The association between MHS use and T2 problems was not confounded by any of the before-mentioned risk or protective factors (Table 2).

12.3.3 RESULTS APPROACH 2

Figure 1 shows the differences between uncorrected and propensity-adjusted mean CBCL scores at T1 and T2 of TRAILS participants with and without MHS use. As can be seen in Figure 1a, MHS users had high initial problem scores which had only marginally decreased at T2, whereas non-users have lower initial scores which had decreased more at T2. Figure 1b shows the results based on the propensity score matching. The initial CBCL scores of MHS users and non-users were approximately the same (non-significant difference), but the scores of non-users had decreased remarkably at T2 while they continued to be high in the MHS users.

Figure 2 displays the problem scores across the three waves after having divided the matched initial MHS users and non-users into four groups, based on further MHS use. Future MHS users, as well as initial users who continued to use MHS, appeared to have higher initial (T1) CBCL scores than non-users and participants with MHS use between T1 and T2 only. Furthermore, adolescents who never used MHS but had equal propensity scores as the MHS users showed the largest reduction in emotional and behavioural problems over time (mean reduction from T1–T3 0.11, t = 6.327, df 87, p-value<0.001). Adolescents who had accessed MHS only between T1 and T2 started with slightly higher problem scores which also decreased in time (mean reduction from T1–T3 0.09, t = 4.6, df 66, p-value<0.001). Adolescents who had accessed MHS only between T2 and T3 showed a significant reduction in problem score before they started using MHS (mean reduction 0.19, t = 4.54, df 20, p-value<0.001), after which their problem scores increased, although this change was not statistically significant. Adolescents who used MHS continuously, i.e. between T1 and T2 as well as between T2 and T3, stayed on a high problem level throughout the three waves, with no significant increase or decrease in problem levels.

12.3.4 RESULTS APPROACH 3

Repeating the multivariable regression analysis with self-reported problem score as outcome measure showed comparable results. Likewise, using data from the T2–T3 time period did not alter the results, neither for parent-reported nor for self-reported problem scores as outcome measure. When we used only clinical mental health care (and covariates) as predictor of parent-reported problem scores, the effect size became smaller and non-significant (β 0.03, SE 0.13, n.s.). With outpatient mental health care only, the effect size increased and remained statistically significant (β 0.26, SE 0.12, p-value = 0.027). For mental health care use between T2 and T3, the effect sizes decreased for both clinical care (β 0.13) and outpatient care (β 0.03), and none of the effects reached statistical significance. The multivariate regression analysis with self-reported problems as outcome measure yielded similar results for clinical and outpatient care separately as for total MHS use for the T1–T2 period. For the T2–T3 time period, the effect of clinical mental health care on self-reported problems was not significant (β −0.09, SE 0.14, n.s.), while for outpatient care, the effect increased (β 0.36, SE 0.14, p-value = 0.013).

TABLE 1: Univariate regression analyses with CBCL scores at T2 as dependent variable (standardised regression coefficients with standard errors).

		β (SE)
CBCL score T1		0.68 (0.02)***
MHS use between T1 and T2		0.38 (0.02)***
Gender (male)		0.04 (0.02)
IQ		−0.14 (0.02)***
Socioeconomic position		−0.16 (0.02)***
Familial vulnerability behavioral disorder		0.16 (0.02)***
Familial vulnerability emotional disorder		0.23 (0.02)***
Temperament	Effortful control	−0.43 (0.02)***
	Affiliation	−0.09 (0.02)***
	Fearfulness	0.24 (0.02)***
	Frustration	0.42 (0.02)***
	Surgency	−0.07 (0.02)**
	Shyness	0.05 (0.02)**
	Aggression	0.41 (0.02)***
	Depressed mood	0.42 (0.02)***
Preschool Behavior	Anxiety	0.16 (0.02)***
	Motor behavior	−0.14 (0.02)***
	Aggression	0.25 (0.02)***
	Social behavior	−0.13 (0.02)***
	Concentration	−0.29 (0.02)***
Previous MHS Use		0.33 (0.02)***
Self-esteem	Learning	−0.06 (0.03)**
	Friends	−0.16 (0.03)***
	Sport	−0.03 (0.02)
	Appearance	0.07 (0.03)*
	Behavior	−0.13 (0.03)***
	General	−0.20 (0.03)**
Social Skills	Cooperation (t)	−0.07 (0.03)*
	Assertion (t)	−0.02 (0.03)
	Self-control (t)	−0.07 (0.04)
	Cooperation (p)	−0.11 (0.03)***
	Responsibility (p)	0.15 (0.03)***
	Assertion (p)	−0.18 (0.03)***

TABLE 1: *Cont.*

		β (SE)
	Self-control (p)	−0.34 (0.03)***
Peer acceptance		−0.15 (0.02)***
Peer rejection		0.16 (0.03)***
Emotional warmth of parents		−0.13 (0.03)***
Parental overprotection		0.13 (0.02)***
Parental rejection		0.21 (0.02)***
Life events past two years		0.22 (0.02)***

*CBCL, Child Behaviour Checklist; MHS, Mental Health Service, IQ, intelligence quotient; EXT, externalizing disorder; INT, internalizing disorder; (t) teacher and (p) parent rating. *p<0.05, **p<0.01, ***p<0.001*

TABLE 2: CBCL scores at T2 predicted by MHS use between T1 and T2, adjusted for baseline severity of symptoms (model 1); baseline severity and markers of adolescents vulnerability and resilience (model 2); and baseline severity, markers of adolescent vulnerability and resilience, and stressful life events (model 3).

		Model 1	Model 2	Model 3
		β (SE)	β (SE)	β (SE)
MHS use between T1 and T2		0.21 (0.02)***	0.21 (0.03)***	0.20 (0.03)***
Total problem scores (CBCL) T1		0.62 (0.02)***	0.48 (0.04)***	0.48 (0.04)***
Gender (male)			−0.03 (0.03)	−0.01 (0.03)
IQ			−0.03 (0.03)	−0.02 (0.03)
Socioeconomic position			−0.05 (0.03)	−0.04 (0.03)
Familial vulnerability behavioral disorder			0.02 (0.03)	0.01 (0.03)
Familial vulnerability emotional disorder			0.10 (0.03)***	0.11 (0.03)***
Temperament	Effortful control		−0.06 (0.04)	−0.06 (0.04)
	Affiliation		−0.01 (0.03)	−0.01 (0.04)
	Fear		−0.02 (0.03)	−0.00 (0.03)
	Frustration		−0.03 (0.04)	−0.03 (0.04)
	Surgency		−0.00 (0.03)	−0.01 (0.03)

TABLE 2: *Cont.*

		Model 1 β (SE)	Model 2 β (SE)	Model 3 β (SE)
	Shyness		−0.01 (0.04)	−0.01 (0.04)
	Aggression		0.09 (0.04)*	0.07 (0.04)
	Depressed mood		0.00 (0.04)	−0.00 (0.04)
Preschool Behavior	Anxiety		−0.05 (0.04)	−0.06 (0.04)
	Motor behavior		−0.06 (0.03)	−0.07 (0.03)*
	Aggression		0.06 (0.04)	0.07 (0.04)
	Social behavior		0.03 (0.03)	0.02 (0.03)
	Concentration		0.03 (0.04)	0.04 (0.04)
Previous MHS use			0.01 (0.03)	−0.00 (0.03)
Self-esteem	Learning		−0.00 (0.04)	−0.01 (0.04)
	Friends		−0.05 (0.04)	−0.04 (0.04)
	Sport		−0.04 (0.03)	−0.04 (0.03)
	Appearance		−0.03 (0.04)	−0.01 (0.04)
	Behavior		−0.04 (0.03)	−0.05 (0.03)
	General		0.05 (0.05)	0.04 (0.05)
Social Skills	Cooperation (t)		0.03 (0.04)	0.06 (0.04)
	Assertion (t)		−0.01 (0.04)	−0.01 (0.04)
	Self-control (t)		0.02 (0.04)	−0.00 (0.05)
	Cooperation (p)		−0.03 (0.04)	−0.04 (0.04)
	Responsibility (p)		0.05 (0.04)	0.05 (0.04)
	Assertion (p)		−0.01 (0.04)	−0.01 (0.04)
	Self-control (p)		−0.01 (0.04)	−0.03 (0.04)
Peer Acceptance			0.00 (0.03)	−0.01 (0.03)
Peer Rejection			0.01 (0.03)	−0.00 (0.03)
Emotional Warmth of Parents			−0.00 (0.03)	−0.01 (0.03)
Parental Overprotection			0.01 (0.03)	−0.00 (0.03)
Parental Rejection			0.05 (0.04)	0.04 (0.04)
Life Events Past Two Years				0.14 (0.03)

*Standardized regression coefficients (β) and standard errors (SE) are presented. CBCL, Child Behaviour Checklist; MHS, Mental Health Service, IQ, intelligence quotient; (t) teacher and (p) parent rating. Adjusted R^2 model 1: 0.51, model 2: 0.52, model 3: 0.52. *p<0.05, **p<0.01, ***p<0.001*

A

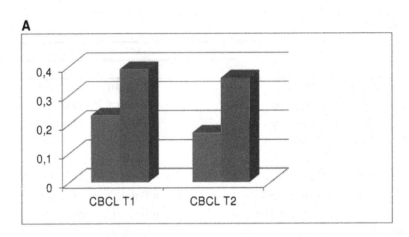

B

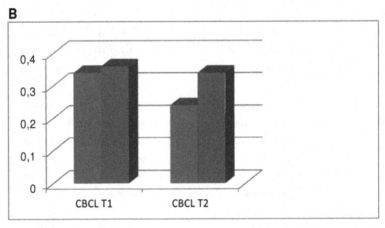

FIGURE 1: A and B. Uncorrected and propensity adjusted mean CBCL-scores of TRAILS participants with and without MHS use. In figure 1A, mean total problem scores (CBCL) are displayed of TRAILS participants with and without MHS use at baseline (T1) and follow up (T2). In figure 1B, mean total problem scores (CBCL) are displayed of propensity matched TRAILS participants with and without MHS use. The participants who did not use MHS had, at baseline, the same propensity (i.e. likelihood) to receive MHS as the participants who actually used MHS. Legend A: Square on right denotes TRAILS participants with MHS use (N = 188). Square on left denotes TRAILS participants without MHS use (N = 1692). CBCL: Child Behaviour Checklist, total problem score. MHS: Mental health services. Legend B: Square on right denotes TRAILS participants with MHS use (N = 167). Square on left denotes propensity score matched TRAILS participants without MHS use (N = 167). CBCL: Child Behaviour Checklist, total problem score. MHS: Mental health services.

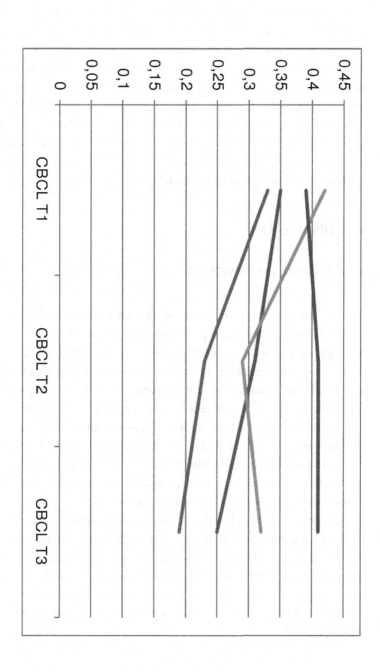

FIGURE 2: MHS use and CBCL scores across the three measurement waves. In this figure, mean CBCL total problem scores are displayed of propensity matched TRAILS participants that did or did not use MHS during a certain time period.

Using self-reported emotional and behavioural problems as outcome measure in the propensity score matching approach yielded slightly deviating results for the group of adolescents that used MHS continuously. Their problem score first increased during T2, then decreased during T3, when it fell slightly below the T1 level. This effect is not seen in the parent-reported problem score for this group. The course of problems for all other groups was similar to what was found with parent-reported problems as outcome measure. The dataset with imputed missing values yielded equivalent results as the ones presented here. More details on any of these analyses are available upon request.

12.4 DISCUSSION

12.4.1 MAIN FINDINGS

In our general population study, adolescents who used MHS had more emotional and behavioural problems than those who did not use MHS, as might be expected. However, MHS use also predicted high problem scores at follow up, and this association was not confounded by any measured marker of adolescent vulnerability or resilience, nor by baseline problem severity. The results were regardless of the informant (i.e. parent- or self-reported problems). Regarding the type of mental health care (clinical or outpatient), the results seem to indicate that these effects are more pronounced for outpatient care than for clinical care, however, in both cases, there is no evidence that the problem scores of the treated group improved more at follow-up than the problem scores of the non-treated group. The propensity score method enabled us to compare the course of mental health problems of a group of treatment users and non-users with comparable likelihood to receive treatment at baseline. The results showed that follow-up problem scores decreased for both non-users and short-term users, but more strongly for non-users. Problem scores of adolescents who use MHS persistently across all waves did not decrease at all.

12.4.2 STRENGTHS AND WEAKNESSES

Studying the outcome of interventions in a naturalistic setting is hampered by the absence of randomisation. The propensity score matching method compensates for that omission by comparing individuals with an equal likelihood of accessing health care services, based on a number of factors that have been shown to influence help seeking behaviour [2], [5]. The matching allowed us to compare the course of emotional and behavioural problems of adolescents with and without MHS use who were, at baseline, equally likely to access MHS based on their propensity score. As opposed to RCTs, which include only adolescents meeting certain inclusion criteria, our respondents came from the general population, reflecting all naturally occurring co-morbidity patterns. This increases the external validity of the results. The propensity score method has proven to be a valuable method to assess treatment effectiveness when randomisation is not possible, or desirable, such as in the situation where one wants to compare the course of problems of treatment users versus non-users. The propensity score method allowed us to balance all measured covariates equally among users and non-users. The large amount of data collected in the TRAILS cohort made it possible to control for a wide range of possible confounders, among which markers of adolescent vulnerability and resilience. The multiple assessment waves enabled the comparison of outcomes over 6 years, with interventions starting and ending at different time points. The multi-informant character of the TRAILS cohort enabled us to use both parent-reported and child-reported measures.

The findings and interpretations as presented in this paper should be regarded in the context of a number of limitations. First, although we adjusted for a wide range of confounders in the multivariate regression analyses and used an equally wide range of variables to calculate the propensity scores, the outcome may have been influenced by variables that were unobserved or difficult to measure. Possible unmeasured differences between treated and untreated adolescents could be, for instance, the clinical view of gatekeepers deciding whether or not to refer adolescents to specialist care, the (perceived) distance to specialist mental health services, (un)favourable past experiences with mental health services, or social support. We did adjust for socioeconomic position, parental education and parental psychopathology, which probably encompass at least part of the bias due to these factors, but may not have been able to exclude all possible bias. Second, information on MHS use was limited in our study: we know which mental health services were visited, but have no information on the duration or intensity of the treatment. Like in regular clinical practice, participants received a variety of specialist mental health care services. We should like to emphasise that, although for research purposes this heterogeneity might be a limitation, an overall (beneficial) effect of MHS use seems absent.

12.4.3 INTERPRETATION OF THE FINDINGS

Confounding by indication, i.e. prognostic factors influencing treatment choices as well as the outcome of treatment, cannot be completely excluded, even though we used sophisticated methods in trying to control for it. However, it might be worthwhile to explore alternative explanations of the findings. For instance, Weisz et al. [8] may have been right in signalling that "care as usual" appears to lack effectiveness. This lack of effect may be caused by the diverse, complex reality of everyday settings, compared to the controlled situation of RCTs. It is possible that evidence-based treatments are not implemented or are implemented for the wrong target group. Alternatively, evidence-based treatments may not be feasible in everyday settings due to a shortage or inadequate schooling of staff [47].

Another possible explanation may be that adolescents using MHS have parents that are more concerned or more troubled by the behaviour of their child compared to parents of adolescents without MHS use. These worries may result in a stronger tendency to access MHS as well as in more severe ratings of their child's behaviour. These speculations are supported by the higher overall explained variance of the model where MHS use is associated with parent-reported problem scores ($R^2 = 0.52$) than of the model predicting self-reported problem scores ($R^2 = 0.46$). On the other hand, use of self-reported problem scores still resulted in a positive association with MHS use, so mono-informant bias is unlikely to explain the association between MHS use and mental health problems completely.

A final explanation for our findings may be sought in unmeasured variance in the duration of treatment. Angold et al. [48] have shown a dose-response relation with regard to the effectiveness of MHS. Adjusted for severity of problems, they showed that psychiatric symptoms started to decrease only after nine therapy sessions. Possibly, our sample contained a group of adolescents with high MHS needs who dropped out of treatment too soon. In a study by Laratatou et al, for instance, approximately 60% of children and adolescents did not comply with treatment, with almost half of them leaving after the first appointment [49]. Early treatment dropout may worsen problem scores. On the other hand, adolescents with relatively mild symptoms who stay in treatment too long may have increasing problems as well, because mental health care visits can lead to (self) stigmatisation [50]. MHS use may support adolescents in dealing with emotional and behavioural problems but also give them the impression that they are needy and weak, incapable of solving their own problems. Unfortunately, we did not collect detailed information on the duration of the MHS use in our study, but future studies should investigate whether these factors possibly increase emotional and behavioural problems rather than decrease them.

12.5 CONCLUSION

Although residual confounding by indication cannot be excluded, our findings urge for a critical analysis of treatment practices in everyday settings. Are evidence-based treatments implemented, and, if they are not, what are the obstacles? If they are implemented, are they effective in real world settings? Is it possible that MHS have adverse effects for some adolescents, and if so, who are these adolescents? However, before such implications are considered, replication studies are necessary to reveal whether or not an artefact is responsible for the results.

REFERENCES

1. Dahl RE, Gunnar MR (2009) Heightened stress responsiveness and emotional reactivity during pubertal maturation: Implications for psychopathology. Dev Psychopathol 21(1):1–6. doi: 10.1017/s0954579409000017

2. Andersen R, Newman JF (1973) Societal and individual determinants of medical care utilization in the united states. Milbank Mem Fund Q Health Soc 51(1):95–124. doi: 10.2307/3349613

3. Sayal K (2006) Annotation: Pathways to care for children with mental health problems. J Child Psychol Psychiatry 47(7):649–659. doi: 10.1111/j.1469-7610.2005.01543.x

4. Verhulst FC, Van der EJ (1992) Agreement between parents' reports and adolescents' self-reports of problem behavior. J Child Psychol Psychiatry 33(6):1011–1023. doi: 10.1111/j.1469-7610.1992.tb00922.x

5. Zwaanswijk M, Verhaak PF, Bensing JM, Van der EJ, Verhulst FC (2003) Help seeking for emotional and behavioural problems in children and adolescents: A review of recent literature. Eur Child Adolesc Psychiatry 12(4):153–161. doi: 10.1007/s00787-003-0322-6

6. Garralda EM (2009) Accountability of specialist child and adolescent mental health services. Br J Psychiatry 194(5):389–391. doi: 10.1192/bjp.bp.108.059477

7. National Institute for Health and Clinical Excellence (NICE) (2005) NICE clinical guideline: Depression in children and young people: Identification and management in primary, community and secondary care.

8. Weisz JR, Jensen-Doss A, Hawley KM (2006) Evidence-based youth psychotherapies versus usual clinical care: A meta-analysis of direct comparisons. Am Psychol 61(7):671–689. doi: 10.1037/0003-066x.61.7.671

9. Weersing VR, Weisz JR (2002) Community clinic treatment of depressed youth: Benchmarking usual care against CBT clinical trials. J Consult Clin Psychol 70(2):299–310. doi: 10.1037/0022-006x.70.2.299

10. Zwaanswijk M, Verhaak PF, Van der EJ, Bensing JM, Verhulst FC (2006) Change in children's emotional and behavioural problems over a one-year period: Associations with parental problem recognition and service use. Eur Child Adolesc Psychiatry 15(3):127–131. doi: 10.1007/s00787-005-0513-4

11. Huisman M, Oldehinkel AJ, de Winter A, Minderaa RB, de Bildt A, et al. (2008) Cohort profile: The dutch 'TRacking adolescents' individual lives' survey'; TRAILS. Int J Epidemiol 37(6):1227–1235. doi: 10.1093/ije/dym273

12. de Winter AF, Oldehinkel AJ, Veenstra R, Brunnekreef JA, Verhulst FC, et al. (2005) Evaluation of non-response bias in mental health determinants and outcomes in a large sample of pre-adolescents. Eur J Epidemiol 20(2):173–181. doi: 10.1007/s10654-004-4948-6

13. Achenbach TM (1991) Manual for the child behavior checklist/4–18 and 1991 profile. Burlington, VT: University of Vermont, Vermont.

14. Achenbach TM (1991) Manual of the youth self-report and 1991 profile. Burlington, VT: University of Vermont, Vermont.

15. Putnam SP, Ellis LK, Rothbart MK (2001) The structure of temperament from infancy through adolescence. In: Eliasz A., Angleiter A, editors. Advances/proceedings in research on temperament. Germany: Pabst Scientist Publisher. pp. 165–182.

16. Oldehinkel AJ, Hartman CA, de Winter AF, Veenstra R, Ormel J (2004) Temperament profiles associated with internalizing and externalizing problems in preadolescence. Dev Psychopathol 16(2):421–440. doi: 10.1017/s0954579404044591

17. Ormel J, Oldehinkel AJ, Ferdinand RF, Hartman CA, de Winter AF, et al. (2005) Internalizing and externalizing problems in adolescence: General and dimension-specific effects of familial loadings and preadolescent temperament traits. Psychol Med 35(12):1825–1835. doi: 10.1017/s0033291705005829

18. Oldehinkel AJ, Hartman CA, Ferdinand RF, Verhulst FC, Ormel J (2007) Effortful control as modifier of the association between negative emotionality and adolescents' mental health problems. Dev Psychopathol 19(2):523–539. doi: 10.1017/s0954579407070253

19. Emond A, Ormel J, Veenstra R, Oldehinkel AJ (2007) Preschool behavioral and social-cognitive problems as predictors of (pre)adolescent disruptive behavior. Child Psychiatry Hum Dev 38(3):221–236. doi: 10.1007/s10578-007-0058-5

20. Spijker J, Graaf R, Bijl RV, Beekman AT, Ormel J, et al. (2004) Functional disability and depression in the general population. results from the netherlands mental health survey and incidence study (NEMESIS). Acta Psychiatr Scand 110(3):208–214. doi: 10.1111/j.1600-0447.2004.00335.x

21. Ganzeboom HBG, Treiman DJ (1996) Internationally comparable measures of occupational status for the 1988 international standard classification of occupations. Soc Sci Res 25: 201–239. doi: 10.1006/ssre.1996.0010

22. Brunnekreef AJ, de Sonneville LM, Althaus M, Minderaa RB, Oldehinkel AJ, et al. (2007) Information processing profiles of internalizing and externalizing behavior problems: Evidence from a population-based sample of preadolescents. J Child Psychol Psychiatry 48(2):185–193. doi: 10.1111/j.1469-7610.2006.01695.x

23. Caspi A, Moffitt TE, Thornton A, Freedman D, Amell JW, et al. (1996) The life history calendar: A research and clinical assessment method for collecting retrospective event-history data. International Journal of Methods in Psychiatric Research 6: 101–114. doi: 10.1002/(sici)1234-988x(199607)6:2<101::aid-mpr156>3.3.co;2-e

24. Harter S (1982) The perceived competence scale for children. Child Development 53(1):87–97. doi: 10.2307/1129640

25. Muris P, Meesters C, Fijen P (2003) The self-perception profile for children: Further evidence for its factor structure, reliability, and validity. Personality and Individual Differences 35: 1791–1802. doi: 10.1016/s0191-8869(03)00004-7

26. Gresham FM, Elliott SN (1990) Social skills rating system. Circle Pines, MN: American Guidance Service.

27. Bakker MB, Ormel J, Lindenberg S, Verhulst FC, Oldehinkel AJ (2011) Generation of interpersonal stressful events: The role of poor social skills and early physical maturation in young adolescents. the TRAILS study. Journal of Early Adolescence 31(5):633–655. doi: 10.1177/0272431610366251

28. Kupersmidt JB, Coie JD (1990) Preadolescent peer status, aggression, and school adjustment as predictors of externalizing problems in adolescence. Child Dev 61(5):1350–1362. doi: 10.2307/1130747

29. Oldehinkel AJ, Rosmalen JG, Veenstra R, Dijkstra JK, Ormel J (2007) Being admired or being liked: Classroom social status and depressive problems in early adolescent girls and boys. J Abnorm Child Psychol 35(3):417–427. doi: 10.1007/s10802-007-9100-0

30. Markus M, Lindhout I, Boer F, Hoogendijk T, Arrindell W (2003) Factors of perceived parental rearing styles: The EMBU-C examined in a sample of dutch primary school children. Pers Individ Differ 34(3):503–519. doi: 10.1016/s0191-8869(02)00090-9

31. Muris P, Meesters C, van Brakel A (2003) Assessment of anxious rearing behaviors with a modified version of "egna minnen betraffande uppfostran" questionnaire for children. J Psychopathol Behav Assess 25(4):229–237.

32. Sentse M, Lindenberg S, Omvlee A, Ormel J, Veenstra R (2010) Rejection and acceptance across contexts: Parents and peers as risks and buffers for early adolescent psychopathology. the TRAILS study. J Abnorm Child Psychol 38(1):119–130. doi: 10.1007/s10802-009-9351-z

33. Black N (1996) Why we need observational studies to evaluate the effectiveness of health care. Br Med J 312(7040):1215–1218. doi: 10.1136/bmj.312.7040.1215

34. de Maat S, Dekker J, Schroevers R, de Jonge F (2007) The effectiveness of long-term psychotherapy: Methodological research issues. Psychotherapy Research 17(1):59–65. doi: 10.1080/10503300600607605

35. Brewin CR, Bradley C (1989) Patient preferences and randomised clinical trials. Br Med J 298(6694):313–315. doi: 10.1136/bmj.299.6694.313

36. Rubin DB (1997) Estimating causal effects from large data sets using propensity scores. Ann Intern Med 127(8):757–763. doi: 10.7326/0003-4819-127-8_part_2-199710151-00064

37. Amone-P'Olak K, Ormel J, Oldehinkel AJ, Reijneveld SA, Verhulst FC, et al. (2010) Socioeconomic position predicts specialty mental health service use independent of clinical severity: The TRAILS study. J Am Acad Child Adolesc Psychiatry 49(7):647–655. doi: 10.1097/00004583-201007000-00005

38. Sentse M, Veenstra R, Lindenberg S, Verhulst FC, Ormel J (2009) Buffers and risks in temperament and family for early adolescent psychopathology: Generic, conditional, or domain-specific effects? the trails study. Dev Psychol 45(2):419–430. doi: 10.1037/a0014072

39. Bouma EM, Ormel J, Verhulst FC, Oldehinkel AJ (2008) Stressful life events and depressive problems in early adolescent boys and girls: The influence of parental depression, temperament and family environment. J Affect Disord 105(0165–0327; 1–3):185–193. doi: 10.1016/j.jad.2007.05.007

40. D'Agostino RB Jr (1998) Propensity score methods for bias reduction in the comparison of a treatment to a non-randomized control group. Stat Med 17(19):2265–2281. doi: 10.1002/(sici)1097-0258(19981015)17:19<2265::aid-sim918>3.0.co;2-b

41. Bartak A, Spreeuwenberg MD, Andrea H, Busschbach JJ, Croon MA, et al. (2009) The use of propensity score methods in psychotherapy research. A practical application. Psychother Psychosom 78(1):26–34. doi: 10.1159/000162298

42. Goodin DS, Jones J, Li D, Traboulsee A, Reder AT, et al. (2011) Establishing long-term efficacy in chronic disease: Use of recursive partitioning and propensity score

adjustment to estimate outcome in MS. PLoS ONE 6(11). doi: 10.1371/journal.
pone.0022444

43. Moroi M, Yamashina A, Tsukamoto K, Nishimura T (2012) Coronary revascular-
ization does not decrease cardiac events in patients with stable ischemic heart disease but might do in those who showed moderate to severe ischemia. Int J Cardiol
158(2):246–252. doi: 10.1016/j.ijcard.2011.01.040

44. Eisner M, Nagin D, Ribeaud D, Malti T (2012) Effects of a universal parenting program for highly adherent parents: A propensity score matching approach. Prevention
Science 13(3):252–266. doi: 10.1007/s11121-011-0266-x

45. Bartak A, Andrea H, Spreeuwenberg MD, Thunnissen M, Ziegler UM, et al. (2011)
Patients with cluster a personality disorders in psychotherapy: An effectiveness
study. Psychother Psychosom 80(2):88–99. doi: 10.1159/000320587

46. Rubin DB (2004) Multiple imputation for nonresponse in surveys. New York: John
Wiley and Sons.

47. McHugh RK, Barlow DH (2010) The dissemination and implementation of evidence-based psychological treatments. A review of current efforts. Am Psychol
65(2):73–84. doi: 10.1037/a0018121

48. Angold A, Costello E, Burns B, Erkanli A, Farmer E (2000) Effectiveness of
nonresidential specialty mental health services for children and adolescents
in the "real world". J Am Acad Child Adolesc Psychiatry 39(2):154–160. doi:
10.1097/00004583-200002000-00013

49. Lazaratou H, Vlassopoulos M, Dellatolas G (2000) Factors affecting compliance
with treatment in an outpatient child psychiatric practice: A retrospective study in a
community mental health centre in athens. Psychother Psychosom 69(1):42–49. doi:
10.1159/000012365

50. Pescosolido BA, Perry BL, Martin JK, McLeod JD, Jensen PS (2007) Stigmatizing
attitudes and beliefs about treatment and psychiatric medications for children with
mental illness. Psychiatr Serv 58(5):613–618. doi: 10.1176/appi.ps.58.5.613

CHAPTER 13

DIALECTICAL BEHAVIOR THERAPY FOR THE TREATMENT OF EMOTION DYSREGULATION AND TRAUMA SYMPTOMS IN SELF-INJURIOUS AND SUICIDAL ADOLESCENT FEMALES: A PILOT PROGRAM WITHIN A COMMUNITY-BASED CHILD AND ADOLESCENT MENTAL HEALTH SERVICE

KEREN GEDDES, SUZANNE DZIURAWIEC, AND CHRISTOPHER WILLIAM LEE

13.1 INTRODUCTION

A large percentage of adolescents present at community-based mental health clinics following acts of nonsuicidal self-injury, such as cutting or burning, due to significant difficulties with self-regulation of their emotions [1–4]. These adolescents often report using self-injury strategies to

Dialectical Behaviour Therapy for the Treatment of Emotion Dysregulation and Trauma Symptoms in Self-Injurious and Suicidal Adolescent Females: A Pilot Programme within a Community-Based Child and Adolescent Mental Health Service. Geddes K, Dziurawiec S, and Lee CW. Psychiatry Journal, 2013 (2013), http://dx.doi.org/10.1155/2013/145219. *Licensed under Creative Commons Attribution 3.0 Unported License, http://creativecommons.org/licenses/by/3.0/.*

overcome emotional numbing [3], and many experience ongoing suicidal ideation, while some go on to make at least one and often more suicide attempts [3, 5, 6]. Given the nature of their presenting difficulties, many would argue that these adolescents have an "emerging borderline personality structure" [7–10].

These distressed adolescents, and the family systems in which they have been developed, have been shown to be remarkably difficult to treat [11], so that many will graduate from child and adolescent mental health settings to become long-term patients of adult mental health services, with multiple hospital admissions due to high levels of dysfunction, extreme management issues, and treatment resistance [3, 12]. The challenges to government-funded health services, both in the public and private sectors within Australia and, indeed, internationally, are compelling [13].

There is a well-established body of literature linking NSSI and suicidal behaviours with emotional dysregulation [3, 14–16] and childhood traumatic experiences, such as physical and sexual abuse [17]. In fact, it has been argued that these behaviours are used as a compensation strategy in posttrauma adaptation, functioning to assist with intra- and interpersonal regulations [17]. Thus, emotion dysregulation and childhood trauma are argued to be intimately linked aspects of the developmental process underpinning NSSI and suicidal behaviours. Support for the primacy of emotional dysregulation as a mediator of self-injury was provided in a randomised controlled trial of cognitive behavioural therapy (CBT) for 15- to 35-year-olds presenting with these difficulties [18]. Results indicated that emotion regulation difficulties, specifically, impulse control and goal-directed behaviours, partially mediated significant reductions in self-injury; however, in contrast, measures of depression, anxiety, and suicidal thoughts played no mediating role. It was recommended, therefore, that interventions aimed at reducing self-injury need to specifically target emotional dysregulation, in preference to other associated mental health disorders.

A promising intervention aimed at improving emotional regulation is dialectical behaviour therapy (DBT), developed by Marsha Linehan [14, 19] to treat chronically suicidal women diagnosed with borderline personality disorder (BPD). Linehan's biosocial theory, central to this intervention, argues that BPD is principally the result of a dysfunctional emotion regulation system associated with instability of thoughts, emotions, behaviours, relationships, and self-image. The original programme [20] was conducted over a one-year period, was highly structured, and included four specific treatment components: weekly individual psychotherapy; weekly group skills-based training; telephone consultation between sessions; and weekly team consultation-supervision meetings. Using principles and strategies drawn from behaviour therapy and Zen Buddhism, DBT is recognised as the first empirically validated treatment developed for adults with BPD [21] and has been accepted as an efficacious way of treating various populations experiencing emotional dysregulation difficulties [22, 23].

Research to date suggests that adult women diagnosed with BPD show improvements following DBT intervention. Specifically, DBT has been found to be effective in reducing targeted problem behaviours, such as self-injury and suicidality, thereby reducing hospital admissions and reducing treatment dropout rates in severely impaired populations. In less severe populations, DBT also appears to produce specific improvements in suicidal ideation, depression, and hopelessness [20, 23, 24].

In 1997, the adult DBT programme was modified (DBT-A) to suit 13- to 19-year-old suicidal adolescents presenting with borderline personality traits [25]. Treatment was reduced from one year to 12 weeks to enhance completion, and weekly individual psychotherapy was also provided, with family members included when family issues predominated. A family member was also included within the skills-training group to act as a coach, improve generalisation of treatment effects, and reduce family dysfunction. The number of skills taught was reduced and the language was simplified to improve learning within 12 weeks. A fifth skills module, "Walking the Middle Path," was also added. Adolescents who completed the programme were also offered a 12-week follow-up patient consultation group, which relied on peer teaching and reinforcement, so that adolescents were able to help each other strengthen the skills learnt in the first three months of the programme.

At the time of the current study development, only three clinical trials of the DBT-A group had been conducted on adolescents presenting with suicidal and self-injury behaviours. The first was a nonrandomised controlled trial for adolescents, aged 14–19 years, who were predominantly females, and compared a DBT group with a treatment-as-usual group [26]. The DBT-A group included adolescents who had attempted suicide and who also presented with a minimum of three additional borderline features. The treatment-as-usual group included suicide attempters only. No difference was found between the groups on rates of suicide attempts; however, DBT-A adolescents had a lower rate of treatment dropout and fewer days of inpatient care. Within the DBT-A group, significant reductions in suicidal ideation, anxiety, and depression were shown. Significant reductions were also found in self-reported BPD symptoms in the areas of confusion about self, impulsivity, emotional dysregulation, and interpersonal problems [26].

Another nonrandomised controlled trial was conducted with adolescent girls residing in three juvenile rehabilitation units [27]. This four-week adaptation of DBT found mixed results when comparing measures of behavioural problems and staff punitive responsiveness between groups of adolescents receiving DBT in a mental health unit with those receiving DBT in a general population unit, against a treatment-as-usual group. Notably, no inclusion or exclusion criteria were used and adolescents in the two DBT comparison groups were distinctly different from each other in terms of behavioural problems, with the mental health adolescent group presenting with more severe mood and thought disturbance. Not unexpectedly, the mental health group showed a marked reduction in problem behaviours following the four-week DBT intervention; however, the general population group showed no reduction in problem behaviours.

In the third trial, adolescents aged between 14 and 17 years were treated with a two-week adaptation of the original DBT-A programme [25] in an inpatient psychiatric unit [28]. Comparisons were made with a treatment-as-usual group and indicated similar improvements in depression, suicidal ideation, and hopelessness for both groups. However, the DBT-A group also showed significantly reduced behavioural incidents on the ward.

A review of the above studies highlighted that the quality of the data was highly questionable due to factors of selection bias, confounding variables, difficulties with outcome measures, and measurement errors [29]. The review concluded that the efficacy of DBT-A in reducing mental health symptoms in adolescents was yet to be established. Specific recommendations for future research were made: firstly, that treatment needed to occur in outpatient settings to minimise the influence of confounding environmental factors on treatment outcome, as can occur in hospital-based settings; and secondly, that more developmentally appropriate measures be used, as all studies incorporated adult and/or child measures that were likely to have been clinically insensitive to the symptomatology of adolescent presentations.

Apart from these three trials, there has also been a study using a within-case design to test DBT with adolescent females, aged between 13 and 19 years, presenting with nonsuicidal self-injurious, and suicidal behaviour within an outpatient setting [30]. The programme consisted of weekly individual therapy, a weekly multifamily skills group, and telephone support, conducted over a 16–24-week period. Results from this study were promising, with adolescents showing reductions in nonsuicidal, self-injurious, and suicidal behaviour, as well as improvements in interpersonal relationships, identity disturbance, impulsivity, and depression over the course of the treatment and at one-year followup. However, given the lack of a supervision/consultation group, it could be argued that treatment integrity was somewhat problematic, given this was one of the four treatment components specified in the original model [25]. More recently, it has also been noted that without treatment adherence ratings, it is difficult to assess whether or not patients actually receive DBT-A treatment [21]. In this regard, it is noteworthy that the most recent study to date [30] did not address the issue of treatment adherence.

The aim of the present study was to develop and pilot a DBT-A programme, based on the original adolescent programme [25], and assess its feasibility and efficacy in treating a community-based outpatient population of adolescents presenting with NSSI and suicidality. Based on the literature, two specific research questions were addressed: (1) does DBT-A lead to improvements in adolescents' capacity to regulate their emotions? and, given the links between emotion dysregulation, borderline personality symptoms, and early trauma experiences, (2) would improvements in emotion regulation produce comparable reductions in trauma-related symptoms, self-injurious behaviours, and suicidality? From the outset, attention was paid to ensure that the measures were appropriate to the age group. In addition, all measures were collected by independent assessors to evaluate outcome.

Importantly, emotional dysregulation was operationalized within the present study as the "fear of losing control over one's emotions or of one's behavioural reactions to emotions" [31, page 241] and relates to the measure of emotional regulation developed for the current study, the Modified Affective Control Scale for Adolescents (MACS-A) [32]. In the development of the original adult measure, the Affective Control Scale (ACS) [31], the fear of fear concept was extended to include the fear of other strong emotions, specifically, depression, positive emotion, and anger, with the focus on attention to internal events, and the perceived ability of individuals to cope with strong emotions. Reflection on the original work of Linehan [14] reveals her acknowledgement of the part played by the fear of anger and of losing control over anger in self-injuring borderline patients, stating "In almost all cases, the under expressive borderline individuals have a marked fear and anxiety about anger expression; at times they fear that they will lose control if they express even the slightest anger, and at other times they fear that targets of even minor anger expression will retaliate" (page 16). Indeed, research in adult populations has found that the fear of one's own emotions is associated with maladaptive psychological outcomes, such as posttraumatic stress disorder, generalized anxiety disorder, and symptoms of borderline personality disorder [33–35].

Two predictions were generated within the present study. First, it was predicted that 14- to 16-year-old adolescents presenting at a community-based Child and Adolescent Mental Health Service with NSSI and suicidality would report a decrease in trauma-based symptoms on the Trauma Symptom Checklist for Children [36] and reduced acts of self-injury and suicidal thoughts, following participation in a 26-week DBT-A programme. Second, it was predicted that a reduction in trauma symptoms, self-injury and suicidal thoughts would be associated with improvements in emotion regulation as measured by a decrease in scores on the Modified Affective Control Scale for Adolescents (MACS-A).

13.2 METHOD

13.2.1 ETHICAL CONSIDERATIONS

This study received joint approval from the Human Research Ethics Committee at Murdoch University, Perth, WA, Australia, and the Human Research Ethics Committee of the South Metropolitan Area Health Service, WA, Australia. All adolescents and their parents participating in this research did so voluntarily.

13.2.2 PARTICIPANTS

Six female adolescents aged between 14.6 years and 15.7 years, with a mean age of 15.1 years, participated in this pilot programme. Three adolescents were current clients of the Child and Adolescent Mental Health Service (CAMHS), while the remaining three adolescents had been recently referred to CAMHS. A parent accompanied all adolescents to the family skills-training component, so that the final group included four mothers and two fathers. Of the six dyads participating, four dyads completed the entire 26-week programme and the remaining two dyads were withdrawn from the programme by their parents, three weeks prior to treatment completion. All six dyads were available for posttreatment (t2) assessments, while five dyads were available for three-month followup (t3).

Adolescents were considered appropriate for the DBT-A programme based on the following criteria:

Inclusion Criteria
1. Aged between 13 and 18 years.
2. Average cognitive ability (clinician's notes, school records) and established reading level (year 5), as measured by the Neale Analysis of Reading Ability [37].
3. Referred to the service because of deliberate self-harm and/or suicidal ideation in the previous 12 months.
4. A minimum of three BPD features, as determined by clinician assessment and according to DSM-IV criteria.

Exclusion Criteria
1. A primary diagnosis of a psychotic disorder.
2. A primary diagnosis of substance abuse.
3. An intellectual disability.

13.2.3 DESIGN

The process of implementation and assessment of this 26-week pilot group was as follows:

1. 8-week engagement and commitment to DBT-A: treatment contracts signed by adolescents and parents, and individual and group clinicians. (t1) Pretreatment measures administered prior to engagement.
2. 18-week DBT-A treatment: (t2) posttreatment measures administered at completion of programme.
3. Followup: (t3) 3-month follow-up measures administered.

13.2.4 MEASURES

13.2.4.1 INTAKE MEASURES

Assessment of Borderline Personality Features. Past researchers [25] investigating the effectiveness of DBT-A in the treatment of suicidal adolescents presenting with borderline features have used a structured clinical interview, the SCID-11 [38], to determine suitability for the DBT-A programme. However, the SCID-11 was designed for use with individuals aged 18 years and older and its construct validity and predictive ability with adolescents has been challenged [7]. Therefore, assessment of borderline features for the purposes of this study was determined in a clinical interview, by reference to criteria set out in the Diagnostic and Statistical Manual IV (1994).

Neale Analysis of Reading Ability [37]. Adolescents were screened individually on this measure of reading ability. The Neale Analysis is a standardised measure of both reading accuracy (word recognition in context) and reading comprehension (assessed by the ability to answer a series of questions about a passage). A reading age equivalent of age 10 was needed to understand programme content.

13.2.4.2 OUTCOME MEASURES

Self-Harm/Suicidal Thoughts Questionnaire: Parent and Adolescent Versions. A self-report questionnaire, developed specifically for this programme, consisted of three sections: section one assessed various forms of self-injurious behaviours, inclusive of abuse of medications, burning, scratching or cutting, and hitting or punching the self; section two assessed the extent of each self-injurious behaviour, including age when commenced, frequency, and seriousness (requiring medical treatment); section three assessed frequency of suicidality.

Modified Affective Control Scale for Adolescents (MACS-A) [32]. This 41-item self-report questionnaire was developed specifically for the current programme as a measure of adolescent's capacity to regulate their emotions and is a reworded version of an adult measure of emotion regulation, the Affective Control Scale (ACS) [39]. This scale consists of four subscales that measure fear of anger (8 items), fear of depression (8 items), fear of anxiety (13 items), and fear of positive emotion (12 items). Participants rate each item on a 7-point Likert scale, from "very strongly disagree" to "very strongly agree," with a neutral midpoint. Individual subscale scores are computed as the mean of the total number of items contained in the subscale. An overall scale score is computed as the mean of all 41 responses, with the higher the mean score, the higher the perceived fear of emotion/s and the greater the difficulty in emotional regulation. The MACS-A was found to be internally consistent in both clinic and nonclinic adolescent samples and to effectively discriminate between these two groups, with the exception of the fear of positive emotion subscale [32]. For this reason, results from this subscale were not included in the current analysis.

Trauma Symptom Checklist for Children (TSCC) [36]. This 54-item self-report measure assesses a variety of symptoms associated with trauma experiences in children, aged between 8 and 16 years. Participants rate each item on a 5-point Likert scale, from "not at all characteristic" to "very characteristic" of themselves. The measure has two validity scales (underresponding and overresponding) and six clinical scales: anxiety, depression, anger, posttraumatic stress, sexual concerns and dissociation. There are also two additional subscales: sexual concerns (sexual preoccupation and sexual distress) and dissociation (overt dissociation, fantasy). The reliability and validity of the TSCC were independently examined in a clinical sample of adolescents, including a percentage with a history of sexual abuse [40]. These researchers found that all six scales and four subscales of the TSCC were a reliable and valid measure of distress in a psychiatric adolescent sample. The current study does not report on results from dissociation (fantasy) or the sexual concerns subscales.

13.3 PROCEDURE

Both parent/s and adolescent attended an initial appointment with the programme coordinator. Programme content and commitments were explained, and consent forms were completed including consent for the videotaping of all individual and group sessions.

13.3.1 DBT-A PROGRAMME DEVELOPMENT (LIFE SURFING)

This programme was developed over the course of 2005 and 2006, based on a previous adaptation of DBT for adolescents [25] that was modified from adult programme content [14, 19].

Similar to previous versions [25], there were four treatment components: individual therapy, a multifamily skills-training group, phone consultation, and a therapist supervision/consultation group. All four components were built into this pilot programme, entitled "Life-Surfing," with the exception of the out-of-hours phone consultation, due to lack of clinician indemnity. In addition, the family skills group ran for 18 weeks, whereas the original DBT-A programme [25] ran for 12 weeks. The following is a description of the components of the DBT-A, "Life-Surfing" programme.

(1) Individual Therapy. Adolescents were seen weekly (twice weekly, if needed) for the length of the programme. The structure of individual treat-

ment was in line with the standard DBT protocol [14], which set out a prescriptive treatment hierarchy consisting of four stages:

1. a pretreatment stage involved orienting the client to treatment, gaining commitment, and agreeing on the goals of treatment;
2. first stage focused on client stability, connection, and safety and structured with a specific subhierarchy of therapeutic goals:
3. decrease life-threatening behaviours;
4. decrease therapy-interfering behaviours;
5. decrease quality-of-life interfering behaviours;
6. increase behavioural skills;
7. second stage involved exposure and emotional processing of the past;
8. third stage looked at increasing respect for the self- and individual goals.

As recommended [25], family members were invited to join individual sessions when systemic issues dominated.

(2) Family Skills Training Group. This group was highly structured and ran for two hours each week. Sessions were psychoeducational in focus with an emphasis on acquisition and practicing of new skills. There were five modules written for the DBT-A programme: Core Mindfulness, Distress Tolerance, Emotion Regulation, Interpersonal Skills, and Middle Path. Modules were presented in the above sequence, and each module ran for four weeks, with the exception of the core mindfulness module, which ran for two weeks. Core mindfulness skills were revisited throughout the length of the programme, and, by the ninth week of the skills training group, adolescents and/or parents volunteered to run the mindfulness exercise that commenced each week's group skills-training session. The family skills-training group ran for 18 weeks.

(3) Phone Consultation. Provided during business hours and focused on helping adolescents use skills learnt during the programme.

(4) Supervision/Consultation Team. A group of interested CAMHS clinicians formed the supervision/consultation team. This team met every week for two hours during the initial stages of the programme development, and then throughout the length of the programme implementation. This was a multidisciplinary team consisting of individuals trained in clinical psychology, social work, and psychiatry. Initially, the purpose of this team was to develop the programme content and structure, including programme viability, funding, ethical considerations, and clinical concerns, as well as to provide ongoing education regarding the implementation of the DBT model. Once treatment commenced, this group provided clinical supervision and addressed treatment integrity through the review of videotaped individual and group skills-training sessions, as recommended [14].

13.3.2 PROGRAMME COMMITMENTS

Adolescents, parents, individual and group skills clinicians, and supervision/consultation team members made formal commitments to the DBT-A programme prior to its commencement. These commitments formed the basis of the programme contracts signed by adolescents, parents, and clinicians as follows:

Adolescents agreed to
1. weekly individual therapy for the length of the programme (26 weeks);
2. weekly family skills-training group (18 weeks);
3. videotaping of all individual and group sessions.

Parents agreed to
1. weekly family skills-training group (18 weeks);
2. videotaping of all group sessions.

Clinicians agreed to work with clients for 6 months which included
1. weekly individual therapy: 26 weeks (individual therapists);
2. weekly family skills group: 18 weeks (group therapists);
3. clinical consultation/supervision group (2 hrs/week);

4. videotaping of all therapy sessions.

Individual and group clinicians also agreed to take no more than two weeks leave within the six-month period of the programme.

13.3.3 CLINICIAN EXPERIENCE AND TRAINING

All members of the team received one full day of in-house DBT training, conducted by two clinical psychologists who were members of the DBT consultation/supervision team. One of these clinicians had attended a five-day intensive training workshop on DBT conducted by Linehan's training organization, Behavior Tech., while the other clinician was at that time co-ordinating an adult DBT programme and was also a coleader of the group skills-training component of that programme.

13.3.4 TREATMENT ADHERENCE CHECK

An estimate of individual and group therapist adherence to the basic strategies of DBT was conducted by rating a random sample of five recorded individual therapy sessions and five recorded group skills-training sessions against a DBT adherence rating scale. The third author, who is a recognised trainer in DBT, rated these sessions. The mean adherence rating was 4.0 out of a possible 5.0, with a range of between 3.5 and 4.5.

13.4 RESULTS

The effect of the programme was investigated by using group mean scores to calculate the Wilcoxon signed-rank test at t1 (pretreatment), t2 (posttreatment), and t3 (three-month followup), on the TSCC and MACS-A. Effect size (r) was also calculated, based on the standardised difference between two means for dependent groups. Initial interpretation of effect size (r), set out below, used the general convention provided by Cohen [41] as follows: r: small > 0.10, medium > 0.3, large > 0.5. However, in interpreting the meaningfulness of effect sizes, it has been noted that a practically significant result is one that has meaning in the real world, and interpretation is a complex and subjective process [42].

TABLE 1: Pre- (t1) and posttreatment (t2) comparisons on the TSCC for the 6 participants.

	Pretreatment (t1)		Posttreatment (t2)		Statistics (t1 to t2)	
TSCC	Mean	SD	Mean	SD	Wilcoxon's test	Effect size
Anxiety	58	9.01	48.5	6.25	P = 0.046*	0.6
Depression	64	9.21	58.33	9.70	P = 0.038*	0.59
Anger	68	11.63	58.17	8.66	P = 0.042*	0.58
PTS	60	10.71	53.83	10.61	P = 0.043*	0.58
Dissociation	63	16.9	61.17	18.43	P = 0.92	0.03

sig < 0.05 (2 tailed).

13.4.1 CHANGES IN SUICIDAL THOUGHTS AND DELIBERATE SELF-HARM BEHAVIOURS

Prior to commencement of therapy, all six adolescents were reporting suicidal thoughts at a minimum of twice weekly to a maximum of several times a day. One adolescent had also attempted suicide on more than one occasion. During treatment, and 12 months after treatment, no adolescent attempted suicide. At the end of the programme, one adolescent reported continuing suicidal thoughts once a week, one other adolescent reported suicidal thoughts once a month, while the remaining four adolescents reported no further suicidal ideation.

All adolescents reported regular DSH for at least three months prior to entry to DBT-A treatment. At the end of the programme, five of the six adolescents had ceased to self-harm over the course of treatment, while the remaining adolescent reported a 50% reduction in DSH events.

13.4.2 COMPARISON BETWEEN TRAUMA-RELATED SYMPTOMS AT PRETREATMENT (T1), POSTTREATMENT (T2), AND 3-MONTH FOLLOWUP (T3)

All participants produced valid TSCC protocols at t1, t2, and t3, as indicated by nonsignificant levels of over- and underresponding. Table 1 presents pre- and posttreatment comparisons on subscale scores of the TSCC, revealing large and statistically significant decreases in mean scores on self-reported anxiety ($z = -2.07$, $P < 0.05$, $r = 0.60$), depression ($z = -2.03$, $P < 0.05$, $r = 0.59$), anger ($z = -2.0$, $P < 0.05$, $r = 0.58$), and posttraumatic stress ($z = -2.02$, $P < 0.05$, $r = 0.58$).

Table 2 presents pretreatment (t1) and three-month (t3) followup comparisons on subscale scores of the TSCC, revealing large and significant decreases in mean scores on self-reported anxiety ($z = -2.02$, $P < 0.05$, $r = 0.64$), depression ($z = -2.02$, $P < 0.05$, $r = 0.64$), and posttraumatic stress ($z = -2.02$, $P < 0.05$, $r = 0.64$). There was also a large decrease in mean scores at three-month followup on self-reported anger; however, this decrease was nonsignificant ($z = -1.83$, $P < 0.05$, $r = 0.58$).

TABLE 2: Pre- (t1) and three-month follow-up (t3) comparisons on the TSCC (n = 5).

TSCC	Pretreatment (t1)		3-month followup (t3)		Statistics (t1–t3)	
	Mean	SD	Mean	SD	Wilcoxon's test	Effect size
Anxiety	67	5.4	49	9.06	P = 0.043*	0.64
Depression	71	10.07	51.4	11.78	P = 0.043*	0.64
Anger	60	8.46	48	6.44	P = 0.068	0.58
PTS	64	6.52	49.6	12.34	P = 0.043*	0.64
Dissociation	68	13.01	54.6	9.5	P = 0.138	0.47

sig < 0.05 (2 tailed).

13.4.3 COMPARISON BETWEEN EMOTIONAL REGULATION AT PRETREATMENT (T1), POSTTREATMENT (T2), AND 3-MONTH FOLLOWUP (T3)

Table 3 presents pre- and posttreatment comparisons on the whole-scale and subscale scores of the MACS-A. On the whole-scale measure of fear of emotion, there was a large but statistically nonsignificant decrease in mean scores ($z = -1.78$, $P > 0.05$, $r = -0.51$) from pretreatment to posttreatment. Comparison of subscale mean scores revealed a large and statistically significant decrease in self-reported fear of anger between pretreatment and posttreatment ($z = -2.20$, $P < 0.05$, $r = -0.64$) and a small but nonsignificant decrease in fear of depression ($z = -0.95$, $r = -0.28$); however, the decrease in fear of anxiety was both negligible and nonsignificant ($z = -0.21$, $P > 0.05$, $r = -0.06$).

TABLE 3: Pre- (t1) and posttreatment (t2) comparisons on the MACS-A ($n = 6$).

MACS-A	Pretreatment (t1)		Posttreatment (t2)		Statistics (t1 to t2)	
	Mean	SD	Mean	SD	Wilcoxon's test	Effect size
Fear of Anxiety	4.57	1.27	3.32	1.22	P = 0.833	−0.06
Fear of Anger	3.86	0.69	3.73	0.45	P = 0.028*	−0.64
Fear of Depression	4.07	1.24	3.33	0.91	P = 0.34	−0.28
Fear of Emotion	4.00	0.83	3.40	0.55	P = 0.075	−0.51

sig < 0.05 (2 tailed).

Table 4 presents pretreatment (t1) and three-month follow-up (t3) comparisons on the whole-scale and subscale scores of the MACS-A. Results from the whole-scale measure of fear of emotion indicate a moderate decrease in mean scores from pretreatment to three-month posttreatment; however, this change was not statistically significant ($z = -1.21$, $P > 0.05$, $r = -0.38$). With regard to the subscales, results reveal a large and statistically significant decrease in self-reported fear of depression ($z = -1.21$, $P > 0.05$, $r = -0.64$) three months after treatment. There was also a moderate but nonsignificant decrease in self-reported fear of anger ($z = -0.1.48$, $P > 0.05$, $r = -0.47$) and fear of anxiety ($z = -1.21$, $P < 0.05$, $z = -0.38$) three months after treatment.

TABLE 4: Pre- (t1) and three-month follow-up (t3) comparisons on the MACS-A (n = 5).

MACS-A	Pretreatment (t1)		3-month followup (t3)		Statistics (t1 to t3)	
	Mean	SD	Mean	SD	Wilcoxon's test	Effect size
Fear of Anxiety	3.9	0.76	3	1.11	P = 0.225	−0.38
Fear of Anger	4.6	1.41	3.36	0.96	P = 0.138	−0.47
Fear of Depression	4.4	1.03	2.88	0.73	P = 0.042*	−0.64
Fear of Emotion	4.01	0.91	3.1	0.8	P = 0.225	−0.38

sig < 0.05 (2 tailed).

13.5 DISCUSSION

The overarching goal of the current study was to develop and pilot a DBT-A programme, based on the work of Miller et al. [25], and to assess both its feasibility and efficacy in a community-based population of adolescent females presenting with DSH and suicidal thoughts. A further focus was to assess the central tenet of Linehan's [14] biosocial theory, which argues that emotional dysregulation underpins the DSH and suicidal behaviours associated with a borderline personality.

In discussing the results of the present study, recognition is given to recent requests for scientifically valid and practical research [43]. When interpreting the practical significance of findings, the majority of studies reporting on effect sizes fail to interpret them in meaningful ways, with three important factors being highlighted when considering interpretation [42, page 34]:

1. context: small effects may be linked to large consequences and that small effects may be cumulative;

2. contribution to knowledge when conducted in real-world settings;
3. Cohen's criteria.

Certainly, when looking at the practical significance of the current findings, it is important to emphasise the difficulties of engaging with and treating this population of adolescents. Effective early interventions are needed, given the high costs of multiple hospital admissions and the likely probability of continued treatment through to adulthood. Given this, it could be argued that even small effect sizes, whereby one or two adolescents respond well to treatment, can be considered practically significant over a longer term.

Results of the current study provided support for our initial hypothesis that adolescents participating in the DBT-A programme would report a decrease in trauma-based symptoms on the TSCC and reduced acts of self-injury and suicidal thoughts. Adolescents reported large and significant reductions in their symptoms of anxiety, anger, depression, and posttraumatic stress immediately following DBT-A treatment. Three months following the end of treatment, adolescents continued to report significantly large reductions in anxiety, depression, and posttraumatic stress symptoms and a large reduction in anger symptoms. While there was no meaningful reduction in dissociative symptoms immediately following treatment, moderate reductions were reported three months after treatment completion. These results are consistent with earlier research where significant reductions in anger, depression, and dissociative symptoms, as measured by the TSCC, were found in a group of self-harming and suicidal adolescents following DBT-A treatment at a community outpatient clinic [44]. Furthermore, the present study findings regarding the cessation of self-harm and reduction in suicidal thoughts by the end of the programme are consistent with earlier DBT-A research [45].

Results from the present study also provided support for our second hypothesis that adolescents participating in the DBT-A programme would show an improved capacity to regulate their emotions, as measured by the MACS-A. Importantly, on average, adolescents reported a large reduction in their fear of emotion following treatment, and this decrease was maintained, albeit more moderately, three months following treatment. On the fear of anger subscale scores of the MACS-A, adolescents reported a large a decrease following treatment, but this was not maintained three months after treatment. On average, adolescents also reported a small reduction in their fear of depression immediately following treatment, and, encouragingly, this reduction became both large and significant three months after treatment completion. Although there were no reported meaningful improvements in adolescents' fear of anxiety on completion of treatment, moderate reductions were reported three months later.

Overall, these results suggest that this group of adolescents reported an improved capacity to manage their strong emotions following participation in the DBT-A programme, and that these gains were maintained in varying degrees three months later. In particular, they reported that their fear of depression and fear of anxiety continued to decrease over the three-month period following the end of all treatments. This result supports previous findings [46] that treatment gains made by self-harming adolescent females following DBT intervention were not only maintained six months after treatment, but continued to show further improvement. Given the importance of the therapy relationship as a container of emotion, particularly in this population [47], the finding that adolescents participating in the current programme were able to report continuing reductions in their fear of depression and anxiety three months after the cessation of all treatment is encouraging.

Importantly, specific recommendations made in a review [29] of the data from past clinical trials were addressed within the current study. First, treatment occurred within a community-based outpatient setting, reducing the confounding effects of environmental factors that are likely to occur within an inpatient setting. Second, the current study used developmentally appropriate measures of outcome, including the development of a measure that specifically assessed emotional regulation in adolescents in the form of perceived fear of emotions, shown by past studies to be linked to problematic mental health outcomes, including borderline personality symptoms. Finally, attention was paid to treatment fidelity. The present study determined an acceptable level of DBT treatment adherence from rating a random sample of taped individual and group sessions.

Confidence in the findings from the present study was also increased by the use of an independent researcher to collect pre-, post-, and follow-up measures, thereby minimising the potential for bias that has occurred in other studies [30]. Furthermore, determining adolescents' capacity to understand the programme material through formal assessment of their reading level and comprehension has not occurred in previous studies and adds to the reliability of the current results.

From a service provision perspective, this study contains some other specific strengths. Of the six adolescents participating in the programme, only one remained in therapy following the end of the programme. Notably, one other adolescent, who had been treated at the clinic at various times since she was six years of age, did not return for any further treatment following the ending of the DBT-A programme, with followups revealing that she had moved into full-time work and training. Given that long waiting lists for admission to CAMHS clinics is a common problem, combined with the high probability for these adolescents to move into adult mental health services, this finding is of great practical significance.

The current study also had some limitations inherent within its design. Specifically, as a pilot study, it lacked a control group, and, therefore, specific conclusions about the effectiveness of the programme cannot be made. Neither can it be concluded that the DBT-A programme was more effective than treatment-as-usual. However, it can be said that four of the six adolescents completed the programme, which is comparable to the 62% completion rate of other studies [45]. Given the high rates of treatment dropout usual for this population, this finding provides some support for the potential effectiveness of DBT-A with these adolescents. A further limitation of this study was the potential influence of demand characteristics on self-report measures. Future studies would benefit from the collection of more objective markers of treatment effectiveness, for instance, collateral information from parents and schools.

13.6 CONCLUSIONS

In this pilot programme, we found preliminary evidence that DBT-A for the treatment of NSSI and suicidality in adolescents was both feasible and efficacious. Despite limited funding for this project, a DBT-A programme was successfully developed and piloted in the community setting in which these high-risk adolescents are most likely to seek initial treatment. Furthermore, results suggest that emotional regulation and trauma symptoms are important constructs to be monitored over time.

REFERENCES

4. S. A. Fortune and K. Hawton, "Deliberate self-harm in children and adolescents: a research update," Current Opinion in Psychiatry, vol. 18, no. 4, pp. 401–406, 2005.
5. R. Best, "Deliberate self-harm in adolescence: a challenge for schools," British Journal of Guidance and Counselling, vol. 34, no. 2, pp. 161–175, 2006.
6. A. L. Miller, J. H. Rathus, and M. M. Linehan, Dialectical Behavior Therapy with Suicidal Adolescents, The Guilford Press, New York, NY, USA, 2007.
7. M. K. Nixon, L. McLagan, S. Landell, A. Carter, and M. Deshaw, "Developing and piloting community-based self-injury treatment groups for adolescents and their parents," The Canadian Child and Adolescent Psychiatry Review, vol. 13, pp. 62–67, 2004.
8. M. S. Gould, T. Greenberg, D. M. Velting, and D. Shaffer, "Youth suicide risk and preventive interventions: a review of the past 10 years," Journal of the American Academy of Child and Adolescent Psychiatry, vol. 42, no. 4, pp. 386–405, 2003.
9. J. Cooper, N. Kapur, R. Webb et al., "Suicide after deliberate self-harm: a 4-year cohort study," American Journal of Psychiatry, vol. 162, no. 2, pp. 297–303, 2005.
10. H. Boudurant, B. Greenfield, and M. T. Sze, "Construct validity of the adolescent Borderline Personality Disorder: a review," The Canadian Child and Adolescent Psychiatry Review, vol. 13, pp. 53–557, 2004.
11. R. Bradley, C. Z. Conklin, and D. Westen, "The borderline personality diagnosis in adolescents: gender differences and subtypes," Journal of Child Psychology and Psychiatry and Allied Disciplines, vol. 46, no. 9, pp. 1006–1019, 2005.
12. M. J. Harman, "Children at-risk for borderline personality disorder," Journal of Contemporary Psychotherapy, vol. 34, no. 3, pp. 279–290, 2004.
13. A. James, "Borderline personality disorder: a study in adolescence," European Child and Adolescent Psychiatry, vol. 5, no. 1, pp. 11–17, 1996.
14. A. L. Miller, J. Glinski, K. A. Woodberry, A. G. Mitchell, and J. Indik, "Family therapy and dialectical behavior therapy with adolescents—part I: proposing a clinical synthesis," American Journal of Psychotherapy, vol. 56, no. 4, pp. 568–584, 2002.
15. A. M. Chanen, L. K. McCutcheon, M. Jovev, H. J. Jackson, and P. D. McGorry, "Prevention and early intervention for borderline personality disorder," The Medical Journal of Australia, vol. 187, no. 7, pp. S18–S21, 2007.
16. N. Pasieczny and J. Connor, "The effectiveness of dialectical behaviour therapy in routine public mental health settings: an Australian controlled trial," Behaviour Research and Therapy, vol. 49, no. 1, pp. 4–10, 2011.
17. M. M. Linehan, Cognitive-Behavioral Treament of Borderline Personality Disorder, The Guilford Press, New York, NY, USA, 1993.
18. A. M. Kring and K. H. Werner, "Emotion regulation and psychopathology," in The Regulation of Emotion, P. Phillippot and R. S. Feldman, Eds., pp. 359–385, Lawrence Erlbaum Associates, Mahwah, NJ, USA, 2004.

19. J. Paris, Ed., The Psychiatric Clinics of North America: Borderline Personality Disorder, W.B. Saunders, Philadelphia, Pa, USA, 2000.

20. T. M. Yates, "The developmental psychopathology of self-injurious behavior: compensatory regulation in posttraumatic adaptation," Clinical Psychology Review, vol. 24, no. 1, pp. 35–74, 2004.

21. N. Slee, P. Spinhoven, N. Garnefski, and E. Arensman, "Emotion regulation as mediator of treatment outcome in therapy for deliberate self-harm," Clinical Psychology and Psychotherapy, vol. 15, no. 4, pp. 205–216, 2008.

22. M. M. Linehan, Skills Training Manual for Treating Borderline Personality Disorder, Guildfor Press, New York, NY, USA, 1993.

23. M. M. Linehan, H. E. Armstrong, A. Suarez, D. Allmon, and H. L. Heard, "Cognitive-behavioral treatment of chronically parasuicidal borderline patients," Archives of General Psychiatry, vol. 48, no. 12, pp. 1060–1064, 1991.

24. S. Groves, H. S. Backer, W. van den Bosch, and A. Miller, "Dialectical behaviour therapy with adolescents: a review," Child and Adolescent Mental Health, vol. 17, no. 2, pp. 65–75, 2012.

25. C. J. Robins and A. L. Chapman, "Dialectical behavior therapy: current status, recent developments, and future directions," Journal of Personality Disorders, vol. 18, no. 1, pp. 73–89, 2004.

26. M. Swales, H. L. Heard, and J. M. G. Williams, "Linehan's Dialectical Behaviour Therapy (DBT) for borderline personality disorder: overview and adaptation," Journal of Mental Health, vol. 9, no. 1, pp. 7–23, 2000.

27. M. M. Linehan, D. A. Tutek, H. L. Heard, and H. E. Armstrong, "Interpersonal outcome of cognitive behavioral treatment for chronically suicidal borderline patients," American Journal of Psychiatry, vol. 151, no. 12, pp. 1771–1776, 1994.

28. A. L. Miller, J. H. Rathus, M. N. Linehan, S. Wetzler, and E. Leigh, "Dialectical behavior therapy adapted for suicidal adolescents," Journal of Practical Psychiatry and Behavioral Health, vol. 3, no. 2, pp. 78–86, 1997.

29. A. L. Miller, S. E. Wyman, J. D. Huppert, S. L. Glassman, and J. H. Rathus, "Analysis of behavioral skills utilized by suicidal adolescents receiving dialectical behavior therapy," Cognitive and Behavioral Practice, vol. 7, no. 2, pp. 183–187, 2000.

30. E. W. Trupin, D. G. Stewart, B. Beach, and L. Boesky, "Effectiveness of a dialectical behaviour therapy program for incarcerated female juvenile offenders," Child and Adolescent Mental Health, vol. 7, pp. 121–127, 2002.

31. L. Y. Katz, B. J. Cox, S. Gunasekara, and A. L. Miller, "Feasibility of dialectical behavior therapy for suicidal adolescent inpatients," Journal of the American Academy of Child and Adolescent Psychiatry, vol. 43, no. 3, pp. 276–282, 2004.

32. C. R. Quinn, "Efficacy of dialectical behaviour therapy for adolescents," Australian Journal of Psychology, vol. 61, no. 3, pp. 156–166, 2009.

33. C. Fleischhaker, R. Böhme, B. Sixt, C. Brück, C. Schneider, and E. Schulz, "Dialectical Behavioral Therapy for Adolescents (DBT-A): a clinical Trial for Patients with suicidal and self-injurious Behavior and Borderline Symptoms with a one-year Follow-up," Child and Adolescent Psychiatry and Mental Health, vol. 5, article 3, 2011.

34. K. E. Williams, D. L. Chambless, and A. Ahrens, "Are emotions frightening? An extension of the fear of fear construct," Behaviour Research and Therapy, vol. 35, no. 3, pp. 239–248, 1997.

35. K. Geddes, S. Dziurawiec, and C. Lee, "The modified affective control scale for adolescents (MACS-A): internal consistency and discriminative ability in matched clinic and non-clinic samples," in Proceedings of the 5th World Congress of Behavioural and Cognitive Therapies, Barcelona, Spain, 2007.

36. L. Roemer, K. Salters, S. D. Raffa, and S. M. Orsillo, "Fear and avoidance of internal experiences in GAD: preliminary tests of a conceptual model," Cognitive Therapy and Research, vol. 29, no. 1, pp. 71–88, 2005.

37. S. Yen, C. Zlotnick, and E. Costello, "Affect regulation in women with borderline personality disorder traits," Journal of Nervous and Mental Disease, vol. 190, no. 10, pp. 693–696, 2002.

38. J. L. Price, C. M. Monson, K. Callahan, and B. F. Rodriguez, "The role of emotional functioning in military-related PTSD and its treatment," Journal of Anxiety Disorders, vol. 20, no. 5, pp. 661–674, 2006.

39. J. Briere, Trauma Symptom Checklist for Children (TSCC) Professional Manual, Psychological Assessment Resources, Odessa, Fla, USA, 1996.

40. M. D. Neale, Neale Analysis of Reading Ability, ACER Press, Australian Council for Educational Research Limited, 3rd edition, 1999.

41. R. L. Spitzer, J. B. W. Williams, M. Gibbon, and M. B. First, "The structured clinical interview for DSM-III-R personality disorders (SCID-II)—part I: description," Journal of Personality Disorders, vol. 9, no. 2, pp. 83–91, 1995.

42. K. E. Williams and D. L. Chambless, An Analogue Study of Panic Onset, American University, Washington, DC, USA, 1992.

43. C. M. Sadowski, "Psychometric properties of the trauma symptom checklist for children (TSCC) with psychiatrically hospitalized adolescents," Child Maltreatment, vol. 5, no. 4, pp. 364–372, 2000.

44. J. Cohen, Statistical Analysis for the Behavioural Sciences, Lawrence Erlbsum Associates, Hillsdale, NJ, USA, 2nd edition, 1988.

45. P. D. Ellis, The Essential Guide to Effect Sizes: Statistical Power, Meta-Analysis and the Interpretation of Research Results, Cambridge University Press, Cambridge, UK, 2010.

46. G. Cumming, F. Fidler, M. Leonard et al., "Statistical reform in psychology is anything changing?" Psychological Science, vol. 18, no. 3, pp. 230–232, 2007.

47. K. A. Woodberry and E. J. Popenoe, "Implementing dialectical behavior therapy with adolescents and their families in a community outpatient clinic," Cognitive and Behavioral Practice, vol. 15, no. 3, pp. 277–286, 2008.

48. J. H. Rathus and A. L. Miller, "Dialectical behavior therapy adapted for suicidal adolescents," Suicide and Life-Threatening Behavior, vol. 32, no. 2, pp. 146–157, 2002.

49. A. C. James, A. Taylor, L. Winmill, and K. Alfoadari, "A preliminary community study of dialectical behaviour therapy (DBT) with adolescent females demonstrating persistent, deliberate self-harm (DSH)," Child and Adolescent Mental Health, vol. 13, no. 3, pp. 148–152, 2008.

50. A. W. Wagner, "A behavioral approach to the case of Ms. S," Journal of Psychotherapy Integration, vol. 15, no. 1, pp. 101–114, 2005.

CHAPTER 14

CONSUMER FEEDBACK FOLLOWING PARTICIPATION IN A FAMILY-BASED INTERVENTION FOR YOUTH MENTAL HEALTH

ANDREW J. LEWIS, MELANIE D. BERTINO,
NARELLE ROBERTSON, TESS KNIGHT,
AND JOHN W. TOUMBOUROU

14.1 INTRODUCTION

There is an increasing recognition of the need for early identification and intervention for youth mental health problems such as depression, anxiety, and substance use. These problems are of growing community concern given their high prevalence [1–3]. The field of youth mental health research now faces a major task of translating a growing body of research into effective clinical practice and service development [4, 5]. Youth mental health disorders are associated with increased health problems, and with problems in family functioning [6–10]. Recent estimates of treatment for depression suggest that only 20% to 30% of the years lived with disability due to depression are averted by current treatment programs, suggesting room for substantial improvement in either service delivery or

Consumer Feedback following Participation in a Family-Based Intervention for Youth Mental Health.
© *Lewis AJ, Bertino MD, Robertson N, Knight T, and Toumbourou JW.* Depression Research and Treatment, ***2012** (2012), http://dx.doi.org/10.1155/2012/235646. Licensed under Creative Commons Attribution 3.0 Unported License, http://creativecommons.org/licenses/by/3.0/.*

effective prevention of new cases of depression [11, 12]. One means of enhancing the efficacy of interventions is to shift the focus from outcomes to issues of implementation which arise in the translation of clinical findings to service delivery systems. In doing so interventions can be developed in directions which are well aligned with relevant government policy, as well as being acceptable and engaging for client groups.

The current paper reports on implementation issues in the "Deakin Family Options" (DFO) multicentre randomised controlled trial (RCT) which compared two interventions for youth depression, anxiety, and substance use. We report qualitative information gathered from participants following the completion of their psychological treatment in the DFO trial. The two treatments in the trial were both designed to reduce adolescent depression and substance use and included an individual CBT program and a family-based program known as "BEST-Plus" (Behaviour Exchange Systems Training for parents "Plus" youth) [13]. The aim of the paper is to evaluate participant feedback on the intervention experience, particularly within BEST-Plus; in order to assess treatment fidelity, effective treatment mechanisms, and potential future program modifications.

Traditionally, RCTs have been concerned with clinical efficacy. However, evaluation of the real world effectiveness of interventions delivered in community settings requires examination of direct feedback from those undertaking the interventions [14, 15]. In addition to the traditional RCT outcomes such as quantitative statistical analyses of group differences, collecting, and analysing qualitative data on individual consumer experiences can provide useful insights. Qualitative data collected from participants undergoing psychological treatments can be used to aid in the translation of research into practice. By capturing the lived experiences of study participants, researchers can gather information on the perceived mechanisms and barriers to change, and suggest further ideas for improving and enhancing interventions [16, 17].

The DFO trial was delivered in a community setting and designed in a manner that attempted to enhance its relevance to parents in the general community who had concerns about the mental health of their adolescents. As such, the DFO trial adopted inclusion criteria which were directly aligned with clinical referral patterns by recruiting young people (aged 12 to 25 years) if they presented with depression and/or anxiety and/or substance use problems. Both the age range of participants and the presenting issues were as inclusive as possible to fit directly with the Australian service delivery system for youth mental health. The purpose of the trial was to evaluate the relative efficacy of three treatments: (1) a family-based treatment program (BEST-Plus); (2) a cognitive-behavioural therapy (CBT), individual treatment program for the youth; (3) receiving both interventions. This paper primarily focuses on families' experiences of BEST-Plus. Much of the data from the consumer focus groups is based on these parent's experiences in the BEST-Plus groups, including their feedback and insights into the perceived mechanisms and barriers for change in themselves and their young person.

The BEST-Plus program is based on an earlier version of the program known simply as BEST, developed by Toumbourou, Bamberg, and colleagues [18]. It was initially developed as a professionally led, multifamily group education program for parents, with content focussed on alcohol and drug use by adolescents. The BEST program was shown to reduce parental mental health symptoms and family stresses [19]. To increase program efficacy, the second stage of development (BEST-Plus) included all family members and focused on inviting siblings, who joined their parents in the group for the final four weeks of the eight-week program. Evaluations showed that additional positive changes in the family system were produced in mental health and stress symptoms, family cohesion, and increases in action by young people to address their substance use and thus improve their mental health [20, 21].

Family-based interventions are less common in the mental health system than psychological therapies focussed on individuals. However, family-based interventions have a number of potential advantages for adolescents in terms of engagement and capacity to address the impact of mental health problems in the family's transition across key developmental periods. There are many circumstances where, for a variety of reasons, an adolescent refuses to participate in a mental health service; this poor uptake of services by youth is extremely common in current Australian youth mental health services [22]. One of the primary aims of the current study was to evaluate how a family-based intervention model can be used to address legitimate concerns raised by parents about the mental health of their adolescent to the benefit of the family as a whole.

Our research questions for this evaluation focused on participant's responses to the BEST-Plus interventions. We were interested in examining how these groups might have benefited parents, and the mechanisms which participants identified as being effective. We were also interested in attempting to understand how family-based groups helped parents to address the mental health needs of their young person, and whether these mechanisms and interventions had been faithful to the treatment manual for BEST-Plus. Finally, we were interested in new ideas that parents in particular had to improve the efficacy of this intervention approach.

14.2 METHOD

14.2.1 STUDY DESIGN AND SAMPLE

While the overarching DFO study was designed as a RCT, the current paper reports mainly on the qualitative data collected from participants during focus groups held 6 months after their treatment in the DFO study. Participants were invited to the focus groups if they completed one of the trial interventions. The experimental treatment was the BEST-Plus program which is a fully manualised treatment. It consists of an eight-week, professionally-led group program designed to assist parents concerned with youth substance use-related problems. The parent/s receive 4 sessions of weekly intervention and then the parent/s, sibling/s, and young person complete 4 sessions of a weekly intervention together, where the family members are willing to attend. The control condition was the CBT intervention for the young person alone. Only one participant in the focus groups received the combined treatment arm (such that they received both the BEST-Plus intervention for the family, and the individual CBT treatment for the young person), and therefore, these results were combined with the results of the rest of the attendees who had participated in the BEST-Plus treatment arm. All interventions were delivered by trained and supervised clinical psychology trainees who were undertaking Masters level training. All therapists received supervision, training; and therapy manuals. A total, of n = 186 individuals participated in the DFO trial which consisted of n = 71 adolescents (38.2%); n = 70 mothers (37.6%); n = 29 fathers (15.6%); n = 13 siblings (7.0%) and n = 3 step-parents. In total n = 86 family units were recruited, of which 13 families participated in the focus groups. Participants in focus groups were compensated with vouchers for their time. Compared to the families who did not participate in the focus groups, the current sample were not significantly different in level of family income, level of education, or in terms of the type of family member who participated (mother or father), but did differ significantly in terms of being more likely to be intact families (married) and more likely to have completed all study questionnaires.

14.2.2 MEASURES

A set of ten questions were used in the focus groups as prompts for group discussion. These questions were as follows: (Q1) What were the most valuable aspects of being a participant in the BEST-Plus group? (Q2) Were there any negative aspects of being a participant in the BEST-Plus group? (Q3) How did your initial expectations relate to what the BEST-Plus group delivered for you? (Q4) Has what you learned from the group impacted the way you parent your young person? (If so, how?) (Q5) Is there anything you would like to see included or changed to improve the program? (Q6) Would you recommend the program to other parents? (Q7) When invited, did your young person or other children in the family attend the BEST-Plus group at session four; if so, what might have helped to allow the young person to attend? (Q8) What aspects of the group did you implement in your family life? (Q9) What additional services, if any, have you accessed since your involvement in the study? (Q10) How are things at present in your family?

Quantitative measures were also administered. At the commencement of focus group meetings, participants were also asked to fill out a brief feedback survey. This consisted of questions concerning the intervention received and the level of satisfaction with (1) the intervention received, (2) improvements in your family/home life since completing the program (3) overall satisfaction with the experience of the Deakin Family Options program; each rated on a scale of 1 to 10, where 10 represents complete satisfaction. Participants were also asked whether they were still implementing the skills and knowledge gained from the program in their daily lives and "Did you feel the program adequately addressed your needs?" and "Would you recommend participating in this program to a friend experiencing similar problems" with Yes/No response options.

14.2.3 PROCEDURES

Three consumer-reference groups were run at the end of 2011 with 7 or 8 participants in each group. Groups were facilitated by the same people that had facilitated the BEST-Plus group. The focus groups ran for 1.5 hours. The focus groups were recorded with consent and transcribed and verified by two observing researchers. Participants were also asked to fill out a brief feedback survey. Most participants (n = 21) in the focus groups were referring to the time they spent in the BEST-Plus groups. In one focus group, two young people from the same family attended with their parents.

14.2.4 DATA ANALYSIS

Descriptive statistics were used to report quantitative data derived from a consumer satisfaction survey and data collected on treatment engagement. The analytical approach we took to the qualitative data was broadly phenomenological in that the emphasis was on the subjective experience and personal interpretation. In line with the phenomenological theory of qualitative research, we were particularly interested in allowing the voices to be heard in order to gain insight into what motivated and engaged the participants [23, 24]. The interviews were transcribed verbatim for analysis, which initially entailed reading the transcripts several times to capture the essence of the data. This process was completed by two members of the research team who then reread the text to draw out emerging themes or meanings embedded in the participants words and discussed their findings to reach consensus on any of the points where disagreement occurred.

TABLE 1: Demographic features of participants in the consumer reference groups (n = 21).

Demographic feature	M	SD
Age of participant (yrs)	48.8	9.04
	n	%
Family member		
Mother	12	4.8
Father	8	57.1
Youth (male)	1	38.1
Marital status		
Married	13	61.9
Divorced	3	14.3
Separated	1	4.8
Family annual income		
Less than $50000	3	14.3
$50000–$80000	3	14.3
Over $80000	9	42.9
Missing	6	28.6
Level of education		
Completed year 10	2	9.5
TAFE diploma or certificate	5	23.8
Undergraduate degree	3	14.3
Postgraduate degree	1	4.8
Other	3	14.3
Missing	7	33.3
Number of BEST-Plus sessions attended		
1	1	4.8
3	2	9.5
4	1	4.8
5	1	4.8
6	1	4.8
7	10	47.6
8	5	23.8

14.3 FINDINGS

Sample characteristics of participants in the reference groups are present-ed in Table 1.

14.3.1 ENGAGEMENT OF YOUNG PEOPLE IN MENTAL HEALTH SERVICES

All participants in the focus groups received the BEST-Plus intervention and engagement rates are presented in Table 2. Overall, 53% of participants engaged in a treatment offered to them after an assessment. Engagement in the present context refers to completing the majority of treatment ses-sions. This figure may seem low but includes many circumstances where a parent would agree to participate, that is, their adolescent randomised to enter the CBT service, but the young person in their family would refuse to participate.

TABLE 2: Cross tabulation of engagement in treatment and type of family member.

	Did not engage in treatment	Engaged in treatment
Identified Youth	47 (66%)	24 (34%)
Sibling	9 (69%)	4 (31%)
Father	6 (21%)	23 (79%)
Mother	22 (31%)	48 (69%)

As presented in Table 2, young people were disproportionately less likely to engage in treatment (i.e., 60–70%) versus parents (20–30%) who do not engage. This difference was statistically significant ($\chi^2(5) = 28.8$, $P < 0.001$). It is also interesting to note that although a larger number of mothers than fathers presented for service within the study, those fathers who did present were more likely to be engaged in a given treatment.

14.3.2 FOCUS GROUP THEMES

14.3.2.1 WE ARE NOT ALONE...

Participants enjoyed the collegial atmosphere of the BEST-Plus groups where they felt that the group process and sharing of experiences helped them to feel that that they were "not alone". Parents considered this to be helpful in that it showed them that other young people went through similar experiences. Participants also commented that they appreciated the safe space that was created by the facilitators so that they could talk and contribute their experiences. The contribution of their own understanding to try to help others in the group was also a key aspect of the group experience. Participants noted that groups worked well when they were very participatory, making the groups a "give-and-take" experience. Parents felt that they learned most from each other. The most common benefits that were mentioned in both focus groups were the advantage of being with others with similar issues, the support, and advice they were able to give and receive as well as not feeling so isolated and alone. This exchange of experiences and help, some participants felt, also helped in reducing levels of self-blame and guilt.

> *I was just feeling so beaten up and battered...so coming here on my own and listening to the other stories of parents, their stories, I felt I wasn't as really as bad as I'd escalated it into my head...I just felt really secure and um, able to say what I felt and felt supported... and It is quite hard for me to let go.*

14.3.2.2 IT IS THEIR JOURNEY

A dominant theme that ran through both of the focus groups was learning to let go and allow the young person to take responsibility for their own life journey. The group had helped parents to understand the importance of separation and individuation in the family developmental process. The way this was expressed was in terms of the ability to "stand back and let go". Parents described how prior to this realisation there was a sense of helplessness, not knowing what to do for, or how to be with their young person, and being constantly caught up in conflict with their young person. They found that by stepping back and allowing young people to experience consequences it helped to defuse the "weapons" (as one participant called them) that their child would use to provoke them. Parents considered that one of the key processes through which they changed their relationship with their adolescent was learning to act rather than always reacting to a situation. This suggested an increased confidence and a greater focus on more authoritative and proactive parenting. Parents also realised that such changes occurred as they experienced reduced levels of distress and anxiety. Letting go also gave rise to opportunities for parents to take time out and to consider their own needs.

> *I felt that what we got out of the group was the letting go part and realising that it is their (the young person's) journey. I think we also approach things in a much different way than what we did... and Just more time out. More time out.*

14.2.3.3 SELF-CARE

The group spoke about the importance of self-care. It was suggested in the focus groups that self-care was something that parents were still implementing after the course had finished; that despite their situation, they recognised the need to look after themselves in order to better care for their child. This recognition emerged from the understanding that, no matter how much they wanted to help make everything better for their child, that ultimately their child needed to own his/her life and embark on that journey, the process was not always easy and the need to intervene often overwhelming. One woman related how her daughter would say "everythings ok ... and then she'll tell me she's not great—and I'm just ... my stomach drops". In the past, what might have led the parent to want to step in and take over became a recognition that she needed to support her child, to be there, but in order to do that she needed to attend to her own well-being.

But I had the chance to go away on my own, which was nice and think just about myself and I keep thinking about what (facilitator) said—that it's her journey and that's probably the most helpful thing I took out of it [the program]. It's her journey and I need to be there, but ultimately it's her life—it's not my life.

14.2.3.4 METAPHORS TO LIVE BY

One of the notable features of the BEST-Plus program is the use of several metaphoric parables which are presented by group facilitators, often with an illustration, designed to evoke themes relevant to the key developmental processes and challenges facing a family during their children's adolescence.

It sounds flippant, but it's funny to think that such a small diagram can put you in a mindset to think yes, we did launch off on our own when we were young, and kids have to do that...

This quotation from a parent exemplifies the power of the metaphor. Having one's situation that seemed so insular likened to a familiar and shared situation helped participants picture their own world from a different perspective. Participants in the focus groups found the metaphors employed in the BEST-Plus groups gave them a new outlook that they were able to continue to employ. They still remembered them and still found them useful. The use of the metaphor tied their situation to something more positive, helped give them context, and make the situation more concrete.

14.2.3.5 THE YOUNG PERSON'S PERSPECTIVE

There were two young people from one family who attended the Melbourne focus group with their parents. One of the young people who had been through the CBT arm of the program reflected that the self-initiated effect of gaining independence by moving out of home had been the most significant thing for him. As well, both felt that they now addressed issues with their parents in a more upfront manner, which they felt was positive. They also felt that their parents had changed how they "dealt" with them.

If I have a problem I address it now, like if they have a problem with me they address it straight up, we get it over with, so yeah it might be a bit confrontational but it gets it over and done with.

The BEST-Plus program consists of eight sessions. In the first four sessions the focus is exclusively on the parents. In the final four sessions parents invite their children to attend. One of the issues raised by group attendees was the low-levels of participation of the young people in the second half of the BEST-Plus groups, although this was mitigated to an extent by some parents engaging their young people within family discussions about their attendance at the group. Such discussion was done primarily so that the young person would know that they were being proactive about finding solutions to the family challenges. This reflects a proactive change in parenting styles that was commented on by many participants.

Many participants would also have liked some continuation of the group because they found the parental support to be very valuable. Some parents suggested that running parent support groups that they could transition into would be beneficial. Generally, participants mentioned that they had started the group with the idea of changing the behaviour of their young person. For many this initial goal had given way to parents thinking that the greatest benefit of the groups was rearranging how they parented and changing their ways of handling family situations and challenges.

14.3.2.6 PROGRAM DEVELOPMENT

Participants offered a number of suggestions on what needs to change to make the BEST-Plus program more relevant to their own and their adolescent's mental health. Parents commented that there was too much information in the groups focused on managing "externalising" behavioural issues such as violence and crime in their young people, and some parents with young people that had depressive or anxious children sometimes found that the information about challenging behaviour was less relevant to their situation.

There was such a diverse range of problems in the group. I found that a lot of the problems and strategies were for behavioural issues where as we are dealing [with] mental illness. The group did not really cater for mental illness.

However, parents generally acknowledged that they derived considerable benefit from the program. All of the participants of the focus group would recommend the Deakin Family Options program to others. Some even felt the BEST-Plus group was better than they had expected.

One other thing I think I had, we approached another school counsellor and then another school counsellor and then we were referred onto 1, 2, 3 places so that's five lots of people, so I had very low expectations of actually like, anything actually engaging with our reality so I was a bit blown away that it did and it did it in a way, not quite the way we expected...

14.3.2.7 PARTICIPANT DIRECT RECOMMENDATIONS

1. Weekly sessions should be longer; some participants felt that 2 hours was not long enough. Participants would have liked an extra half an hour or so to extend their discussions.
2. Participants would like on-going support; the majority of the participants would have liked the group to continue beyond the 8-week program. Some considered follow-up sessions once a month would be valuable.
3. There needs to be an improved balance in the focus on behavioural versus mental health issues. All participants felt that they had gained something from the BEST-Plus program, but parents whose young person had depressive and anxious disorders would have liked some of the weekly group focus directly on how to address

these issues rather than spending too much time on behavioural and drug use issues.

4. Earlier intervention was highly recommended. Interventions need to be offered to parents before major problems arise. Participants felt that having something set up as an early intervention would be very helpful to them. This would help them to address parenting and potential challenges with adolescents before the problems arise. Parents suggested that similar content would be helpful if it commenced in early primary school years and was offered within a school setting.

TABLE 3: Results of consumer satisfaction survey for parents participating in BEST-Plus (n = 20).

Satisfaction			Range	
	M	SD	High	Low
With the intervention received	7.66	1.58	10	3
With any improvements in your family/home life	6.64	1.65	10	3
Overall satisfaction with program	8.30	1.49	10	4
			n	%
Felt the program adequately addressed your needs		(yes)	12	57.1
		(somewhat	8	38.1
Would recommend participating in this program to a friend		(yes)	20	95.2
Is still implementing the skills and knowledge from the program		(yes)	20	95.2

14.4 RESULTS FROM THE FEEDBACK SURVEY

Results from the consumer satisfaction surveys completed on the same evening as the focus groups are presented in Table 3. The young person in attendance did not complete the questionnaire. Overall most participants were satisfied both with the intervention and their experience of the Deakin Family Options program. Satisfaction with the improvements in their family life since completing the program scored slightly lower. However, when asked the question, "would you recommend participating in this program to a friend experiencing similar problems?" all participants (n = 20) answered yes. The majority of parents felt that the Deakin Family Options program had adequately addressed their needs, for others, the lack of behavioural change by their young person impacted on their satisfaction with the program. No participant responded that the program had not addressed their needs at all. Nearly all (n = 20) participants were still implementing the skills and knowledge that they gained from the program in their daily life approximately six months after completing the intervention.

14.5 DISCUSSION

There were four major themes that consistently came out of the focus groups. Participants pointed to the advantage of meeting with like-situated parents and being able to safely share their experiences under facilitation. The advantage of this was to break down the sense of isolation. From the weekly sessions, the participants felt they learned or relearned the skill of taking a step back from the situation. Acknowledging the responsibility their young person had to take for their own lives and actions was also a powerful therapeutic moment for many parents. This helped alleviate the guilt and sense of helplessness that was a common experience described by participants. Further, participants took away the idea of the importance of self-care. The role of metaphor within the program was also confirmed as a valuable element, helping parents to situate themselves and their young person in a developmental context with the hope of a positive outcome. Each of these themes are congruent with themes that have consistently been reported by BEST-Plus participants, from the initial implementation of the program over a decade ago [18].

In terms of evaluating the BEST-Plus groups within the RCT, these findings suggest that parents received many of the key features of the intervention as presented in the BEST-Plus manual and training materials. The consumer feedback consistently suggests that what parents received corresponds closely with what the manual intended. In this sense, the findings presented add to the probability that the intervention was delivered in a way that was consistent with the treatment manual. These findings also add to the evidence that the BEST-Plus training and supervision provide an effective transmission of the program logic to a diverse range of mental health clinicians. The effective implementation of the program logic can be seen in terms of the changes in parenting style reported by a majority of the focus group participants. However, given the small sample who participated in these focus groups, it remains unknown the degree to which this finding can be generalised to the full RCT sample, or to other groups who undergo BEST-Plus programs. Often parents had expected a change in the behaviour of their young person through participation in the group but generally they found the greatest change was in how they viewed situations and how they responded to their young people. This illustrates the systemic mechanism through which change is often achieved in family-based interventions.

The DFO study was designed as a multicentre trial, and included a wide range of referrals from clinical services, community services, and community organisations such as schools; to further enhance generalizability of findings. The study design was initially developed under the expectation that the referred youth would be motivated to attend a treatment, and that their parents would enter the treatments if they were randomly allocated to the family intervention. Unexpectedly, many of the referrals to the DFO study came from concerned parents where the young person was unwilling to initially engage in a treatment program for their depression. Rather than excluding these families, the research team decided to allow the parents to access the only possible treatment (BEST-Plus, as it can be completed with the parents alone or with whole families), and to evaluate the outcomes for these families following the program. This was an attempt to prevent the exclusion of a relevant and large cohort of needy families, who appear to be underresearched and underserviced under the current Australian mental health system, given the reluctance of the young person to attend a standard treatment [22, 25].

The current study has a number of implications for the effective implementation of family-based interventions for youth mental health. Diagnostically, the current sample shows considerable heterogeneity in youth mental health issues, with both internalizing and externalizing profiles represented. This reflects the common referral patterns of clinical practice. Typically, referral to mental health services in this age group is initiated by parents, or at the very least strongly encouraged by parental support. Both intake and initial assessment procedures in youth mental health could thus benefit from a stronger family focus to reflect this common circumstance. The other key finding from our study is the clear capacity to achieve considerable transformation of family functioning within a relatively brief, intensive, and highly structured group format. Feedback from parents suggests that developmental themes of separation individuation remain highly salient, and that many families are receptive to interventions designed to facilitate the transition from adolescence to early adulthood.

One of the key outcomes of the DFO study was that the BEST-Plus model was modified to encourage the identified youth to attend the program with their parents and siblings, and to provide support for families whose young person presents more of an internalizing profile (where depression and anxiety are the dominant presenting issues). Previous versions of BEST tended to focus more on externalizing problems associated with substance use and employed behavioural management techniques and boundary setting. Focus group participants as well as the research team were also concerned by the high rate of nonparticipation of the young people in the second half of the BEST-Plus group. However, nonattendance was mitigated by parents engaging their children in discussion about the group and the flow on effect by their changed parenting styles and view of their situation. Many participants would also have liked some continuation of the group because they found the parental support valuable. They also felt that this sort of program should become more preventative, acting as an early intervention in schools. The Deakin Family Options program, and in particular, the BEST-Plus group, led to a number of positive changes according to the focus group participants.

Based on the findings in the DFO study, and the feedback from consumers described in the current paper, the BEST-Plus program has subsequently been extended to a third stage of development, known as BEST-MOOD [26]. The BEST-MOOD program has integrated much of the feedback presented in this paper and is aimed at addressing the problem of engaging young people in mental health treatments via the family system, and delivering relevant and effective interventions in the community. Notably there was a departure from the stated intention of the BEST-Plus manual in terms of young people directly impacted by mental health issues attending the youth component of the groups in the DFO study. This was consistently adopted across the interventions in the DFO trial and then integrated into the current revised BEST-MOOD model, so it is less of a "limitation" as perhaps a development that occurred within the DFO trial.

There are a number of important limitations to the present study that should be considered when appraising its findings. The findings do not explore the perspective of families that did not engage and thus may miss an important contrary perspective. There was limited information available from young people whose parents were in BEST-Plus and the findings are based mostly on the views of parents. It is also notable that the BEST-Plus facilitator was in many cases also focus group leader which may have biased discussion in a positive direction—and yet it is notable that significant suggestions and criticisms of the program were still forthcoming. In general, it should be noted that while a focus group is an effective way of gathering a large number of views, there is always the possibility that a large group may not allow dissenting voices to be expressed.

14.6 CONCLUSIONS

There is a clear recognition by governments that the cost of depression is high and effective depression prevention and early intervention programs are likely to be worth implementing (1). However, to implement these plans of action, there needs to be substantial investment to build the knowledge and infrastructure for prevention and early intervention including research capacity, prevention, and early intervention program development, evaluation and implementation frameworks. Our experience with gaining qualitative evaluation of consumer experiences within a RCT convinces us that such evaluation ought to be routinely used for gathering and analysing participant feedback in order to improve treatments.

REFERENCES

1.   N. Roxon, J. Macklin, and M. Butler, Budget: National Mental Health Reform Ministerial Statement, Can Print Communications, Canberra, Australia, 2011.

2. P. D. McGorry, A. G. Parker, and R. Purcell, "Youth mental health services," In-
    Psych Bulletin, 2006, http://www.psychology.org.au/publications/inpsych/youth_
    mental_health.
3. Australian Bureau of Statistics, "Mental health of young people," Cat 4840.0.55.001,
    Australian Bureau of Statistics, Canberra, Australia, 2007.
4. I. B. Hickie, "Youth mental health: we know where we are and we can now say
    where we need to go next," Early Intervention in Psychiatry, vol. 5, no. 1, pp. 63–69,
    2011.
5. B. McDermott, M. Baigent, and A. Chanen, beyondblue Expert Working Committee
    Clinical Practice Guidelines: Depression in Adolescents and Young Adults, Beyond-
    blue: The National Depression Initiative, Melbourne, Australia, 2010.
6. A. Angold, E. J. Costello, and C. M. Worthman, "Puberty and depression: the roles
    of age, pubertal status and pubertal timing," Psychological Medicine, vol. 28, no. 1,
    pp. 51–61, 1998.
7. D. A. Brent, J. A. Perper, G. Moritz et al., "Psychiatric risk factors for adolescent
    suicide: a case-control study," Journal of the American Academy of Child and Ado-
    lescent Psychiatry, vol. 32, no. 3, pp. 521–529, 1993.
8. D. M. Fergusson, L. J. Horwood, E. M. Ridder, and A. L. Beautrais, "Sexual orienta-
    tion and mental health in a birth cohort of young adults," Psychological Medicine,
    vol. 35, no. 7, pp. 971–981, 2005.
9. G. Parker and K. Roy, "Adolescent depression: a review," Australian and New Zea-
    land Journal of Psychiatry, vol. 35, no. 5, pp. 572–580, 2001.
10. G. Saluja, R. Iachan, P. C. Scheidt, M. D. Overpeck, W. Sun, and J. N. Giedd, "Prev-
    alence of and risk factors for depressive symptoms among young adolescents," Ar-
    chives of Pediatrics and Adolescent Medicine, vol. 158, no. 8, pp. 760–765, 2004.
11. G. Andrews, C. Issakidis, K. Sanderson, J. Corry, and H. Lapsley, "Utilising survey
    data to inform public policy: comparison of the cost-effectiveness of treatment of
    ten mental disorders," British Journal of Psychiatry, vol. 184, pp. 526–533, 2004.
12. D. Chisholm, K. Sanderson, J. L. Ayuso-Mateos, and S. Saxena, "Reducing the glob-
    al burden of depression: population-level analysis of intervention cost-effectiveness
    in 14 world regions," British Journal of Psychiatry, vol. 184, pp. 393–403, 2004.
13. J. Toumbourou and J. Bamberg, "Behaviour Exchange and Systems Training-Plus,"
    Unpublished Manual. 2010.
14. D. A. Chambers, H. Ringeisen, and E. E. Hickman, "Federal, state, and foundation
    initiatives around evidence-based practices for child and adolescent mental health,"
    Child and Adolescent Psychiatric Clinics of North America, vol. 14, no. 2, pp. 307–
    327, 2005.
15. J. R. Weisz, I. N. Sandler, J. A. Durlak, and B. S. Anton, "Promoting and protecting
    youth mental health through evidence-based prevention and treatment," American
    Psychologist, vol. 60, no. 6, pp. 628–648, 2005.
16. L. W. Green and R. E. Glasgow, "Evaluating the relevance, generalization, and ap-
    plicability of research: issues in external validation and translation methodology,"
    Evaluation and the Health Professions, vol. 29, no. 1, pp. 126–153, 2006.
17. R. Grol and R. Jones, "Twenty years of implementation research," Family Practice,
    vol. 17, no. 1, pp. S32–S35, 2000.

18. J. Toumbourou, A. Blyth, J. Bamberg, G. Bowes, and T. Douvos, "Behaviour exchange systems training: the "BEST-Plus" approach for parents stressed by adolescent drug problems," Australian and New Zealand Journal of Family Therapy, vol. 18, no. 2, pp. 92–98, 1997.

19. A. Blyth, J. H. Bamberg, and J. W. Toumbourou, BEST-Plus Behaviour Exchange Systems Training: A Program for Parents Stressed by Adolescent Substance Abuse, Acer Press, Camberwell, Victoria, 2000.

20. J. H. Bamberg, J. W. Toumbourou, and R. Marks, "Including the siblings of youth substance abusers in a parent-focused intervention: A pilot test of the BEST-Plus program," Journal of Psychoactive Drugs, vol. 40, no. 3, pp. 281–291, 2008.

21. J. W. Toumbourou and J. H. Bamberg, "Including the siblings of youth substance abusers in a parent-focused intervention: a pilot test of the BEST-Plus program," Substance Use & Misuse, vol. 43, no. 3, pp. 1829–1843, 2008.

22. M. G. Sawyer, F. M. Arney, P. A. Baghurst et al., "The mental health of young people in Australia: Key findings from the child and adolescent component of the national survey of mental health and well-being," Australian and New Zealand Journal of Psychiatry, vol. 35, no. 6, pp. 806–814, 2001.

23. M. Bloor, J. Frankland, M. Thomas, and cRobson, Focus Groups in Social Research, Sage, London, UK, 2001.

24. T. Groenewald, "A phenomenological research design illustrated1," International Journal of Qualitative Methods, vol. 3, pp. 110–143, 2004.

25. T. J. Nehmy, "School-based prevention of depression and anxiety in Australia: Current state and future directions," Clinical Psychologist, vol. 14, no. 3, pp. 74–83, 2010.

26. A. J. Lewis, M. D. Bertino, J. Toumbourou, R. Pryor, and T. Knight, "Behaviour Exchange and Systems Training-MOOD," Unpublished Manual. 2012.

AUTHOR NOTES

CHAPTER 1

Funding
The Robert Wood Johnson Foundation Physician Faculty Scholars Program and National Institutes of Health K23 (K23 HD057130) awards funded this study. Mei-Po Kwan was supported by the following grants while writing this article: NSF BCS-1244691 and NSFC 41228001. The funders had no role in study design, data collection and analysis, decision to publish, or preparation of the manuscript.

Competing Interests
The authors have declared that no competing interests exist.

Acknowledgments
We thank Bwana L. Brooks for coordinating this study, Shawn Hoch for his valuable input on the geospatial representation of the data including producing Figure 1B/C, Aaron Burgess for his help with geospatial data management, Amy L. Gilbert for help editing the manuscript, and the Pearl Grlz participants and our Near West Indianapolis community partners for their collective support.

Author Contributions
Conceived and designed the experiments: SEW MPK JW JDF. Performed the experiments: SEW. Analyzed the data: SEW. Contributed reagents/materials/analysis tools: SEW MPK JW JDF. Wrote the paper: SEW MPK JW JDF.

CHAPTER 2

Conflict of Interest

The authors declare that there is no conflict of interests regarding the publication of this paper.

CHAPTER 3

Competing Interests

The author declares that he has no competing interest.

Author Contributions

The data were collected as a part of the Nord-Trøndelag Health Study (HUNT) by the HUNT Research Center. JDD did the analyses, interpreted the data and wrote the paper.

Acknowledgements

The Nord-Trøndelag Health Study (HUNT) is a product of the collaboration between the HUNT Research Centre, the Faculty of Medicine at the Norwegian University of Science and Technology (NTNU, Levanger), the Norwegian Institute of Public Health and the Nord-Trøndelag County Council. This study was financed by the Norwegian Foundation for Health and Rehabilitation through the Norwegian Council for Mental Health.

CHAPTER 4

Funding

This project was funded by a Doctoral scholarship provided by the Centre for Research into Disability and Society and the School of Occupational Therapy and Social Work, Curtin University, Perth, Australia. It was part of a larger study that was awarded the 2007 Social Determinants for Health Research award by Healthway Australia. The funders had no role in study design, data collection and analysis, decision to publish, or preparation of the manuscript.

Competing Interests

The authors have declared that no competing interests exist.

Author Contributions

Conceived and designed the experiments: SV AEP. Performed the experiments: SV. Analysed the data: SV RP. Contributed reagents/materials/ analysis tools: SV AEP. Wrote the manuscript: SV TF RP MF AEP. Critically reviewed the manuscript: TF RP MF.

CHAPTER 5

Funding

This research is part of the TRacking Adolescents' Individual Lives Survey (TRAILS). TRAILS has been financially supported by various grants from the Netherlands Organization for Scientific Research NWO (Medical Research Council program grant GB-MW 940-38-011; ZonMW Brainpower grant 100-001-004; ZonMw Risk Behavior and Dependence grants 60-60600-97-118; ZonMw Culture and Health grant 261-98-710; Social Sciences Council medium-sized investment grants GBMaGW 480-01-006 and GB-MaGW 480-07-001; Social Sciences Council project grants GB-MaGW 452-04-314 and GB-MaGW 452-06-004; NWO large-sized investment grant 175.010.2003.005; NWO Longitudinal Survey and Panel Funding 481-08-013), the Dutch Ministry of Justice (WODC), the European Science Foundation (EuroSTRESS project FP-006), Biobanking and Biomolecular Resources Research Infrastructure BBMRI-NL (CP 32), and the participating universities. The funders had no role in study design, data collection and analysis, decision to publish, or preparation of the manuscript.

Competing Interests

Dr Verhulst is head of the department of Child and Adolescent Psychiatry at Erasmus MC, which publishes ASEBA materials and from which he receives remuneration. This does not alter our adherence to PLOS ONE policies on sharing data and materials. Ms Veldman and Drs Bültmann, Stewart, Ormel, and Reijneveld report no biomedical financial interests or potential conflicts of interest.

Acknowledgments

This research is part of the TRacking Adolescents' Individual Lives Survey (TRAILS). Participating centers of TRAILS include various departments of the University Medical Center and University of Groningen, the Erasmus University Medical Center Rotterdam, the University of Utrecht, the Radboud Medical Center Nijmegen, and the Parnassia Bavo group, all in the Netherlands. The authors are grateful to all adolescents, their parents, and teachers who participated in this research, and to everyone who worked on this project and made it possible.

Author Contributions
Conceived and designed the experiments: KV UB SAR JO FCV. Performed the experiments: KV RES. Analyzed the data: KV RES. Contributed reagents/materials/analysis tools: JO FCV. Wrote the paper: KV.

CHAPTER 6

Funding
This project was financed by the Swiss National Science Foundation (SNSF, to MT, project no. PZ00P1_137023). GM received SNSF funding under project no. 100014_135328. The funders had no role in study design, data collection and analysis, decision to publish, or preparation of the manuscript. The National Comorbidity Survey Replication Adolescent Supplement (NCS-A) was funded by: United States Department of Health and Human Services, National Institutes of Health, National Institute of Mental Health (U01-MH60220); United States Department of Health and Human Services, National Institutes of Health, National Institute of Drug Abuse (R01-DA12058-05); United States Department of Health and Human Services, Substance Abuse and Mental Health Services Administration; Robert Wood Johnson Foundation (Grant 044780); John W. Alden Trust.

Competing Interests
The authors have declared that no competing interests exist.

Acknowledgments
Disclaimer: Hereby, we acknowledge that the original collector of the data, ICPSR, and the relevant funding agency bear no responsibility for use of the data or for interpretations or inferences based upon such uses.

Author Contributions

Conceived and designed the experiments: MT GM. Analyzed the data: MT ES AB GM. Wrote the paper: MT. Conceptualization and design of the study: MT GM. Data acquisition: MT ES GM. Statistical analyses: MT AB GM. Interpretation and analysis of data: MT ES AB GM. Draft of initial manuscript: MT. Critical review of the manuscript: MT ES AB GM. Approval of the final version of the manuscript: MT ES AB GM.

CHAPTER 7

Competing Interests

The authors declare that they have no competing interests.

Author Contributions

All four authors participated in the design, interpretation of data, and writing of the paper. AL and OH did the analyses. All authors read and approved the final manuscript.

Acknowledgements

We wish to thank the school nurses, school headmasters, teachers and parents who contributed, and a special thanks to the children. The survey was financially supported by the National Education Office, Møre og Romsdal County.

CHAPTER 8

Funding

The publication of this study was supported by the Netherlands Organization for Scientific Research (NWO). This funder had no role in study design, data collection and analysis, decision to publish, or preparation of the manuscript.

Competing Interests

The authors have declared that no competing interests exist.

Acknowledgments
The authors thank the Municipal Public Health Service Rotterdam area for providing research data.

Author Contributions
Conceived and designed the experiments: RB SB PL FW HR. Performed the experiments: RB SB. Analyzed the data: RB SB HR. Contributed reagents/materials/analysis tools: RB SB PL FW HR. Wrote the paper: RB SB.

CHAPTER 9

Funding
The publication of this study was supported by a grant of the Netherlands Organization for Scientific Research (NWO). This funder had no role in study design, data collection and analysis, decision to publish, or preparation of the manuscript.

Competing Interests
The authors have declared that no competing interests exist.

Acknowledgments
The authors thank the Municipal Public Health Service Rotterdam area for providing research data.

Author Contributions
Conceived and designed the experiments: RB SB PL HR. Analyzed the data: RB SB HR. Contributed reagents/materials/analysis tools: RB PL. Wrote the paper: RB SB.

CHAPTER 10

Competing Interests
Dr Consoli reported receiving travel support from Bristol-Myers Squibb and Dr. Cohen reported past consultation for or the receipt of honoraria from Schering-Plough, Bristol-Myers Squibb, Otsuka, Janssen, Shire, and Sanofi-Aventis. Dr Revah-Levy, Moro, Peyre, Speranza, Falissard, Mme Hassler, Touchette have no relationships that might have interest in the

submitted work. No authors have any non-financial interests that may be relevant to the submitted work.

Author Contributions
Study concept and design: ARL, ET, AC, HP, BF. Acquisition of data: CH, ARL, HP, ET. Statistical analysis: BF, DC, HP, CH. Interpretation of data: all authors. Drafting the manuscript: AC, ARL, DC. Critical revision of the manuscript revision for important intellectual content: MRM, ARL, MS, DC, BF. Final draft: all authors. All authors read and approved the final manuscript.

Acknowledgments
We acknowledge the considerable contribution of the coordinators of the French Monitoring Center for drugs and drug addiction and the tireless work of the French Armed Forces responsible for the survey administration. We also thank Stephane Legleye, Angela Swaine-Verdier for revising the English and of course all the French adolescents who completed this survey.

Funding
This survey was funded by the French Monitoring Center for Drugs and Drug Addiction. Grants from the Foundation Pfizer funded AC for this research. Funding agencies were not involved in the study design, collection, analysis and interpretation of data, writing of the paper, and/or the decision to submit for publication.

CHAPTER 11

Competing Interests
The authors declare that they have no competing interests.

Author Contributions
MB designed the study and AC performed the data search; MB and AC reviewed the studies and carried out the quality assessment ratings; RJ and VP contributed to the interpretation of the data and the drafting of the manuscript. All authors read and approved the final manuscript.

Acknowledgments
The authors wish to acknowledge the support of the WHO Task Force on Mainstreaming Health Promotion Evidence Project led by Dr Gauden

Galea at WHO Geneva, who commisioned the original evidence review on which this paper is based. We are grateful to Dr Taghi Mohammad Yasamy, WHO Department of Mental Health and Substance Abuse, who acted as WHO focal point, and Professor Elizabeth Waters, Coordinating Editor of the Cochrane Public Health Group and Consulting Editor for the Mainstreaming Health Promotion Evidence Project, for their technical guidance and comments on the original review. We also acknowledge the assistance of a number of study authors globally who supplied us with additional information on the interventions and their evaluation. The views expressed in this paper are solely those of the authors and do not necessarily reflect the views of WHO. The authors have declared that no competing interests exist. VP is supported by a Wellcome Trust Senior Research Fellowship in Tropical Medicine. His work with young people is additionally supported by the MacArthur Foundation.

CHAPTER 12

Funding

This research is part of the TRacking Adolescents' Individual Lives Survey (TRAILS). Participating centres of TRAILS include various departments of the University Medical Centre and University of Groningen, the Erasmus University Medical Centre Rotterdam, the University of Utrecht, the Radboud Medical Centre Nijmegen, and the Parnassia Bavo group, all in the Netherlands. TRAILS has been financially supported by various grants from the Netherlands Organization for Scientific Research NWO (Medical Research Council program grant GB-MW 940-38-011; ZonMW Brainpower grant 100-001-004; ZonMw Risk Behavior and Dependence grants 60-60600-98-018 and 60-60600-97-118; ZonMw Culture and Health grant 261-98-710; Social Sciences Council medium-sized investment grants GB-MaGW 480-01-006 and GB-MaGW 480-07-001; Social Sciences Council project grants GB-MaGW 457-03-018, GB-MaGW 452-04-314, and GB-MaGW 452-06-004; NWO large-sized investment grant 175.010.2003.005; NWO Longitudinal Survey and Panel Funding 481-08-013); the Sophia Foundation for Medical Research (projects 301 and 393), the Dutch Ministry of Justice (WODC), the European Science Foundation (EuroSTRESS project FP-006), and the participating universities. The funders had no role in study design, data collection and analysis, decision to publish, or preparation of the manuscript.

Competing Interests
The authors have declared that no competing interests exist.

Acknowledgments
This research is part of the TRacking Adolescents' Individual Lives Survey (TRAILS). Participating centres of TRAILS include various departments of the University Medical Centre and University of Groningen, the Erasmus University Medical Centre Rotterdam, the University of Utrecht, the Radboud Medical Centre Nijmegen, and the Parnassia Bavo group, all in the Netherlands. We are grateful to all adolescents, their parents and teachers who participated in this research and to everyone who worked on this project and made it possible.

Data Sharing
TRAILS data of the T1 and T2 measurement waves are deposited in DANS-KNAW and can be accessed at www.dans.knaw.nl.

Author Contributions
Analyzed the data: FJ JO AJO. Wrote the paper: FJ. Interpretation of the results and commented on youth mental health care issues: SAR DEMCJ FCV Provided critical comments on earlier versions of the report: AJO JO DEMCJ SAR FCV.

CHAPTER 13

Conflict of Interests
The authors declare that they have no conflict of interests.

CHAPTER 14

Acknowledgments
This paper uses data from the Deakin Family Options study which was funded by beyondblue: the national depression initiative and the Centre for Mental Health and Well Being, Deakin University. The DFO study was

a partnership between Deakin University and drummond street services. The authors would like to thank Louise McDonald and Reima Pryor for their assistance with data collection, transcription and data management and Jaclyn Danaher, Gabrielle Connell, Ian Shephard, Karen Richens, Daniel Condon, Sophie McIntosh, Catherine Bull, Jenni Shannahan, Olivia Morrow and Helen Rimmington.

INDEX

Printed in the United States
by Baker & Taylor Publisher Services